DORLAND'S
LABORATORY/PATHOLOGY WORD BOOK FOR MEDICAL TRANSCRIPTIONISTS

D1249945

DORLAND'S LABORATORY/PATHOLOGY WORD BOOK FOR MEDICAL TRANSCRIPTIONISTS

Series Editor:
SHARON B. RHODES, CMT, RHIT

Edited & Reviewed by:
Arlaine Walsh, CMT

SAUNDERS

SAUNDERS
An Imprint of Elsevier Science

11830 Westline Industrial Drive
St. Louis, Missouri 63146

DORLAND'S LABORATORY/PATHOLOGY WORD BOOK FOR
MEDICAL TRANSCRIPTIONISTS   0-7216-9525-6

International Standard Book Number 0-7216-9525-6

Acquisitions Editor: Karen Fabiano
Developmental Editor: Ellen Wurm
Publishing Services Manager: Peggy Fagen
Designer: Ellen Zanolle

KI/MVY
Printed in the United States of America
Last digit is the print number: 9   8   7   6   5   4   3   2   1

PREFACE

I am proud to present the *Dorland's Laboratory/Pathology Word Book for Medical Transcriptionists*—one of the ongoing series of word books being compiled for the professional medical transcriptionist. For one hundred years, W.B. Saunders has published the *Dorland's Illustrated Medical Dictionary*. With the advent of medical transcription, it became the dictionary of choice for medical transcriptionists.

When I was approached several years ago to help develop a series of Dorland's word books for medical transcriptionists, I have to admit the thought absolutely overwhelmed me. The *Dorland's Illustrated Medical Dictionary* was one of my first book purchases when I began my transcription career over thirty years ago. To participate in this project is an honor I could never have imagined for myself!

Transcriptionists need and will continue to need trusted up-to-date resources to help them research difficult terms quickly. In developing the *Dorland's Laboratory/Pathology Word Book for Medical Transcriptionists*, I had access to the entire Dorland's terminology database for the book's foundation. In addition to this immense database, a context editor, Arlaine Walsh, CMT, a recognized leader in the field of medical transcription, was selected to review the material from the database and to remove outdated and obsolete terms. As well, Arlaine spent countless hours researching terms for inclusion in this word book. With Arlaine's extensive research and diligent work, I believe this to be the most up-to-date word book for laboratory and pathology terms available.

In developing the laboratory and pathology word book, I wanted the size to be manageable so the book would be easy to handle, provide a durable long-lasting binding, and use a type font large enough to read while providing extensive terminology not found in other resources available to medical transcriptionists.

A separate index of bacteriology terms has been included as Appendix A to this book. As well, a table of normal values for laboratory tests is included as Appendix B.

Although I have tried to produce the most thorough word book for laboratory and pathology available to medical transcriptionists, it is difficult to include every term. New tests and procedures are developed, and new organisms are found every day. As you discover new terms, please feel free to share them with me for inclusion in the next edition of the *Dorland's Laboratory/Pathology Word Book for Medical Transcriptionists*.

I may be reached at the following e-mail address: Sharon@TheRhodes.com.

SHARON B. RHODES, CMT, RHIT
Brentwood, Tennessee

AA
> AA spectrophotometer

AAA
> androgenic anabolic agent

AAC
> antibiotic-associated colitis

AAH
> atypical adenomatous hyperplasia

AAN
> amino acid nitrogen
> AAN test

AAR
> antigen-antiglobulin reaction

Aarskog-Scott syndrome

Aarskog syndrome

AAS
> aortic arch syndrome
> atomic absorption spectrophotometry

A1AT
> α_1 antitrypsin

AAV
> adeno-associated virus

AB
> Alcian blue
> asbestos body

A/B
> acid-base ratio

abacterial thrombotic endocarditis

abarognosis

abarticular gout

abarticulation

abasia
> a. atactica

abasia (*continued*)
> choreic a.
> paralytic a.
> paroxysmal trepidant a.
> spastic a.
> trembling a.
> a. trepidans

abasic

abatic

Abbé
> A. condenser
> B. test plate

Abbé-Zeiss
> A.-Z. apparatus
> A.-Z. counting chamber

Abbott
> A. Cell-Dyn hematology analyzer
> B. stain for spores

ABC
> avidin-biotin-peroxidase complex
>> ABC Elite staining kit
>> ABC technique

abdominal
> a. dropsy
> a. fibromatosis
> a. fistula
> a. muscle deficiency syndrome

Abell-Kendall method

Abelson murine leukemia virus

Abercrombie syndrome

aberrancy
> acceleration-dependent a.
> bradycardia-dependent a.
> deceleration-dependent a.
> tachycardia-dependent a.

aberrant
> a. ductule

aberrant (*continued*)
    a. ganglion
    a. goiter
    a. hemoglobin
    a. pancreas
    a. renal vessel
    a. rest
    a. tissue

aberratio
    a. testis

aberration
    chromosome a.
    distantial a.
    intraventricular a.
    penta-X chromosomal a.
    tetra-X chromosomal a.
    triple-X chromosomal a.

abetalipoproteinemia
    normotriglyceridemic a.

ABG
    arterial blood gas

abiatrophy

abionergy

abiotrophic

abiotrophy
    retinal a.

abiuret

abiuretic

ABL
    abetalipoproteinemia

ablate

ablastin

ablatio
    a. placentae
    a. retinae

ablation

ablative chemotherapy

ablepharia

ablepharon

ablepharous

ABN, Abn, abn
    abnormal

abnormal
    a. chorion
    a. chorionic villi
    a. endochondral
      ossification
    a. flow
    a. glucose tolerance test
      (AGTT)
    a. mucopolysacchariduria
      (AMPS)
    a. shortening

abnormality
    bone marrow a.
    cytologic a.
    fetal a.
    genetic a.
    morphologic a.
    nonspecific hepatocellular
      a. (NHA)
    no serious a. (NSA)
    no significant a. (NSA)

ABO
    A. antibodies
    B. antigen
    C. blood group
    D. compatibility
    E. factor
    F. hemolytic disease of the
      newborn
    G. incompatibility
    A. typing

Abopon

ABO-Rh typing

aborted ectopic pregnancy

abortus fever

aboulia

abraded wound

Abrams test

Abruptio placentae

Abrus

ABS
    Alkylbenzene sulfonate

abscess
    acute a.
    a. aerobic culture
    alveolar a.
    amebic a. of liver
    anorectal a.
    apical a.
    appendiceal a.
    appendicular a.
    arthrifluent a.
    Bartholin a.
    bartholinian a.
    Bezold's a.
    bicameral a.
    bile duct a.
    biliary a.
    bone a.
    brain a.
    broad ligament a.
    Brodie's a.
    canalicular a.
    caseous a.
    cerebral a.
    cheesy a.
    cholangitic a.
    chronic a.
    circumtonsillar a.
    cold a.
    collar-button a.
    crypt a.
    diffuse a.
    Douglas a.
    dry a.
    Dubois a.
    embolic a.
    epidural a.
    epiploic a.
    extradural a.
    fecal a.
    follicular a.
    frontal a.
    gas a.
    gravitation a.
    gummatous a.

abscess (*continued*)
    hematogenous a.
    hepatic a.
    hot a.
    hypostatic a.
    interlobular a.
    intersphincteric a.
    intradural a.
    intramastoid a.
    ischiorectal a.
    Kogoj a.
    lacrimal a.
    lacunar a.
    lung a.
    mammary a., central
    mammary a.,
      interlobular
    mammary a., periductal
    mastoid a.
    metastatic a.
    migrating a.
    miliary a.
    Munro a.
    mycotic a.
    orbital a.
    otic a.
    parafrenal a.
    parametrial a.
    parametric a.
    parametritic a.
    paranephric a.
    parotid a.
    Pautrier a.
    pelvic a.
    pelvirectal a.
    perforating a.
    perianal a.
    periapical a.
    periappendiceal a.
    periarticular a.
    periductal a.
    perinephric a.
    perirectal a.
    peritoneal a.
    peritonsillar a.
    periureteral a.
    periurethral a.
    phlegmonous a.

abscess (*continued*)
  Pott a.
  premammary a.
  psoas a.
  pulp a.
  pulpal a.
  pyemic a.
  renal a.
  residual a.
  retrobulbar a.
  retrocecal a.
  retromammary a.
  retroperitoneal a.
  retropharyngeal a.
  retrotonsillar a.
  ring a.
  satellite a.
  septicemic a.
  serous a.
  shirt-stud a.
  spermatic a.
  splenic a.
  stellate a.
  stercoraceous a.
  stercoral a.
  sterile a.
  stitch a.
  strumous a.
  subacute a.
  subaponeurotic a.
  subareolar a.
  subcutaneous a.
  subdiaphragmatic a.
  subdural a.
  subepidermal a.
  subfascial a.
  subgaleal a.
  subhepatic a.
  submammary a.
  subpectoral a.
  subperiosteal a.
  subperitoneal a.
  subphrenic a.
  subscapular a.
  subungual a.
  sudoriparous a.
  superficial a.
  suprahepatic a.

abscess (*continued*)
  supralevator a.
  sympathetic a.
  syphilitic a.
  thecal a.
  thymic a.
  Tornwaldt a.
  tropical a.
  tuberculous a.
  tubo-ovarian a.
  tympanitic a.
  tympanocervical a.
  tympanomastoid a.
  urethral a.
  urinary a.
  verminous a.
  vitreous a.
  von Bezold a.
  wandering a.
  Welch a.
  worm a.

abscissa

absence
  congenital a.

Absidia
  A. corymbifera
  A. ramosa

absolute
  a. alcohol
  a. eosinophil count
  a. erythrocytosis
  a. iodine uptake (AIU)
  a. leukocytosis
  a. retention time (ART)
  a. system of units
  a. value
  a. viscosity
  a. zero

absorbency index

absorbent
  carbon dioxide a.

absorptiometer

absorption
  atomic a.

absorption (*continued*)
    a. cavity
    a. coefficient
    a. constant
    disjunctive a.
    a. of erythrocyte antibody
    fat a.
    iron a.
    a. peak
    a. spectrum

absorption-equivalent thickness
    (AET)

absorptive
    a. cell
    a. lipemia
    a. state

absorptivity
    molar a.
    specific a.

abstinence
    alimentary a.

abstriction

abtorsion

abulia

AC
    anticoagulant
    anticomplementary
    anti-inflammatory corticoid

ac
    acute

ACA
    adenocarcinoma

acalculia

acampsia

acanthamebiasis

acanthesthesia

acanthocephaliasis

acanthocyte

acanthocytosis

acanthoid cell

acantholysis

acantholytic

acanthoma
    a. adenoides cysticum
    basal cell a.
    clear cell a.
    pilar sheath a.
    a. verrucosa seborrheica

acanthopodia

acanthor

acanthorrhexis

acanthosis
    glycogen a.
    glycogenic a.
    a. nigricans

acanthotic

acanthrocyte

acanthrocytosis

acapnia

acapnial alkalosis

acarbia

acardiacus

acardius

acariasis

acaricide

acarid

Acarina

acarine

acarinosis

acarodermatitis
    a. urticarioides

acaroid

acarology

acaryote

acatalasemia

acatalasia

acathectic

acathexia

ACC
    acinar cell carcinoma
    adenoid cystic carcinoma

accelerated
    a. reaction
    a. rejection

acceleration
    growth a.

accelerator
    a. factor
    a. globulin
    proserum prothrombin
        conversation a. (PPCA)
    prothrombin a.
    serum a.
    serum prothrombin
        conversion a. (SPCA)
    serum thrombotic a. (STA)

accelerin

accelerometer

accentuator

acceptor
    hydrogen a.
    oxygen a.
    proton a.

access
    exit a.
    multiple a.
    sequential a.
    a. time

accessory
    a. adrenal
    a. atrium
    a. cell
    a. chromosome
    a. molecule
    a. organ

accessory (continued)
    a. pancreas
    a. spleen

accident
    cardiovascular a. (CVA)
    cerebrovascular a. (CVA)
    serum a.

accidental
    a. host
    a. parasite

acclimation

accolé forms

accreta
    placenta a.

accretio
    a. cordis
    a. pericardii

AccuDate Easy glucose meter

accumulation
    a. of carbohydrates
    a. of complex lipids
    a. disease
    a. of glycogen
    intracellular a.
    a. of pigment
    a. of protein

accuracy
    photometric a.
    wavelength a.

ACD
    acid-citrate-dextrose

ACE
    adrenocortical extract

acellular

acelom

acelomate

acentric

acephaline

acephalocyst

acephalous

acervulus

acestoma

acetabuli
    protrusio a.

acetal

acetaldehydase

acetaldehyde

acetamide

acetaminophen
    a. assay
    a. hepatic toxicity

acetate
    cresyl violet a.
    deoxycorticosterone a.
    ethyl a.
    methyl a.

Acetest

acetic
    a. acid-alcohol-formalin
    a. acid and potassium
        ferrocyanide test
    a. aldehyde
    a. anhydride
    a. orcein

acetoacetate

acetoacetic
    a. acid test
    a. aciduria

acetoacetyl

acetoacetyl-CoA
    a.-C reductase
    a.-C thiolase

acetocarmine

acetoin
    a. test

acetolysis

acetone

acetone (*continued*)
    a. body
    a. compound
    a. fixative
    a. test

acetone-insoluble antigen

acetonemia

acetonemic

acetonitrile

acetonumerator

acetonuria

aceto-orcein stain

acetowhite test

aceturate
    diminazene a.

acetylation

acetylcholine receptor antibody

acetylcholinesterase
    a. assay

acetyl-CoA
    a.-C acetyltransferase
    a.-C acyltransferase
    a.-C carboxylase
    a.-C hydrolase
    a.-C synthetase

acetylcoenzyme A

acetylene trichloride

N-acetylgalactosamine

N-acetylglucosamine

N-acetylmannosamine

acetylmethylcarbinol

N-acetylneuraminic

acetylsalicylic acid

acetylstrophanthidin

acetylsulfadiazine

acetylsulfaguanidine

acetylsulfathiazole

acetyltransferase
    acetyl-CoA a.

acetyl value

AcG, ac-g
    accelerator globulin

ACH
    Adrenocortical hormone

achalasia
    biliary a.
    cricopharyngeal a.
    esophageal a.
    pelvirectal a.
    sphincteral a.

Acard syndrome

Acard-Thiers syndrome

achillobursitis

achillodynia

achiral

achiria

achlorhydria
    watery diarrhea,
        hypokalemia a. (WDHA)

achlorhydric enemia

achlorophyllous

Acholeplasmataceae

acholia

acholic
    a. stool

acholuria

acholuric
    a. jaundice

achondrogenesis

achondroplasia
    homozygous a.

achondroplastic
    a. dwarf
    a. dwarfism

achondroplasty

achordal

achrestic enemia

achroacytosis

achrodextrin (*var. of*
    achroodextrin)

achromacyte

achromasia

achromate

achromatic
    a. lens
    a. objective
    a. spindle

achromatin

achromatinic

achromatism

achromatize

achromatocyte

achromatolysis

achromatophil

achromatophilia

achromatopsia

achromatosis

achromatous

achromaturia

achromia
    congenital a.
    cortical a.
    a. parasitica
    a. unguium

achromic

achromin

Achromobacteraceae

achromocyte

achromophil

achromophilic

achromophilous

achromotrichia

Achucárro stain

achylia

achymia

achymosis

acid
    N-acetylaspartate a.
    N-acetylmuramic a.
    acetylsalicylic a.
    adenylic a.
    a. agglutination
    a. alcohol
    aldaric a.
    aldonic a.
    alginic a.
    aliphatic a.
    allantoic a.
    alpha amino a.'s
    amino a.
    aminoacetic a.
    p-aminobenzoic a. (PAB.
      PABA)
    γ-aminobutyric a. (GABA)
    aminoglutaric a.
    p-aminohippuric a. (PAH,
      PAHA)
    aminolevulinic a.
    6-aminopenicillanic a.
    aminosuccinc a.
    a. anhydride method
    arachidonic a.
    aromatic a.
    ascorbic a.
    asparaginic a.
    aspartic a. (Asp)
    aurin tricarboxylic a.
    behenic a.
    benzoic a.
    benzoylaminoacetic a.
    bile a.'s
    binary a.
    boric a.

acid (*continued*)
    Brönsted-Lowry a.
    butanoic a.
    butyric a.
    cacodylic a.
    carbolic a.
    carbonic a.
    carboxylic a.
    carminic a.
    catechinic a.
    catechuic a.
    cerebronic a.
    a. challenge test
    chenodeoxycholic a.
    cholic a.
    chromic a.
    chromotropic a.
    citric a.
    a. clearance test (ACT)
    conjugate a.
    cytidylic a.
    decanoic a.
    dehydroascorbic a.
    deoxyadenylic a.
    deoxycholic a.
    deoxycytidylic a.
    deoxyguanylic a.
    deoxyribonucleic a. (DNA)
    deoxyuridylic a.
    diacetic a.
    dibasic a.
    dicarboxlic a.
    (2,4-dichlorophenoxy)
      acetic a.
    diethylenetriaminepenta-
      acetic a.
    dihydrofolic a.
    dihydroxymandelic a.
      (DHMA, DOMA)
    3,4-dihydroxymandelic a.
    2,5-dihydroxyphenylacetic
      a.
    1-dimethylaminoaphthalene–
      5 sulfonic a. (DANS)
    dipicolinic a.
    a. dye
    edetic a.
    elaidic a.

acid (*continued*)
- a. elution test
- epsilon a.
- essential fatty a.'s (EFA)
- ethacrynic a. (ECA)
- ethanoic a.
- ethylenediaminetetraacetic a. (EDTA)
- ethylene tetraacetic a.
- a. fast (AF)
- fatty a. (FA)
- flavianic a.
- folic a.
- folinic a.
- a. formaldehyde hematin
- formic a.
- formiminoglutamic a. (FIGLU)
- free a. (FA)
- free fatty a.'s (FFA)
- a. fuchsin
- fumaric a.
- gamma-aminobutyric a. (GABA)
- glacial acetic a.
- $_D$-glucaric a.
- glucuronic a.
- glutamic a.
- glutaric a.
- glycochenodeoxycholic a.
- glycocholic a.
- glycodeoxycholic a.
- glycolithocholic a.
- a. glycoprotein
- guanidino-aminovaleric a.
- guanylic a.
- a. hemolysin test
- heparinic a.
- hexanoic a.
- hexuronic a.
- hippuric a.
- homogentistic a. (HGA)
- homovanillic a. (HVA)
- hyaluronic a.
- hydrochloric a.
- hydrocyanic a.
- hydrofluoric a.
- a. hydrolase

acid (*continued*)
- *p*-hydroxybenzoic a.
- 5-hydroxyindoleacetic a.
- *o*-hydroxyphenylacetic a.
- *p*-hydroxyphenyllactic a.
- *p*-hydroxyphenylpyruvic a.
- iduronic a.
- imidazolepyruvic a.
- imino a.
- indolacetic a.
- indolaceturic a.
- inorganic a.
- inosinic a.
- a. intoxication
- iodic a.
- a. ionization constant
- isobutyric a.
- isocitric a.
- isovaleric a.
- keto a.
- lactic a.
- lauric a.
- leukocyte ascorbic a. (LAA)
- Lewis a.
- lignoceric a.
- linolenic a.
- lipoic a.
- lithic a.
- lithocholic a.
- long-chain fatty a. (LCFA)
- a. magenta
- malic a.
- malonic a.
- medium-chain fatty a. (MCFA)
- mercaptoacetic a.
- metaphosphoric a.
- methoxyhydroxymandelic a. (MOMA)
- methylmalonic a.
- monoaminodicarboxylic a.
- monoaminomonocarboxylic a.
- monobasic a.
- monoenoic fatty a.
- a. mucopolysaccharide (AMP)

acid (*continued*)
- a. mucopolysaccharides (AMPS)
- muramic a.
- mycolic a.
- myristic a.
- neuraminic a.
- *p*-nitrophenylic a.
- nitrous a.
- nonesterified fatty a.
- a. number
- octanoic a.
- octulsonic a.
- oleic a.
- a. orcein
- organic a.
- orotic a.
- orthophosphoric a.
- osmic a.
- oxalic a.
- oxaloacetic a.
- oxo a.
- 3-oxobutyric a.
- 2-oxoglutaric a.
- ocolinic a.
- palmitic a.
- palmitoleic a.
- pantothenic a.
- para-aminobenzoic a.
- para-aminohippuric a.
- peracetic a.
- perchloric a.
- performic a.
- a. perfusion test
- periodic a.
- phenaceturic a.
- phenylacetic a.
- phenylpyruvic a.
- a. phosphatase
- a. phosphatase assay
- a. phosphatase stain
- a. phosphatase staining
- a. phosphatase test
- a. phosphatase test for semen
- a. phosphate
- phosphatidic a.
- 6-phosphogluconic a.

acid (*continued*)
- 5-phosphomevalonic a.
- phosphomolybdic a.
- phosphonoacetic a.
- phosphoric a.
- phosphotungstic a. (PTA)
- phthalic a.
- phytanic a.
- phytic a.
- picramic a.
- picric a.
- polyadenylic a.
- polybasic a.
- polyenoic a.
- polyphosphoric a.
- polysialic a.
- polyunsaturated fatty a. (PUFA)
- polyuridylic a.
- pristanic a.
- propanoic a.
- propionic a.
- prostanoic a.
- proton a.
- prussic a.
- pteroic a.
- pteroylglutamic a.
- 4-pyridoxic a.
- pyrophosphoric a.
- pyroracemic a.
- pyruvic a.
- quinolinic a.
- radioiondinated fatty a. (RIFA)
- a. reaction
- a. red 87
- a. red 91
- a. reflux test
- retinoic a.
- rhodanic a.
- ribonucleic a. (RNA)
- ribothymidylic a.
- ricinoleic a.
- *p*-rosolic a.
- rubeanic a.
- saccharic a.
- salicylic a.
- salicylsaliclic a.

acid (*continued*)
  salicylsulfonic a.
  salicyluric a.
  saturated fatty a. (SUA)
  sialic a.
  silicic a.
  soluble ribonucleic a.
    (SRNA)
  stearic a.
  succinic a.
  sugar a.
  sulfanilic a.
  sulfindigotic a.
  sulfinic a.
  sulfonic a.
  sulfosalicylic a. (SSA)
  sulfuric a.
  sulfurous a.
  tannic a.
  tartaric a.
  taurochenodeoxycholic a.
  taurocholic a.
  taurodeoxycholic a.
  ^{99m}Tc pentetic a.
  teichoic a.
  ternary a.
  n-tetracosanoic a.
  tetrahydrofolic a.
  thio a.
  thioctic a.
  thioglycolic a.
  thymidylic a.
  a. tide
  titratable a. (TA)
  toluic a.
  total fatty a.'s (TFA)
  tribasic a.
  tricarboxylic a.
  trichloroacetic a. (TCA)
  (2,4,5-tricholorophenoxy)
    acetic a.
  tuberculostearic a.
  tungstic a.
  UDP-glucuronic a.
  UDP-iduronic a.
  unesterified fatty a.'s
    (UFA)
  uridylic a.

acid (*continued*)
  urobenzoic a.
  urocanic a.
  uronic a.
  ursodeoxycholic a.
  vaccenic a.
  valeric a.
  valporic a.
  a. value
  vanillic a.
  vanillylmandelic a. (VMA)
  vinegar a.
  a. wave
  xanthurenic a.
  xanthylic a.

acid-alcohol-formalin
  acetic a.

acidaminuria

acid-base
  a.-b. balance
  a.-b. diagram
  a.-b. indicator
  a.-b. nomogram
  a.-b. ratio (A/B)

acid-citrate-dextrose (ACD)

acidemia
  argininosuccinic a.
  lactic a.
  methylmalonic a.
  organic a.
  propionic a.

acid-fast
  a.-f. bacillus (AFB)
  a.-f. bacterium
  a.-f. stain
  a.-f. staining method

α-acid glycoprotein

$α_1$-acid glycoprotein

acidic
  a. dye

acidifiable

acidified serum test

acidifier

acidify

acidimetry

acidity
    a. reduction test
    total a. (A, a)

acid-lability test

acid lipase deficiency

acid maltase deficiency

acidocyte

acidocytopenia

acidocytosis

acidogenic

acidophil, acidophile
    a. adenoma
    alpha a.
    a. cell
    epsilon a.
    a. granule

acidophilic
    a. adenoma
    a. body
    a. index
    a. leukocyte
    a. necrosis
    a. normoblast

acidophilus milk

acidosic

acidosis
    carbon dioxide a.
    compensated a.
    diabetic a.
    hypercapnic a.
    hyperchloremic a.
    lactic a.
    metabolic a.
    nonrespiratory a.
    potassium a.
    primary renal tubular a.
    renal hyperchloremia a.

acidosis (*continued*)
    renal tubular a.
    renal tubular a., distal
    renal tubular a., generalized
       distal
    renal tubular a., proximal
    renal tubular a., type 1
    renal tubular a., type 2
    renal tubular a., type 4
    respiratory a.
    respiratory a., compensated
    secondary renal tubular a.
    starvation a.
    a. test
    uncompensated a.
    uremic a.

acidosteophyte

acidotic

acid-Schiff
    periodic a.-S. (PAS)
    a.-S stain

acid-secretion rate

aciduria
    acetoacetic a.
    β-aminoisobutyric a.
    argininosuccinic a.
    beta aminoisoburyric a.
    L-glyceric a.
    glycolic a.
    methylmalonic a.
    organic a.
    orotic a.
    paroxysmal a.
    propionic a.
    xanthurenic a.

acinar

acinesia

acinetic

acinic
    a. cell adenocarcinoma
    a. cell carcinoma
    a. cell tumor
    a. cell tumor of lung

acinic (*continued*)
    a. cell tumor of salivary
      gland

aciniform

acinitis

acinose carcinoma

acinotubular

acinous carcinoma

acinus
    pancreatic a.

acladiosis

aclasia

aclasis
    diaphysial a.
    tarsoepiphyseal a.

aclastic

acne
    a. atrophia
    bromide a.
    chlorine a.
    common a.
    a. conglobata
    conglobate a.
    contact a.
    a. cosmetica
    cystic a.
    a. detergicans
    epidemic a.
    a. estivalis
    excoriated a.
    a. excoriée des filles
    a. excoriée des jeunes filles
    a. frontalis
    a. fulminans
    halogen a.
    a. indurata
    infantile a.
    iodide a.
    a. keloid
    Mallorca a.
    a. mechanica
    mechanical a.

acne (*continued*)
    a. necrotica miliaris
    neonatal a.
    a. neonatorum
    occupational a.
    oil a.
    a. papulosa
    picker's a.
    pomade a.
    premenstrual a.
    a. pustulosa
    a. rosacea
    a. rosacea keratitis
    a. scrofulosorum
    tropical a.
    a. tropicalis
    a. urticata
    a. varioliformis
    a. venenata
    a. vulgaris

acnegen

acnegenic

acneiform

acnemia

acnitis

aconitase

aconitaate hydratase

acoprosis

acoprous

acorea

acoria

Acosta disease

acousmatamnesia

acoustic
    a. coupler
    a. neurilemoma
    a. neurinoma
    a. schwannoma

ACPA
    anticytoplasmic antibody

ACPA (*continued*)
    ACPA test

acquired
    a. agammaglobulinemia
    a. atrophy
    a. character
    a. defect
    a. deformity
    a. dysplasia
    a. hemolytic anemia (AHA)
    a. hemolytic icterus
    a. hypogammaglobulinemia
    a. ichthyosis
    a. immunity
    a. immunodeficiency
      syndrome (AIDS)
    a. leukoderma
    a. leukopathia
    a. methemoglobulinemia
    a. nevus
    a. sensitivity
    a. toxoplasmosis in adults

acquista

acral lentiginous melanoma

acrania

Acrel ganglion

acridine
    a. dye
    a. hydrochloride
    a. orange (AO)
    a. orange method
    a. orange stain
    tetramethyl a.
    a. yellow

acriflavine

acritochromacy

acroagnosis

acroanesthesia

acroarthritis

acroasphyxia

acroblast

acrobrachycephaly

acrobystiolith

acrobystitis

acrocentric

acrocephalia

acrocephalic

acrocephalopolysyndactyly
    a., type I
    a., type II
    a., type III
    a., type IV

acrocephalosyndactylia

acrocephalosyndactylism

acrocephalosyndactyly
    a., type V
    a., type I
    a., type III

acrocephalous

acrocephaly
    a.-syndactyly

acrochordon

acrocinesis

acrocinetic

acrocontracture

acrocyanosis

acrodermatitis
    a. continua
    a. enteropathica
    Hallopeau a.
    infantile a.
    a. papulosa infantum
    a. perstans
    papular a. of childhood

acrodermatosis

acrodolichomelia

acrodynia

acrodysplasia

acroedema

acroesthesia

acrofacial
    a. dysostosis
    a. syndrome

acrogenous

acrohypothermy

acrokeratoelastioidosis

acrokeratosis
    paraneoplastic a.
    a. verruciformis

acrokinesia

acrolein

acromacria

acromastitis

acromegalia

acromegalic

acromegalogigantism

acromegaloidism

acromegaly

acromelalgia

acromesomelia

acrometagenesis

acromicria

acromphalus

acromyotonia

acromyotonus

acroneurosis

acro-osteolysis

acropachy

acropachyderma
    a. with pachyperiostitis

acroparalysis

acroparesthesia

acropathology

acropathy
    ulcerative mutilating a.

acropetal

acropleurogenous

acroposthitis

acropustulosis
    infantile a.

acroscleroderma

acrosclerosis

acrosomal
    a. granule
    a. vesicle

acrosome reaction

acrosphenosyndactylia

acrospiroma

acrostealgia

acrosyndactyly

acrotheca

acrotic

acrotism

acrotrophodynia

acrotrophoneurosis

acrylamide gel electrophoresis

acrylonitrile

ACT
    acid clearance test
    activated coagulation time
    anticoagulant therapy

ACTH
    adrenocorticotropic
        hormone
            ACTH stimulation test

ACTH-producing adenoma

ACTH-RF
    adrenocorticotropic
        hormone-releasing factor

actin
    anti-sarcomeric a.
    anti-smooth muscle a.
    muscle-specific a. (HHF-35)
    sarcomeric a.
    smooth-muscle a.
    α-smooth-muscle a.

actinic
    a. dermatitis
    a. keratosis
    a. porokeratosis
    a. reticuloid

actinin
    α a.
    alpha a.

actinium

actinodermatitis

actinohematin

Actinomycetaceae

Actinomycetales

actinomycetic

actinomycetoma

actinomycin

actinomycosis

actinomycotic
    a. appendicitis
    a. mycetoma

actinomyoma

Actinomyxidia

actinophage

actinophytosis

Actinoplanaceae

action
    buffer a.
    calorigenic a.
    capillary a.
    cumulative a.
    diastasic a.
    law of mass a.

action (*continued*)
    opsonic a.
    specific dynamic a.
    thermogenic a.
    vitaminoid a.

activated
    a. charcoal
    a. coagulation time (ACT)
    a. complex
    a. lymphocyte
    a. macrophage
    a. partial thromboplastin
        substitution test
    a. partial thromboplastin
        time (APTT, aPTT)

activating
    a. agent
    a. enzyme

activation
    allosteric a.
    a. analysis
    complement a.
    cross a.
    a. energy
    lymphocyte a.
    plasma a.
    trans a.
    very late a. (VLA)

activator
    plasminogen a.
    polyclonal a.

active
    a. anaphylaxis
    a. chronic hepatitis
    a. chronic inflammation
    a. elctrode
    a. immunity
    a. immunization
    a. prophylaxis
    a. rosette test
    a. sensitization
    a. transport

activity
    blood granulocyte-specific
        a. (BGSA)

activity (*continued*)
   chemotactic a.
   colony-stimulating a. (CSA)
   continuous muscle a.
   continuous muscle fiber a.
   a. determination
   general gonadotropic a.
      (GGA)
   insulin-like a. (ILA)
   leukemia-associated
      inhibitory a.
   non-suppressible insulin-
      like a. (NSILA)
   plasma insulin a.
   plasma renin a.
   postheparin lipolytic a.
      (PHLA)
   a. ratio
   relative specific a. (RSA)
   renal vein renin a. (RVRA)
   rheumatoid factor-like a.
      (RFLA)
   surface-oriented pinocytic
      a.
   thyrocine-specific a. (T_4SA)
   total antitryptic a. (TAT)
   triggered a.
   tryptic a.

actomyosin

ACTP
   Adrenocorticotropic
      polypeptide

actuate

acuta
   pityriasis lichenoides et
      varioliformis a. (PLEVA)

acute
   a. abscess
   a. anterior poliomyelitis
   a. atropic paralysis
   a. bacterial endocarditis
   a. bulbar poliomyelitis
   a. cardiovascular disease
   a. cellular rejection
   a. and chronic
      inflammation

acute (*continued*)
   a. compression triad
   a. contagious conjunctivitis
   a. crescentic
      glomerulonephritis
   a. diffuse peritonitis
   a. disseminated
      encephalomyelitis
      (ADEM)
   a. disseminated myositis
   a. disseminated lupus
      erythematosus
   a. epidemic conjuctivitis
   a. epidemic infectious
      adenitis
   a. epidemic
      leukoencephalitis
   a. exudative
      glomerulonephritis
   a. febrile jaundice
   a. fibrinous pleuritis
   a. focal hepatitis
   a. follicular conjunctivitis
   a. fulminating
      meningovovval
      septicemia
   a. gangrenous appendicitis
   a. gastritis
   a. gelatinous pneumonia
   a. glomerulonephritis
      (AGN)
   a. goiter
   a. granulocytic leukemia
      (AGL)
   a. hemolytic transfusion
      reaction
   a. hemorrhagic
      bronchopneumonia
   a. hemorrhagic cholecystitis
   a. hemorrhagic cystitis
   a. hemorrhagic encephalitis
   a. hemorrhagic
      glomerulonephritis
   a. hemorrhagic
      inflammation
   a. hemorrhagic
      leukoencephalititis
      (AHLE)

acute (*continued*)
  a. hemorrhagic pancreatitis
  a. hemorrhagic ulcer
  a. hemorrhagic ulceration
  a. idiopathic polyneuritis
  a. infarct
  a. infectious disease (AID)
  a. infectious nonbacterial
    gastroenteritis
  a. infective endocarditis
  a. inflammatory exudate
  a. inflammatory infiltrate
  a. inflammatory membrane
  a. inflammatory necrosis
  a. inflammatory transudate
  a. intermittent porphyria
    (AIP)
  a. interstitial nephritis (AIN)
  a. isolated myocarditis
  a. lymphoblastic leukemia
    (ALL)
  a. lymphocytic leukemia
    (ALL)
  a. mastitis
  a. megakaryoblastic
    leukema
  a. miliary tuberculosis
  a. monoblastic leukemia
    (AML, AMoL)
  a. monocytic leukemia
    (AML, AMoL, MLa)
  a. myelocytic leukemia
    (AML)
  a. myelomonocytic
    leukemia (AMML)
  a. myocardial infarction
    (AMI)
  a. necrotizing encephalitis
  a. necrotizing enterocolitis
  a. necrotizing hemorrhagic
    encephalomyelitis
  a. necrotizing myelitis
  a. nephritis
  a. nephrosis
  a. nonlymphocytic leukemia
    (ANLL)
  otitis media, purulent, a.
    (OMPA)

acute (*continued*)
  a. parenchymatous
    hepatitis
  a. paroxysmal
    myoglobinuria
  a. phase protein
  a. phase reactant
  a. phase reaction
  a. posthemorrhagic anemia
  a. post-streptococcal
    glomerulonephritis
  a. primary hemorrhagic
    meningoencephalitis
  a. proliferative (AP)
  a. promyelocytic leukemia
    (APL)
  a. pulmonary alveolitis
  a. pyelonephritis
  a. pyogenic membrane
  a. recurrent rhabdomyolysis
  a. renal failure (ARF)
  a. respiratory disease (ARD)
  a. respiratory distress
    syndrome (ARDS)
  a. respiratory failure (ARF)
  a. rheumatic arthritis
  a. rhinitis
  a. rickets
  a. salivary adenitis
  a. serous synovitis
  a. splenic tumor
  a. splenitis
  a. suppurative appendicitis
  a. thyroiditis
  a. transverse myelitis
  a. tubular necrosis (ATN)
  a. ulcerative colitis
  a. undifferentiated
    leukemia (AUL)
  a. uric acid nephropathy
  a. viral hepatitis (AVH)
  a. yellow atrophy
  a. yellow atrophy of liver

ACVD
  Acute cardiovascular
    disease

acyanotic

acyl
    a. carrier protein
    a. peroxide

acyl-CoA
    a. dehydrogenase
    long-chain a.
        dehydrogenase (LCAD)
        deficiency
    medium-chain a.
        dehydrogenase (MCAD)
        deficiency
    short-chain a.
        dehydrogenase (SCAD)
        deficiency
    a. synthetase

acyloxy group

N-acylsphingosine

acylsphingosine deacylase

acyltransferase
    acetyl-CoA a.
    lecithin-cholesterol a.
        (LCAT)
    phosphatidylcholine-
        cholesterol a.

acystia

AD
    Aleutian disease
    Average deviation

ADA
    adenosine deaminase

adactylia

adactylism

adactylous

adactyly

Adair-Dighton syndrome

1-adamantanamine

adamantine prism

adamantinoma
    a. of long bones
    pituitary a.

adamantoblast

Adamkiewicz test

Adams-Stokes
    A.-S. attack (ASA)
    A.-S. disease (AS)

adaption
    cellular a.
    enzymatic a.
    genetic a.
    phenotypic a.

adaptive
    a. enzyme
    a. hormone
    a. hypertrophy

ADCC
    Antibody-dependent cell-
        mediated cytotoxicity

Addis
    A. count
    A. test

Addison
    A. anemia
    A. disease
    A. keloid

Addison-Biermer disease

addisonian
    a. anemia
    a. crisis
    a. syndrome

addisonism

addition
    binary a.
    a. polymer
    a. reaction

addition-deletion mutation

adressin

adelomorphic

adelomorphous

ADEM
    acute disseminated
        encephalomyelitis

adenalgia

adenectopia

adendric

adendritic

adenectopia

Aden fever

adenia

adenine arabinoside

adenine
  phosphoribosyltransferase
  deficiency

adenitis
  acute epidemic infectious
    a.
  acute salivary a.
  Bartholin a.
  cervical a.
  cervical a., tuberculous
  mesenteric a.
  phlegmonous a.
  a. tropicalis
  vestibular a.

adenoacanthoma

adenoameloblastoma

adeno-associated virus (AAV)

adenocarcinoma (ACA)
  acinic cell.
  alveolar a.
  anaplastic a.
  bronchiolar a.
  bronchioloalveolar a.
  clear cell a.
  colloid a.
  endometrial a.
  follicular a.
  gelatinous a.
  infiltrating duct a.
  inflammatory a.
  lobular a.
  Lucké
  medullary a.

adenocarcinoma (*continued*)
  mesonephric a.
  mixed squamous cell
    carcinoma and a.
  a. of Moll
  mucinous a.
  mucoid a.
  oxyphilic endometrioid a.
  papillary a.
  renal a.
  sebaceous a.
  signet ring a.
  a. in situ
  sweat gland a.
  trabecular a.
  undifferentiated a.

adenoblast

adenocarcinoma
  a. of infantile testis

adenocellulitis

adenochondroma

adenocyte

adenocystic carcinoma

adenocystoma

adenodiastasis

adenodynia

adenoepithelioma

adenofibroma

adenofibromyoma

adenofibrosis

adenohypophyseal hormone

adenohypophysis

adenohypophysitis

adenoid
  a. cystic carcinoma (ACC)
  a. face
  a. facies
  a. squamous cell
    carcinoma

adenoid (*continued*)
  a. tumor

adenoidal-pharyngeal-
  conjunctival (APC)

adenoidism

adenoiditis

adenoleiomyofibroma

adenolipomatosis
  symmetric a.

adenologaditis

adenolymphitis

adenolymphocele

adenolymphoma

adenoma
  acidophil a.
  acidophilic a.
  ACTH-producing a.
  adnexal a.
  adrenocortical a.
  aldosterone-producing a.
  apocrine a.
  basal cell a.
  basophil a.
  benign a.
  bile duct a.
  bronchial a.
  carcinoma ex pleomorphic
    a.
  ceruminous a.
  chief cell a.
  chromophil a.
  chromophobe a.
  clear cell a.
  colloid a.
  depressed a.
  embryonal a.
  eosinophil a.
  fetal a.
  fibroid a.
  fibrous a.
  Fuchs a.
  gonadotropin-
    producing a.

adenoma (*continued*)
  growth hormone-producing
    a.
  hepatic a.
  hepatocellular a.
  Hürthle a.
  islet a.
  lactating a.
  liver cell a.
  Leydig a.
  macrofollicular a.
  malignant a.
  mammosomatotropic a.
  microfollicular a.
  monomorphic a.
  multiple a.
  nephrogenic a.
  a. of nipple
  null cell a.
  onocytic a.
  ovarian tubular a.
  oxyphil a.
  papillary cystic a.
  papillary a. of large
    intestine
  parathyroid a.
  Pick testicular a.
  Pick tubular a.
  pituitary a.
  pleomorphic a.
  polypoid a.
  prolactin-producing a.
  prostatic a.
  renal cortical a.
  sebaceous a.
  a. sebaceum
  somatroph a.
  sweat duct a.
  sweat gland a.
  testicular tubular a.
  toxic a.
  trabecular a.
  tubovillous a.
  tubular a.
  undifferentiated cell a.
  villous a.

adenomalacia

adenomatoid
    a. odontogenic tumor

adenomatosis
    endocrine a.
    erosive a. of nipple
    familial multiple endocrine
      a., type 1, 2
    fibrosing a.
    multiple endocrine a.
      (MEA)
    pluriglandular a.
    polyendocrine a.
    pulmonary a.

adenomatous
    a. crypt
    a. goiter
    a. hyperplasia
    a. polyp

adenomegaly

adenomyoepithelial adenosis

adenomyoepithelioma

adenomyofibroma
    atypical polyoid a. (APA)

adenomyoma
    atypical polyoid a. (APA)

adenomyometritis

adenomyosarcoma

adenomyosis
    a. externa
    stromal a.
    a. tubae
    a. uteri

adenoncus

adenopathy

adenopharyngitis

adenophlegmon

Adenophorasida

Adenophorea

adenophthalmia

adenophyma

adenopituicyte

adenosalpingitis

adenosarcoma
    müllerain a.

adenosatellite virus

adenosclerosis

adenosine
    a. 3′,5′-cylic
      monophosphate
    a. 3′,5′-cylic phosphate
      (cyclic AMP) (cAMP)
    a. deaminase (ADA)
    a. deaminase assay
    a. deaminase deficiency
    a. diphosphate
    a. 5′-diphosphate (ADP)
    a. monophosphate (AMP)
    a. triphosphatase (ATPase)
    a. triphosphate (ATP)

adenosis
    adenomyoepithelial a.
    apocrine a.
    blunt duct a.
    fibrosing a.
    mammary sclerosing a.
    microglandular a.
    sclerosing a.
    sclerosing a. of breast
    secretory a.
    simple a.
    a. vaginae
    vaginal a.

adenosquamous carcinoma

S-adenosyl$_{-L}$-homocysteine

S-adenosyl$_{-L}$-methionine

Adenoviridae

adenovirus
    canine a. 1
    a. immunofluorescence
    porcine a.

adenylate
　a. cyclase
　a. kinase

adenyl cyclase

adenylic acid

adenylosuccinate

adenylpyrophosphatase

adenylyl

adenylylation

adermia

adermogenesis

ADH
　alcohol dehydrogenase
　antidiuretic hormone
　　ADH assay
　　ADH deficiency

adherence
　bacterial a.
　immune a.
　Treponema pallidum
　　immobilization (immune)
　　a. (TPIA)

Adherens
　zonula a.

adherent
　a. pericarditis
　a. pericardium

adhesins

adhesion
　amniotic a.
　fibrinous a.
　fibrous a.
　a. molecule
　a. phenomenon
　sublabial a.
　a. test

adhesive
　albumin slide a.
　a. arachnoiditis
　a. capsulitis

adhesive (*continued*)
　a. chronic pachymeningitis
　gelatin slide a.
　a. immflammation
　a. pericarditis
　a. peritonitis
　a. phlebitis
　a. pleurisy
　a. vaginitis

adiadochocinesia

adiadochocinesis

adiadochokinesia

adiadochokinesis

adiadokokinesia

adiadokokinesis

Adiantum

adiaspiromycosis

adiaspore

adiasporosis

Adie
　A. pupil
　A. syndrome

adiemorrhysis

Adienida

adiphenine hydrochloride

adipic

adipocele

adipoceratous

adipocere

adipocyte

adipocytic neoplasm

adipohepatic

adipokinesis

adipokinetic hormone

adipolysis

adipolytic

adiponecrosis
    a. subcutanea neonatorum

adiposalgia

adipose
    a. degeneration
    a. infiltration
    a. tissue
    a. tissue extract (ATE)

adiposis
    a. cardiaca
    a. cerebralis
    a. dolorosa
    a. hepatica
    a. orchica
    a. tuberosa simplex
    a. universalis

adipositas
    a. ex vacuo

adipositis

adiposity
    cerebral a.
    pituitary a.

adiposogenital dystrophy

adiposuria

adipsia

aditus

adnexitis

ADPKD

adjusted rate

adjuvant
    Freund complete a.
    Freund incomplete a.
    mycobacterial a.
    a. vaccine

Adler test

AND-B assay

adnexa

adnexal
    a. adenoma
    a. carcinoma
    a. neoplasm

adnexitis

adolescent
    a. albuminuria
    a. round back

adoptive
    a. immunity
    a. immunotherapy

ADP
    adenosine 5′-diphosphate

ADP/ATP ratio

adrenal
    accessory a.
    a. antibody
    a. ascorbic acid depletion
      test
    a. cortex
    a. cortical carcinoma
    a. cortical hyperplasia
    a. crisis
    a. disease
    a. epithelioid angiosarcoma
      (AEA)
    a. feminizing syndrome
    a. function test
    a. gland
    a. gland virilizing syndrome
    a. insufficiency
    Marchand a.'s
    a. medulla
    a. neoplasm
    a. rest
    a. tumor
    a. virilism
    a. virilization

adrenaline

adrenalinemia

adrenalin test

adrenalinuria

adrenalism

adrenalitis

adrenalopathy

adrenarche
   delayed a.
   precocious a.

adrenergic
   a. blocking
   a. blocking agent
   a. neuron blockade
   a. neuron blocking agent

α-adrenergic
   α-a. blockade
   α-a. blocking agent

β-adrenergic
   β-a. antagonist
   β-a. blockade
   β-a. blocking agent

adrenitis

adrenochrome

adrenocortical
   a. adenoma
   a. extract (ACE)
   a. hormone (ACH)
   a. inhibition test
   a. insufficiency
   a. rest tumor

adrenocorticohyperplasia

adrenocorticosteroid

adrenocorticotropic
   a. cell
   a. hormone (ACTH)
   a. hormone assay
   a. hormone-releasing factor
     (ACTH-RF)
   a. hormone stimulation test
   a. hormone suppression
     test
   a. polypeptide (ACTP)

adrenocorticotropin

adrenodoxin

adrenogenital syndrome
   (AGS)

adrenoleukodystrophy

adrenomedullary
   a. hormone
   a. triad

adrenomedullin

adrenomegaly

adrenomyeloneuropathy

adrenopathy

adrenoprival

Adriamycin
   A. cardiomyopathy

adromia

ADS
   antibody deficiency
     syndrome
   antidiurectic substance

adsorb

adsorbate

adsorbed plasma

adsorbent
   gastrointestinal a.

adsorption
   agglutinin a.
   chemical a.
   a. chromatography
   immune a.
   physical a.

adtorsion

adult
   a. celiac disease
   a. cystic teratoma
   a. gonococcal conjunctivitis
   a. granulosa cell tumor
     (AGCT)
   a. hemoglobin
   a. medulloepithrlioma
   a. polycystic disease

adult (*continued*)
   a. respiratory distress
      syndrome (ARDS)
   a. T-cell leukemia (ATL)
   a. T-cell lymphoma (ATL)
   a. tuberculosis

adulteration

adult-onset diabetes

adultorum
   blennorrhea a.

adult-type xanthogranuloma
   (AXG)

adventitia
   aortic tunica a.

adventitial neuritis

adventitious
   a. albuminuria
   a. cyst

adynamia
   a. episodica hereditaria
   hereditary a.

adynamic ileus

AE
   antitoxic unit

AE1
   antikeratin
      AE1 immunoperoxidase
         stain
      AE1 plus CAM

AE1/3 antibody

AE1/AE3 antibody

AEA
   adrenal epithelioid
      angiosarcoma

AEC detection system

AEM
   analytical electron
      microscope

AEq
   age equivalent

aequorin

AER
   aldosterone
      excretion rate

aerated

aeration

aerial mycelium

aeremia

aerobe
   obligate a.

aerobic
   a. and anaerobic blood
      culture
   a. bacterium
   a. diphtheroid
   a. metabolism

aerobiology

aerobiosis

aerobiotic

aerocele
   epidural a.
   intracranial a.

aerocolpos

aerodermectasia

aeroembolism

aerogastria
   blocked a.

aerogen

aerogenesis

aerogenic

aeroperitoneum

aeroperitonia

aerophil, aerophile

aerophilic

aerophilous

aeroplankton

aerosinusitis

aerosis

aerosol generator

aerotaxisis

aerotitis media

aerotolerant

aerotonometer

aerotropism

aestivoautumnal fever

AET
    absorption-equivalent
      thickness

AF
    acid fast
    aldehyde fuchsin
    anti-body forming

AFB
    acid-fast bacillus
      AFB smear
      AFB stain

AFC
    antibody-forming cell

afebrile
    a. abortion

affected
    part a. (Par. aff.)

affinity
    a. antibody
    a. chromatography
    a. constant
    a. label
    testosterone-binding a.
      (TBA)

afibrinogenemia
    congenital a.

AFIP
    Armed Forces Institute of
      Pathology

aflatoxicosis

aflatoxin

AFP
    α-fetoprotein

African
    A. hemorrhagic fever
    A. histoplasmosis
    A. horse sickness
    A. horse sickness virus
    A. sleeping sickness
    A. tick-borne fever
    A. trypanosomiasis

aftercataract

afterchroming

aftergilding

AG
    antiglobulin
    atrial gallop

A/G
    albumin-globulin
      A/G ratio
      A/G ratio test

Ag
    antigen
    silver

AGA
    appropriate for gestational
      age

agalactia

agalactosis

agalactosuria

agalorrhea

agamete

agamic

agammaglobulinemia
    acquired a.
    Bruton type a.
    common variable a.
    congenital a.
    lymphopenic a.
    primary a.

agammaglobulinemia
(*continued*)
   secondary a.
   Swiss-type a.
   transient a.
   X-linked a.
   X-linked infantile a.

agamocytogeny

Agamofilaria

agamogenesis

agamogenetic

agamogony

agamont

agamous

aganglionic
   a. megacolon

aganglionosis
   congenital a.

agar
   ascitic a.
   bile esculin a.
   bile salt a.
   birdseed a.
   bismuth-sulfite a.
   blood a.
   Bordet-Gengou potato
    blood a.
   brain-heart infusion a.
   brilliant green bile salt a.
   casein a.
   CB a.
   chocolate blood a.
   Christensen urea a.
   citrate a.
   Columbia blood a.
   cornmeal a.
   a. cutter
   cystine trypticase a.
   Czapek-Dox a.
   Czapek solution a.
   deep a.
   deoxycholate-citrate a.
    (DCA)

agar (*continued*)
   deoxyribonuclease a.
   a. diffusion method
   DNase a.
   egg-yolk a.
   EMB a.
   Emmon modification of
    Sabouraud dextrose a.
   eosin-methylene
    blue a.
   French proof a.
   Hektoen enteric a.
   inhibitory mold a.
   Kliger iron a. (KIA)
   laked blood a.
   lysine-iron a.
   MacConkey a.
   malt a.
   Martin-Lester a.
   Middlebrook a.
   Mueller-Hinton a.
   mycobiotic a.
   nitrate a.
   nutrient a.
   oatmeal-tomato paste a.
   Pfeiffer blood a.
   phenylethyl alcohol blood
    a.
   a. plate count
   potato dextrose a.
   rabbit blood a.
   rice-Tween a.
   Sabhi a.
   Sabourand dextrose
    and brain heart
    infusion a.
   Salmonella-Shigella a.
   Schaedler blood a.
   serum a.
   sheep blood a.
   Simmons citrate a.
   TCBS a.
   Thayer-Martin a.
   triple sugar iron a.
   trypicase soy a. (TSA)
   tryptic soy a.
   TSI a.
   urea a.

agar (*continued*)
Wilkins-Chilgren a.
XLD a.
xylose-lysine-deoxycholate a.
yeast extract a.

agaric
deadly a.
fly a.

agarose gel electrophoresis

Ag-AS
silver-ammoniacal silver
Ag-AS stain

agastria

agastric

AGCT
adult granulosa cell tumor

age
appropriate for gestational a. (AGA)
chronological a. (CA)
a. equivalent (AEq)
gestational a. (GA)

age-adjusted rate

aged serum

agenesia
a. corticalis

agenesis
callosal a.
cerebellar a.
gonadal a.
nuclear a.
ovarian a.
pure red cell a.
sacral a.
testicular a.
thymic a.

agent
activating a.
adrenergic a.
a-adrenergic blocking a.

agent (*continued*)
adrenergic neuron blocking a.
alkylating a.
androgenic anabolic a.
antibacterial a.
antifungal a.
antiviral a.
bacteriostatic a.
beta-adrenergic blocking a.
biological alkylating a.
Bittner a.
caudalizing a.
chelating a.
chimpanzee coryza a. (CCA)
cholinergic blocking a.
clearing a.
δ a.
delta a.
drying a.
Eaton a.
embedding a.
etiologic a.
F a.
fertility a.
foamy a.
ganglionic blocking a. (GBA)
gonadotropin-releasing a. (GRA)
Gordon a.
Hawaii a.
infectious a.
initiating a.
LDH a.
lysing a.
Marburg a.
Marcy a.
MS-1, -2 a.
nitrosourea a.
Norwalk a.
A. Orange
oxidizing a.
PANTA antimicrobial a.
Pittsburg pneumonia a.
progestational a.
promoting a.

agent (*continued*)
    reducing a.
    reovirus-like a.
    surface-active a.
    thrombolytic a.
    transforming a.
    vacuolating a.
    virus-inactivating a. (VIA)
    wetting a.

age-specific rate

ageusia

ageusic

ageustia

agglutinate

agglutinating antibody

agglutination
    acid a.
    bacterial a. (BA)
    bacteriogenic a.
    chick-cell a.
    cold a.
    cross a.
    direct a. (DA)
    false a.
    group a.
    immune a.
    indirect a.
    intravascular a.
    latex a.
    macroscopic a.
    mediate a.
    microscopic a.
    mixed a.
    nonimmune a.
    O a.
    passive a.
    platelet a.
    reverse a.
    salt a.
    slide latex a.
    spontaneous a.
    T a.
    a. test
    a. titer

agglutination (*continued*)
    Treponema pallidum a. (TPA)
    tube a.
    Vi a.

aggluntinator
    rheumatoid a.

agglutinin
    α a.
    a. adsorption
    alpha a.
    anti-RH a.
    α a.
    beta a.
    blood group a.'s
    chief a.
    cold a.
    cross-reacting a.
    febrile a.
    flagellar a.
    group a.
    H a.
    heterophil a.
    immune a.
    incomplete a.
    latex a.
    leukocyte a.
    major a.
    Mg a.
    minor a.
    O a.
    partial a.
    plant a.
    platelet a.
    Rh a.
    saline a.
    salmonella a.
    serum a.
    somatic a.
    warm a.
    wheat germ a. (WGA)

agglutinogen
    blood groups a.'s
    T a.

agglutinogenic

agglutinophilic

agglutinoscope

agglutogen

agglutogenic

aggregate
    a. anaphylaxis
    cytoplasmic crystalline a.
    cytoplasmic lipid a.
    cytoplasmic
      macromolecule a.
    nuclear crystalline a.
    nuclear lipid a.

aggregated
    a. albumin
    a. microsphere

aggregation

aggregometer

aggrephore

aggressin

aggressive infantile fibromatosis

AGL
    acute granulocytic
      leukemia

aglobulia

aglobuliosis

aglobulism

aglomerular

aglutition

aglycemia

aglycogenosis

aglycone

aglycosuria

aglycosuric

AGN
    acute glomerulonephritis

agnathus

agnea

agnogenic myeloid metaplasia

agnosia
    acoustic a.
    auditory a.
    body-image a.
    face a.
    facial a.
    finger a.
    ideational a.
    tactile a.
    time a.
    visual a.
    visual-spatial a.
    visuospatial a.

agonad

agonadal

agonadism

agonal
    a. leukocytosis
    a. thrombosis
    a. thrombus

agonist

agrammatica

agrammatism

agrammatologia

agranular
    a. endoplasmic reticulum
    a. leukocyte

agranulocyte

agranulocytic angina

agranulocytosis
    feline a.
    infantile genetic a.

agranuloplasia

agranuloplastic

agraphia
    absolute a.
    acoustic a.

agraphia (*continued*)
    a. amnemonica
    a. atactica
    cerebral a.
    jargon a.
    literal a.
    mental a.
    motor a.
    musical a.
    optic a.
    verbal a.

agraphic

agretope

AGS
    adrenogenital syndrome

AGT
    antiglobulin test

AGTT
    adnormal glucose tolerance
        test

ague

AGV
    aniline gentian violet

agyria

agyric

AH
    amenorrhea and hirsutism
    antihyaluronidase
    Arachis hypogaea
    arterial hypertension
        AH assay
        AH titer

AHA
    acquired hemolytic anemia
    autoimmune hemolytic
        anemia

ahaptoglobinemia

ahaustral

AHD
    arteriosclerotic heart
        disease

AHD (*continued*)
    atherosclerotic heart
        disease

AHF
    antihemophilic factor A

AHG
    antihemophilic globulin
    antihuman globulin
        AHG factor

AHH
    analog of histidine

AHLE
    acute hemorrhagic serum

AHLS
    antihuman lymphocyte
        serum

AHT
    antihyaluronidase titer
    augmented histamine test

Ahumada-Del Castillo syndrome

AI
    angiotensin I
    aortic incompetence
    aortic insufficiency

Aicardi syndrome

AID
    acute infectious disease

Aid
    Cryostat Frozen Sectioning
        A.

AIDS
    aquired immunodeficiency
        syndrome
        AIDS serology

AIDS-related
    A.-r. complex (ARC)
    A.-r. virus (ARV)

AIEP
    amount of insulin
        extractable from
        pancreas

AIH
homogous artificial insemination

AIHA
autoimmune hemolytic anemia

AII
angiotensin II

AIII
angiotensin III

AIL
angicentric immunoproliferative lesion

AILD
angioimmunoblastic lymphadenopathy with dysproteinemia

AIN
acute interstitial nephritis

ainhum

AIO
amyloid of immunoglobulin origin

AIP
acute intermittent porphyria
automated immunoprecipotation

air
alveolar a.
a. core
a. dose
a. embolism
a. foil
a. monitor
a. quality standard
a. thermometer

airborne infection

air-dried smear

AITT
arginine insulin tolerance test

AIU
absolute iodine uptake

Akabane virus

akamushi disease

akaryocyte

akaryota

akaryote

akeratosis

akinesia

akinesis

akinesthesia

akinetic

akoria

AKT1 virus

AKT8 retrovirus

Akureyi disease

ALA
aminolevulinic acid
ALA test

alacrima

alactasia

ALAD
aminolevulinic acid dehydrase

alaninemia
hyper-β-a.
hyperbeta-a.

alaninuria

alanyl

alanyl-RNA synthetase

alar chest

AlaSTAT latex allergy test

Alba
Pityriasis a.

Albarrán disease

albedo
   a. retinae

Albers-Schönberg disease

Albert
   A. disease
   B. stain

Albert-Linder bone sectioning

albicans

albiduria

albinism
   albinism I
   albinism II
   Amish a.
   autosomal dominant
     oculocutaneous a.
   brown a.
   complete imperfect a.
   complete perfect a.
   localized a.
   ocular a.
   ocular a., autosomal
     recessive
   ocular a., Forsius-Eriksson
     type
   ocular a.m, Nettleship-Falls
     type
   ocular a., X-linked
     (Nettleship)
   oculocutaneous a.
   partial a.
   red a.
   rufous a.
   tyrosinase-negative (ty-neg)
     oculocutaneous a.
   tyrosinase-positive (ty-pos)
     oculocutaneous a.
   xanthous a.
   yellow mutant (ym)
     oculocutaneous a.

albinismus
   a. circumscriptus

albinoidism
   oculocutaneous a.
   punctate oculocutaneous a.

albinotic

albinuria

Albright-McCune-Sternberg
  syndrome

albunginea

albuginitis

albumimeter

albumin
   a. A
   aggregated a.
   a. assay
   a. B
   Bence Jones a.
   blood a.
   bovine serum a. (BSA)
   chromated Cr 51 serum a.
   a. clearance (C/alb)
   coagulated a.
   crystalline egg a. (CEA)
   derived a.
   a. Ghent
   hematin a.
   human serum a. (HSA)
   iodinated human serum a.
     (IHSA)
   iodinated I–125 serum a.
     (human)
   iodinated I–131 serum a.
     (human)
   iodinated macroaggregated
     a. (IMAA)
   macroaggregated a. (MAA)
   a. Mexica
   a. Naskapi
   native a.
   normal human serum a.
   Patein a.
   a. quotient
   radioactive iodinated
     human serum a. (RIHSA)
   radioactive iodinated serum
     a. (RISA)
   radioiodinated serum a.
   a. Reading
   serum a. (SA)

albumin (*continued*)
    a. slide adhesive
    a. suspension test
    ^{99m}Tc serum a.
    thryoxine-binding a.
    a. X
    a. X_1

albuminaturia

albumin-calcium-magnesium
  (ACM)

albuminemia

albumin-globulin (A/G)

albumininiferous

albuminimeter

albuminimetry

albuminiparous

albuminocholia

albuminocytological

albuminocytologic dissociation

albuminogenous

albuminoid degeneration

albuminometer

albuminoptysis

albuminoreaction

albuminorrhea

albuminous
    a. degeneration
    a. swelling

albuminuretic

albuminuria
    adolescent a.
    adventitious a.
    a. of athletes
    Bamberger a.
    Bence Jones a.
    benign a.
    cardiac a.
    colliquative a.

albuminuria (*continued*)
    cyclic a.
    dietetic a.
    digestive a.
    essential a.
    false a.
    febrile a.
    functional a.
    intermittent a.
    lordotic a.
    march a.
    neuropathic a.
    orthostatic a.
    physiologic a.
    postrenal a.
    postural a.
    prerenal a.
    recurrent a.
    regulatory a.
    transient a.

albumunuric

albumose-free tuberculin (TAF)

ALC
    approxiamate lethal
      concetration

alcaptonuria

alcaptonuric

Alcian
    A. blue (AB)
    A. blue stain

ALCL
    anaplastic large cell
      lymphoma

alcohol
    absolute a.
    acid a.
    a. addiction
    aliphatic a.
    allyl a.
    a. assay
    benzyl a.
    blood a.
    butyl a.
    dehydrated a.

alcohol (*continued*)
    a. dehydrogenase (ADH)
    dihydric a.
    ethyl a.
    a. fixation
    isobutyl a.
    monohydric a.
    polyhydric a.
    polyvinyl a. (PVA)
    propyl a.
    a. thermometer

alcoholemia

alcoholic
    a. cardiomyopathy
    a. cirrhosis
    a. coma
    a. formalin
    a. hepatitis
    a. hyalin
    a. hyaline
    a. hyaline body
    a. myopathy

alcohol-soluble eosin

alcoholuria

aldaric acid

aldehyde
    acetic a.
    a. dehydrogenase
    a. fixative
    formic a.
    a. fuchsin (AF)
    a. oxidase

Alder-Reilly
    A.-R. anomaly
    A.-R. body

aldicarb

adimine

aldofuranose

aldohexose

aldolase
    a. assay
    fructose-bisphosphate a.
    a. test

aldonic acid

aldopentose

aldopyranose

aldose

aldosterone
    a. assay
    a. excretion rate (AER)
    a. excretion defect (ASD)
    a. secretion rate (ASR)
    a. secretory rate (ASR)
    a. stimulation rate
    a. suppression test

aldosterone-producing
  adenoma (APA)

aldosteronism
    primary a.
    pseudoprimary a.
    secondary a.

aldosteronopenia

aldosteronuria

aldotransferase

aldotriose

Aldrich syndrome

aldrin

aleukemia

aleukemic
    a. granulocytic leukemia
    a. lymphocytic leukemia
    a. monocytic leukemia
    a. myelosis

aleukemoid

aleukia
    a. hemorrhagica

aleukocytic

aleukocytosis

aleurioconidium

aleurospore

Aleutian
    A. disease (AD)
    A. mink disease
    A. mink disease virus

Alexander
    A. disease
    A. leukodystrophy

alexia
    cortical a.
    motor a.
    musical a.
    optical a.
    subcortical a.

alexic

alexin
    a. unit

aleydigism

Alezzandrini syndrome

ALG
    antilymphocyte globulin

aldesidystrophy

algesiogenic

algid
    a. malaria
    a. stage

algin

alginate

alginic acid

algiomotor

algiomuscular

algodystrophy

algoid cell

algogenic

ALGOL
    algorithm-oriented
        language

algorithm

algorithm-oriented language

algoscopy

algospasm

Aliber disease

alicyclic
    a. hydrocarbon

alienia

aliesterase

aligned grid

alignment chart

alimentary
    a. abstinence
    a. diabetes
    a. glycosuria
    a. lipemia
    a. osteopathy
    a. pentosuria
    a. tract smear

aliphatic
    a. acid
    a. alcohol
    a. saturated hydrocarbon
    a. unsaturated hydrocarbon

aliquant

aliquot

alizarin
    a. cyanin
    a. indicator
    a. monosulfonate
    a. No. 6
    a. purpurin
    a. red
    a. red S
    a. test
    a. yellow
    a. yellow g

alizarinopurpurin

alkalemia

alkalescence

alkalescent

alkali
- a. denaturation test
- a. metal
- olatile a.
- a. tolerance test

alkalimeter

alkalimetry

alkaline
- a. earth metal
- a. intoxication
- a. phosphatase (alk phos, alk phos)
- a. phosphatase activity of granular leukocyte (APGL)
- a. phosphatase assay
- a. phosphatase isoenzyme
- a. phosphatase isoenzyme elctrophoresis
- a. phosphatase method
- a. phosphatase stain
- a. phosphatase test
- a. reaction
- a. RNase
- a. tide
- a. toluidine blue O
- a. tuberculin (TA)
- a. wave

alkalinization

alkalinize

alkalinuria

alkali-soluble nitrogen (ASN)

alkalization

alkalize

alkaloid test

alkalosis
- acapnial a.
- altitude a.
- compensated a.
- hypochloremic a.
- hypokalemic a.
- metabolic a.

alkalosis (*continued*)
- metabolic a., compensated
- nonrespiratory a.
- potassium a.
- respiratory a.
- respiratory a., compensated
- uncompensated a.

alkalotic

alkaluria

alkane

alkanet

alkannan

alkannin
- a. paper

alkapton body

alkaptonuria test

alkaptonuric

alkene

alkenyl

alkoxide ion

alkoxy

alk phos
- alkaline phosphatase

alkyl
- a. group
- a. peroxide

alkylate

alkylating agent

alkylation

alkylbenzene sulfonate (ABS)

alkyne

ALL
- acute lymphoblastic leukemia
- acute lymphocytic leukemia

allachesthesia
- optical a.

allantoic
    a. acid
    a. cyst

allantoin

allantoinuria

allele
    multiple a.

allele-specific
    a.-s. loss
    a.-s. oligonucleotide (ASO)
    a.-s. oligonucleotide probe
    a.-s. PCR (A-PCR)

allelic
    a. exclusion
    a. gene

Allen
    A. correction
    C. test

Allen-Doisy
    A.-D. test
    A.-D. unit

Allen-Masters syndrome

allergen
    atopic a.

allergenic
    a. extract
    a. protein preparation

allergin-specific IgE anitbody

allergic
    a. asthma
    a. conjunctivitis
    a. coryza
    a. dermatitis
    a. eczema
    a. encephalitis
    a. encephalomyelitis
    a. extract
    a. granulomatous angiitis
    a. inflammation
    a. neuritis
    a. purpura

allergic (*continued*)
    a. reaction
    a. rhinitis
    a. transfusion reaction

allergin

allergization

allergized

allergoid

allergosis

allergy
    atopic a.
    bacterial a.
    cold a.
    contact a.
    delayed a.
    drug a.
    immediate a.
    latent a.
    physical a.
    polyvalent a.

allescheriosis

allesthesia
    visual a.

alligator
    a. clip
    a. skin

alloagglutinin

alloalbuminemia

alloantibody

alloantigen

alloantin-D antibody

allocation
    dynamic storage a.
    static storage a.
    storage a.

allocheiria

allochesthesia

alloschezia, allochetia

allochiral

allochiria

allochroic

allochroism

allochromacy

allochromasia

allodynia

alloesthesia

allogenic, allogeneic
    a. antigen
    a. graft
    a. inhibition
    a. transplantation

allograft
    a. rejection

allogroup

alloimmune

alloimmunization

allometric

allometry

allophanamide

allophenic

allophore

allophthalmia

alloplasia

alloplasmatic

alloplast

alloploidy

allopolyploidy

allopurinol

allorhythmia

allorhythmic

allosensitization

allosome
    paired a.

allosteric
    a. activation
    a. effector
    a. enzyme
    a. inhibition
    a. site

allostery

allotopia

allotopic

allotope

allotopia

allothreonine

allotransplantation

allotriogeustia

allotriosmia

allotrope

allotropic

allotrophy

allotype
    Gm a.
    InV a.
    Km a.

allotypic
    a. determination
    a. marker

alloxan

alloxan-Schiff reaction

alloxantin

alloxuria

allyl alcohol

Almeida disease

Almén test for blood

ALMI
    anterior lateral myocardial
       infarct

alochia

alopecia
    androgenetic a.
    a. androgenetica
    a. areatus
    cicatricial a.
    a. cicatrisata
    a. circumscripta
    congenital sutural a.
    a. congenitalis
    drug a.
    drug-induced a.
    male pattern a.
    moth-eaten a.
    a. mucinosa
    postpartum a.
    premature a.
    pressure a.
    psychogenic a.
    radiation a.
    radiation-induced a.
    a. seborrheica
    stress a.
    syphilitic a.
    a. syphilitica
    a. totalis
    traction a.
    traumatic a.
    traumatic marginal a.
    a. universalis
    x-ray a.

alopecic

ALP
    antilymphocyte plasma

AL patch test

Alpers disease

alpha, α
    a. acid glycoprotein
    a. acidophil
    a. actinin
    a. adrenergic blockade
    a. adrenergic receptor
    a. agglutinin
    a. amino acids
    a. blockade
    a. cell

alpha (*continued*)
    a. cell of hypophysis
    a. cell of pancreas
    a. chain
    a. decay
    a. fetoprotein
    a. globulin antibody
    a. globulins
    1, 4-a. glucan branching
      enzyme
    a. glucan-branching
      glycosyltransferase
    a. granule
    a. heavy-chain disease
    a. helix
    a. hemolysin
    a. hemolysis
    17 a. hydroxyprogesterone
    a. interferon therapy
    a. lipoprotein
    a. metachromasia
    a. motor neuron
    a. naphthol
    a. particle
    a. staphylolysin
    a. streptococcus
    a. substance
    a. thalassemia
    a. thalassemia intermedia
    a. units

alpha-a, α_1
    a. antichymotrypsin
    a. antitrypsin
    a. antitrypsin assay
    a. antitrypsin deficiency
    a. antitrypsin phenotyping
    a. band
    a. fetoglobulin
    a. fetoprotein
    a. fetoprotein assay
    a. globulin
    a. inhibitor
    a. protease inhibitor
    a. seromucoid
    a. trypsin inhibitor

alpha-2, α_2
    a. antiplasmin

alpha-2 (*continued*)
   a. globulin
   a. macroglobulin
   a. macroglobulin inhibitor
   a. neuraminoglycoprotein

aplha-1-acid glycoprotein

alpha-1,4-glucosidase deficiency

alpha cell

alpha chain disease

alphameric

alphanumeric

alphavirus

Alport syndrome

ALS
   amyotropic lateral sclerosis
   antilymphocyte syndrome

Alström syndrome

ALT
   alanine aminotransferase
      ALT test

ALT:AST ratio

alteration
   bone matrix a.
   carilage matrix a.
   chromosome a.
   crystalline macromolecule
      a.
   cyclic tissue a.
   cytologic a.
   cytoplasmic fiber a.
   cytoplasmic fibril a.
   cytoplasmic filament a.
   cytoplasmic lipid droplet a.
   cytoplasmic matrix a.
   decidul a.
   extracellular fibril a.
   extracellular matrix a.
   fibrocartilage matrix a.
   Golgi cavity a.
   Golgi membrane a.
   Golgi vacuole a.

alteration (*continued*)
   Golgi vesicle a.
   hematopoiectic maturation
      a.
   keratohyaline a.
   leukocytic maturation a.
   mitochondrian cristae a.
   mitochondrian matrix a.
   mitochondrian membrane
      a.
   Nissl substance a.
   nuclear-cytoplasmic ratio a.
   nuclear membrane a.
   nuclear pore a.
   nuclear sap a.
   nuclear shape a.
   nuclear size a.
   pH a.
   predecidual a.
   syncytical a.
   verrucopapillary a.

alterative inflammation

alternans
   cardiac a.
   mechanical a.
   pulsus a.
   total a.

alternant
   trace a.

alternate host

alternation
   a. of generations
   a. of the heart

alternative
   a. complement pathway
   a. hypothesis
   a. inheritence
   one-side a.
   two-sided a.

altitude
   a. anoxia
   a. disease

Altmann
   A. anilin-acid fuchsin stain

Altmann (*continued*)
   A. fixative
   A. granule

Altmann-Gersh method

alum
   a. carmine
   chrome a.

alum-hematoxylin

alumina
   a. hydroxide
   a. hydroxide gel
   a. oxide

aluminosis

alum-precipitated
   a.-p. pyridine (APP)
   a.-p. toxoid (APT)

alveobronchiolitis

alveolar
   a. abcess
   a. adenocarcinoma
   a. air
   a. air equation
   a. asthma
   a. cell
   a. cell carcinoma
   a. fenestra
   a. hydatid
   a. hydatid cyst
   a. hydatid disease
   a. macrophage
   a. phagocyte
   a. pneumocyte hyperplasia
   a. pore
   a. proteinosis
   a. rhabdomyosarcoma
   a. soft part sarcoma

alveolar-arterial
   a.-a. carbon dioxide
     difference
   a.-a. oxygen difference

alveolitis
   allergic a.
   cryptogenic fibrosing a.

alveolitis (*continued*)
   extrinsic allergic a.
   fibrosing a.

alveolitis
   acute pulmonary a.
   extrinsic allergic a.

alveoloclasia

alveolus
   pulmonary a.

alvinolith

ALW
   arch-loop-whorl

alymphia

alymphocytosis

alymphoplasia
   thymic a.

AM
   amperemeter

amacrinal

amacrine

Am antigen

amaranth

amastia

amaurosis
   central a.
   a. centralis
   cerebral a.
   a. congenita
   a. congenita of Leber
   congenital a.
   diabetic a.
   a. fugax
   Leber's congenital a.
   a.'s partialis fugax
   reflex a.
   saburral a.
   uremic a.

amaurotic

amazia

ambilevosity

ambilevous

ambiopia

ambisexual

ambisinister

ambisinistrous

amblyaphia

amblychromasia

amblychromatic

amblygeustia

amblyope

amblyopia
color a.
deficiency a.
a. ex anopsia
nocturnal a.
nutritional a.
reflex a.
strabismic a.
traumatic a.
uremic a.

ambosexual

ambustion

ameba
a. verrucosa

amebiasis
a. cutis
hepatic a.
intestinal a.
pulmonary a.

amebocyte

ameboma

ameburia

ameiosis

amelanosis

amelification

ameloblast

amelogenesis
a. imperfecta

amelogenic

amelogenin

amenia

amenorrhea
dysponderal a.
hypothalamic a.
lactation a.
nutritional a.
ovarian a.
physiologic a.
pituitary a.
premenopausal a.
primary a.
relative a.
secondary a.
traumatic a.

amenorrheal

ametachromophil

ametaneutrophil

ametria

ametropia
axial a.
curvature a.
index a.
position a.
refractive a.

ametropic

AMEX processing and
embedding

AMF
automated motility factor

AMG
antimacrophage globulin

AMH
anti-müllerian hormone

AMI
acute myocardial infarction

amianthoid

amicroscopic

amidobenzene

amimia

aminoacidemia

aminoacidopathy

aminoaciduria

α-aminoadipicaciduria

p-aminoazobenzene

aminobenzene

β-aminoisobutyricaciduria

aminosis

aminosuria

aminuria

amitosis

amitotic

AML
    acute monblastic leukemia
    acute monocytic leukemia
    acute myelocytic leukemia

AMLS
    anti-mouse lymphocyte
      serum

AMM
    ammonia

ammeter

AMML
    acute myelomonocytic
      leukemia

ammoaciduria

ammonemia

ammonia
    a. hemate

ammoniemia

ammoniomagnesium
  phosphate

ammonium
    a. oxalate
    a. purpurate
    a. magnesium phosphate

ammoniuria

amniocele

amniocyte

amnionitis

amniorrhea

amniorrhexis

AMoL
    acute monoblastic
      leukemia
    acute monocytic leukemia

amorphosynthesis

amotio
    a. retinae

AMP
    acid mucopolysaccharide
    adenosine monophosphate
      cyclic AMP

amphiaster

amphicyte

amphicytula

amphigastrula

amphigonadism

amphikaryon

amphimorula

amphipyrenin

amphitene

amphochromatophil

amphochromophil

amphocyte

amphodiplopia

amphophil

amphophile

amphophilic
    a.-basophil
    gram-a.
    a.-oxyphil

amphophilous

amphoricity

amphoriloquy

amphorophony

amphoterodiplopia

amphotony

AMPS
    abnormal
        mucopolysacchariduria
    acid mucopolysaccharides

ampullitis

ampullula

AMS
    antimacrophage serum
    automated multiphasic
        screening

amusia
    instrumental a.
    sensory a.
    vocal motor a.

AMV2
    avian myelocytomatosis
        virus

amyelinic

amylasuria

amylemia

amylodyspepsia

amyloid
    a. A
    a. L

amyloidosis
    AA a.
    a. of aging

amyloidosis (*continued*)
    AL a.
    cutaneous a.
    dialysis a.
    familial a.
    hemodialysis-associated a.
    hereditary a.
    hereditary neuropathic a.
    heredofamilial a.
    idiopathic a.
    immunocyte-derived a.
    immunocytic a.
    lichen a.
    light chain-related a.
    macular a.
    nodular a.
    primary a.
    reactive systemic a.
    renal a.
    secondary a.
    senile a.

amylopectinosis

amylorrhea

amylosuria

amyluria

amyoesthesia

amyoesthesis

amyoplasia
    a. congenita

amyostasia

amyostatic

amyotonia

amyotrophia
    neuralgic a.
    a. spinalis progressiva

amyotrophic

amyotrophy

amyous

amyxia

amyxorrhea

ANA
    antinuclear antibody

anacatesthesia

anacidity
    gastric a.

anacousia

anacusis

anadipsia

anadrenalism

anadrenia

anaerobiosis

anakmesis

anakusis

analbuminemia

analgesia
    a. algera
    paretic a.

analgetic

analgia

analgic

analphalipoproteinemia

analysis
    blood gas a.
    chromatographic a.

analyzer
    blood gas a.
    image a.
    oxygen gas a.

anangioid

ANAP
    anionic neutrophil
        activating peptide

anapepsia

anaphase
    flabby a.

anaphia

anaphoresis

anaphoria

anaptic

anarithmia

anarthria

anasarca

anasarcous

anascitic

anastral

anatomicopathological

anatropia

anatropic

ANCA
    antimeutrophil cytoplasmic
        antibody
    antimeutrophil cytoplasmic
        autoantibody

anconagra

anconitis

AND gate

androcyte

androgalactozemia

androgone

androgyne

androgynism

androgynoid

androgynous

androgyny

andropathy

anectasis

anemia
    achrestic a.
    achylic a.
    anhematopoietic a.
    aplastic a.

anemia (*continued*)

Arctic a.
aregenerative a.
congenital aregenerative a.
Bartonella a.
Blackfan-Diamond a.
cameloid a.
a. of chronic disease
a. of chronic disorders
congenital a. of newborn
Cooley's a.
cow's milk a.
deficiency a.
Diamond-Blackfan a.
dilution a.
dimorphic a.
congenital dyserythropoietic a.
elliptocytary a.
elliptocytic a.
elliptocytotic a.
Fanconi's a.
folic acid deficiency a.
goat's milk a.
Heinz body a.
hemolytic a.
autoimmune hemolytic a.
congenital hemolytic a.
congenital nonspherocytic hemolytic a.
drug-induced immune hemolytic a.
immune hemolytic a.
infectious hemolytic a.
nonspherocytic hemolytic a.
toxic hemolytic a.
hemolytic a. of newborn
hemorrhagic a.
hereditary iron-loading a.
hypochromic a.
hypochromic microcytic a.
a. hypochromica sideroachrestica hereditaria
hypoplastic a.
congenital hypoplastic a.
iron deficiency a.

anemia (*continued*)

leukoerythroblastic a.
macrocytic a.
nutritional macrocytic a.
tropical macrocytic a.
Mediterranean a.
megaloblastic a.
megalocytic a.
microangiopathic a.
microcytic a.
milk a.
mountain a.
myelopathic a.
myelophthisic a.
a. neonatorum
refractory normoblastic a.
normochromic a.
normocytic a.
nutritional a.
osteosclerotic a.
pernicious a.
congenital pernicious a.
physiologic a.
polar a.
acute posthemorrhagic a.
posthemorrhagic a. of newborn
pure red cell a.
pyridoxine-responsive a.
a. refractoria sideroblastica
refractory a.
scorbutic a.
sickle cell a.
sideroachrestic a.
acquired sideroachrestic a.
congenital sideroachrestic a.
hereditary sideroachrestic a.
primary acquired sideroblastic a.
X-linked sideroblastic a.
sideropenic a.
spherocytic a.
splenic a.
spur cell a.
microangiopathic hemolytic a.

anemia (*continued*)
    refractory sideroblastic a.
    sideroblastic a.
    hereditary sideroblastic a.
    acquired sideroblastic a.
    immunohemolytic a.
    juvenile pernicious a.

anephric

anepiploic

anerythroplasia

anerythroplastic

anerythropoiesis

anerythroregenerative

anesthecinesia

anesthekinesia

anesthesia
    angiospastic a.
    bulbar a.
    compression a.
    crossed a.
    dissociated a.
    dissociation a.
    a. dolorosa
    facial a.
    gauntlet a.
    girdle a.
    glove a.
    gustatory a.
    muscular a.
    nausea a.
    olfactory a.
    peripheral a.
    pressure a.
    segmental a.
    spinal a.
    tactile a.
    thalamic hyperesthetic a.
    thermal a.
    traumatic a.
    unilateral a.
    visceral a.

anetoderma
    Jadassohn's a.

anetoderma (*continued*)
    Jadassohn-Pellizari a.
    perifollicular a.
    postinflammatory a.
    Schweninger-Buzzi a.

aneugamy

aneuploid

aneuploidy

aneurogenic

aneurysm
    abdominal a.
    abdominal aortic a.
    ampullary a.
    aortic a.
    aortic sinusal a.
    arterial a.
    arteriosclerotic a.m
    arteriovenous a.
    arteriovenous pulmonary a.
    atherosclerotic a.
    axillary a.
    bacterial a.
    berry a.
    brain a.
    cardiac a.
    cerebral a.
    Charcot-Bouchard a.
    cirsoid a.
    compound a.
    congenital cerebral a.
    cylindroid a.
    dissecting a.
    ectatic a.
    embolic a.
    false a.
    fusiform a.
    hernial a.
    infected a.
    innominate a.
    intracranial a.
    lateral a.
    luetic a.
    miliary a.
    mixed a.
    mycotic a.

aneurysm (*continued*)
    Park's a.
    Pott's a.
    racemose a.
    Rasmussen's a.
    renal a.
    Richet's a.
    saccular a.
    sacculated a.
    serpentine a.
    spurious a.
    suprasellar a.
    syphilitic a.
    traumatic a.
    true a.
    tubular a.
    varicose a.
    venous a.
    ventricular a.

aneurysmal

aneurysmatic

angialgia

angiasthenia

angiectasis

angiectatic

angiectopia

angiitis
    allergic granulomatous a.
    granulomatous a. of central
      nervous system
    isolated a. of central
      nervous system
    hypersensitivity a.
    leukocytoclastic a.
    necrotizing a.

anginal

anginiform

anginoid

anginous

angioataxia

angioblast

angioblastic

angioblastoma

angiocarditis

angiocentric

angiocrine

angiocrinosis

angiocyst

angioderm

angiodynia

angiodysplasia

angiodystrophia

angiodystrophy

angioectatic

angioedema

angioedematous

angioelephantiasis

angiogranuloma

angiohemophilia

angiohyalinosis

angioinvasive

angiokeratoma
    a. circumscriptum
    a. corporis diffusum
    diffuse a.
    a. of Fordyce
    a. of Mibelli
    a. of scrotum
    solitary a.

angiokeratosis

angioleucitis

angioleukitis

angiolupoid

angiolymphangioma

angiolymphitis

angioma
    arteriovenous a. of brain
    capillary a.
    a. cavernosum
    cavernous a.
    cherry a.
    a. cutis
    fissural a.
    senile a.
    a. serpiginosum
    spider a.
    a. venosum racemosum

angiomatosis
    cerebroretinal a.
    encephalofacial a.
    encephalotrigeminal a.
    hepatic a.
    a. of retina
    retinocerebral a.

angiomatous

angiomegaly

angionecrosis

angioneuralgia

angioneuropathic

angioneuropathy

angioneurotic

angionoma

angioparalysis

angioparesis

angiopathology

angiopathy
    cerebral amyloid a.
    congophilic a.

angiophakomatosis

angioreticuloma

angiosclerosis

angioscotoma

angiospasm

angiospastic

angiostenosis

angiosteosis

angiotelectasis

angiotome

angitis

angle
    Cobb a.
    kyphotic a.
    squint a.

angor
    a. ocularis
    a. pectoris

angulus
    a. infectiosus

anhaphia

anhidrosis

anhidrotic

anhydremia

anhydrochloric

aniacinamidosis

aniacinosis

anidrosis

anidrotic

anile

aniline

anility

aniridia

aniseikonia

aniseikonic

anisoaccommodation

anisochromasia

anisochromia

anisocoria

anisocytosis

anisodactylous

anisodactyly

anisoiconia

anisokaryosis

anisomastia

anisomelia

anisometrope

anisometropia

anisometropic

anisophoria

anisopia

anisopiesis

anisopoikilocytosis

anisosmotic

anisosthenic

anisuria

ANLL
    acute nonlymphocytic
    leukemia

ankyloblepharon
    a. filiforme adnatum

ankylocheilia

ankylocolpos

ankyloglossia
    complete a.
    partial a.
    a. superior

ankylopoietic

ankylosed

ankyloses

ankylosis
    bony a.is
    cricoarytenoid joint a.
    extracapsular a.

ankylosis (*continued*)
    false a.
    fibrous a.
    intracapsular a.
    spurious a.
    stapedial a.
    true a.

ankylotic

ankylurethria

annulus
    a. of nuclear pore

anochromasia

anodmia

anodontia

anodontism

anomalad
    Robin's a.

anomalotrophy

anomaly
    Alder's a.
    Axenfeld's a.
    Chédiak-Higashi a.
    Chédiak-Steinbrinck-
     Higashi a.
    chromosomal a.
    chromosome a.
    Ebstein's a.
    Freund's a.
    Hegglin's a.
    Jordans' a.
    May-Hegglin a.
    Pelger's nuclear a.
    Pelger-Huët a.
    Pelger-Huët nuclear a.
    Peters' a.
    Poland's a.
    Rieger's a.
    Uhl's a.

anomia

anonychia

anophoria

anorchia

anorchid

anorchidic

anorchidism

anorchism

anorectic

anorectitis

anoretic

anorthography

anorthopia

anosmatic

anosmia
    a. gustatoria
    preferential a.
    a. respiratoria

anosmic

anosognosia

anosphresia

anosteoplasia

anostosis

anotropia

ANOVA
    analysis of variance

anovaria

anovarianism

anovarism

anovular

anovulation

anovulatory

anovulomenorrhea

anoxia
    altitude a.
    anemic a.
    anoxic a.
    myocardial a.

anoxia (*continued*)
    a. neonatorum
    stagnant a.

anoxiate

anoxic

ANS
    antineutrophilic serum
    arterolonephrosclerosis

ansa
    a. nephroni

antagonism
    salt a.

anteflexion

antelocation

antemortem

antephase

anteposition

anteprostatitis

anteversion

anthracene

anthraconecrosis

anthracosilicosis

anthracosis
    a. linguae

anthracotic

anthrax
    cerebral a.
    inhalational a.
    meningeal a.
    pulmonary a.

antibody
    anticardiolipin a.
    antigliadin a.
    anti-La a.
    anti-Ro a.
    anti-SS-A a.
    anti-SS-B a.

antigen
La a.
Ro a.
SS-A a.
SS-B a.

antileukocytic

antimetropia

antimitotic

antimongolism

antimongoloid

antinatriuresis

antinuclear

antiperistalsis

antiperistaltic

antiplastic

antipodal

antipode

antiport

antitemplate

antitrismus

antitubulin

antritis

antrocele

antrodynia

antrophose

anucleated

anulus
a. of spermatozoon

anuresis

anuretic

anuria
angioneurotic a.
calculous a.
obstructive a.
postrenal a.

anuria (*continued*)
prerenal a.
renal a.
suppressive a.

anuric

anus
ectopic a.
imperforate a.
a. vesicalis
a. vestibularis
vulvovaginal a.

anusitis

AOD
arterial occlusive disease

aortalgia

aortitis
Döhle-Heller a.
luetic a.
nummular a.
rheumatic a.
syphilitic a.
a. syphilitica

aortoduodenal

aortoenteric

aortoesophageal

aortogastric

aortopathy

aortosclerosis

AP
acute proliferative
aminopeptidase
angina pectoris

APA
aldosterone-producing
edenoma
aminopenicillanic acid
antipernicious anemia factor
atypical polypoid
adenomyofibroma
atypical polypoid
adenomyoma

apallesthesia

APA-LMP
Atypical polypoid
adenomyofibroma of low
malignant potential

apancrea

apancreatic

aparathyroidism

aparathyrosis

APC
adenoidal-pharyngeal-
conjunctival
APC virus

A-PCR
allele-specific PCR

APE
anterior pituitary extract

APEC glucose analyzer

apeidosis

apellous

aperistalsis

apertometer

APF
anabolism-promoting factor
animal protein factor

APGL
alkaline phosphatase
activity of granular
leukocyte

APH
antepartum hemorrhage
anterior pituitary hormone

aphacia

aphacic

aphagopraxia

aphakia

aphakic

aphalangia

aphasia
acoustic a.
acquired epileptic a.
amnesic a.
amnestic a.
anomic a.
associative a.
auditory a.
Broca's a.
central a.
combined a.
commissural a.
complete a.
conduction a.
expressive a.
expressive-receptive a.
fluent a.
frontocortical a.
gibberish a.
global a.
graphomotor a.
impressive a.
intellectual a.
jargon a.
mixed a.
motor a.
nominal a.
nonfluent a.
receptive a.
semantic a.
sensory a.
syntactical a.
tactile a.
total a.
transcortical a.
true a.
visual a.
Wernicke's a.

aphasiac

aphasic

aphasiology

aphemesthesia

aphemia

aphonogelia

aphose

aphosphagenic

aphotesthesia

APHP
   anti-*Pseudomonas* human
      plasma

aphrasia

aphtha
   Bednar's a.
   Mikulicz's a.
   recurring scarring a.

aphthae

aphthoid

aphthongia

aphthosis

aphthous

API 20 Strep System

apicitis

apituitarism

APL
   acute promyelocytic
      leukemia
   anterior pituitary-like

aplasia
   a. axialis extracorticalis
      congenita
   a. cutis congenita
   hereditary retinal a.
   Michel's a.
   nuclear a.
   pure red cell a.
   retinal a.
   Scheibe's a.
   thymic a.
   thymic-parathyroid a.

aplastic

apleuria

apneumatosis

apneusis

apneustic

apocamnosis

apochromat

apochromatic

apocrinitis

apokamnosis

aponeurositis

apophyseopathy

apoplasmatic

apoplectic

apoplectiform

apoplectoid

apoplexy
   abdominal a.
   adrenal a.
   bulbar a.
   cerebellar a.
   cerebral a.
   embolic a.
   heat a.
   ovarian a.
   pancreatic a.
   pituitary a.
   placental a.
   pontile a.
   pontine a.
   Raymond's a.
   renal a.
   spinal a.
   thrombotic a.
   uteroplacental a.

apoptosis

apoptotic

aposome

aposthia

APP
   alum-precipitated pyridine

apparatus
    central a.
    chromidial a.
    Golgi a.
    juxtaglomerular a.
    spindle a.
    subneural a.
    sucker a.
    Tiselius a.

appearance
    urea nitrogen a.

appendagitis
    epiploic a.

appendicitis
    actinomycotic a.
    acute a.
    amebic a.
    chronic a.
    a. by contiguity
    foreign-body a.
    fulminating a.
    gangrenous a.
    helminthic a.
    left-sided a.
    lumbar a.
    a.s obliterans
    obstructive a.
    perforating a.
    perforative a.
    protective a.
    purulent a.
    recurrent a.
    relapsing a.
    segmental a.
    skip a.
    stercoral a.
    subperitoneal a.
    suppurative a.
    traumatic a.
    verminous a.

appendicocele

appendicolithiasis

appendicopathy

appendolithiasis

applanation

APR
    amebic prevalence rate

apractagnosia

apractic

apraxia
    akinetic a.
    amnestic a.
    Bruns' a. of gait
    buccofacial a.
    classic a.
    Cogan's oculomotor a.
    congenital oculomotor a.
    constructional a.
    dressing a.
    facial a.
    ideational a.
    ideokinetic a.
    ideomotor a.
    innervatory a.
    Liepmann's a.
    motor a.
    sensory a.
    a. of speech
    transcortical a.

apraxic

aproctia

APT
    alum-precipitated toxoid

APTT, aPTT
    activated partial
      thromboplastin time
    APTT test

apt test

aptyalia

aptyalism

APUD
    amine precursor uptake
      and decarboxlation

apyetous

apyknomorphous

apyogenic

apyous

apyrene

aquaporin

AR
   analytical reagent grade
   Argyll Robertson
      AR grade

arabinosuria

arachidic

arachnitis

arachnodactylia

arachnodactyly
   congenital contractural a.

araphia

arbor
   dendritic a.

arborization

ARC
   AIDS-related complex

archamphiaster

arctation

arcuation

ARD
   acute respiratory disease

ARDS
   acute respiratory distress
      syndrome
   adult respiratory distress
      syndrome

ardor
   a. urinae

area
   Bamberger's a.
   a. cerebrovasculosa
   Cohnheim's a.
   a. medullovasculosa
   pressure a.
   watershed a.

areflexia

aregenerative

areolitis

ARF
   acute renal failure
   acute respiratory failure

argamblyopia

argema

argentaffin

argentation

arginase deficiency

argininemia

argininosuccinase deficiency

argininosuccinate synthase
   deficiency

argininosuccinicacidemia

argininosuccinicaciduria

argyremia

argyrophil

ariboflavinosis

ARM
   artificial rupture of
      membranes

arrhaphia

arrhigosis

arrhythmia

arrhythmic

arrhythmogenesis

arrhythmogenic

arrhythmokinesis

ARS
   antirabies serum

ART
   absolute retention time
   automated reagin test

ART (*continued*)
   ART test

arteralgia

arteria
   a. lusoria

arteriectasia

arteriectasis

arteriectopia

arteriolith

arteriolitis
   hyperplastic a.
   necrotizing a.

arteriolonecrosis

arteriolopathy
   calcific uremic a.

arteriolosclerosis
   hyaline a.
   hyperplastic a.

arteriolosclerotic

arterionecrosis

arteriopathy
   hypertensive a.
   plexogenic a.
   plexogenic pulmonary a.y

arteriorrhexis

arteriosclerosis
   cerebral a.
   coronary a.
   hyaline a.
   hypertensive a.
   infantile a.
   intimal a.
   medial a.
   Mönckeberg's a.
   a. obliterans
   peripheral a.
   presenile a.
   senile a.

arteriosclerotic

arteriosteogenesis

arteriostosis

arteritides

arteritis
   aortic arch a.
   brachiocephalic a.
   a. brachiocephalica
   coronary a.
   cranial a.
   giant cell a.
   granulomatous a.
   Horton's a.
   infantile a.
   infectious a.
   localized visceral a.
   necrotizing a.
   a. obliterans
   rheumatic a.
   syphilitic a.
   Takayasu's a.
   temporal a.
   tuberculous a.
   a. umbilicalis

artery
   copper-wire a.

arthrempyesis

arthritide

arthritides

arthrocele

arthrochalasis
   a. multiplex congenita

arthrochondritis

arthroclasia

arthroclisis

arthrodynia

arthrodysplasia

arthroempyesis

arthrogryposis
   congenital multiple a.
   a. multiplex congenita

arthrokatadysis

arthrokleisis

arthrolith

arthrolithiasis

arthromeningitis

arthroncus

arthroneuralgia

arthro-onychodysplasia

arthro-ophthalmopathy
    hereditary progressive a.

arthropathia
    a. ovaripriva
    a. psoriatica

arthropathic

arthropathology

arthropathy
    Charcot's a.
    chondrocalcific a.
    crystal a.
    hemophilic a.
    inflammatory a.
    neurogenic a.
    neuropathic a.
    osteopulmonary a.
    psoriatic a.
    pyrophosphate a.
    static a.
    syphilitic a.
    tabetic a.

arthrophyma

arthrophyte

arthropyosis

arthrosclerosis

arthrosynovitis

ARV
    AIDS-related virus

arylsulfatase A deficiency

arylsulfatase B deficiency

arytenoiditis

AS
    Adams-Stokes disease
    aortic stenosis
    arteriosclerosis
    atherosclerosis

ASA
    Adams-Stokes attack

ASAP Biopsy System

asbestosis

ascariasis
    pulmonary a.

ascites
    a. adiposus
    bile a.
    bloody a.
    chyliform a.
    a. chylosus
    chylous a.
    exudative a.
    fatty a.
    hemorrhagic a.
    hydremic a.
    milky a.
    a. praecox
    preagonal a.
    pseudochylous a.
    transudative a.

ascitic

ascitogenous

ascorbemia

ascorburia

ASCUS
    atypical squamous cells of
      undetermined significance

ASCVD
    arterioclerotic
      cardiovascular disease
    atheroclerotic
      cardiovascular disease

ASD
    aldosterone sercretion test
    atrial septal defect

asemasia

asemia

ASH
    asymmetrical septal
        hypertrophy

asialia

asiderosis

asitia

ASMI
    anteroseptal myocardial
        infarct

ASN
    alkali-soluble nitrogen

Asn
    asparagine

ASO
    allele-specific
        oligonucleotide
    antistreptolysin-O
    arteriosclerosis obliterans
        ASO probe
        ASO test
        ASO titer

asomatognosia

Asp
    aspartic acid

aspartylglucosaminuria

aspartylglycosaminuria

aspergilloma

aspergillosis
    aural a.
    bronchopneumonic a.
    bronchopulmonary a.
    bronchopulmonary a.,
        allergic
    chronic necrotizing a.
    invasive a.
    pulmonary a.

aspermatism

aspermatogenesis

aspermia

asphygmia

asphyxia
    birth a.
    blue a.
    a. cyanotica
    fetal a.
    a. livida
    a. neonatorum
    a.pallida
    perinatal a.
    secondary a.
    traumatic a.
    white a.

asphyxial

asphyxiant

asphyxiate

asphyxiation

aspiration
    meconium a.

asplenia
    functional a.

asplenic

ASR
    aldosterone secretion rate
    aldosterone secretory rate

assay
    competitive protein-binding
        a.
    enzyme-linked
        immunosorbent a.
    four-point a.
    radioligand a.
    radioreceptor a.
    stable isotope dilution a.

AST
    asparate aminotransferase
        AST test

astasia

astatic

asteatodes

asteatosis

aster

astereocognosy

astereognosis

asterixis

asteroid

asthenia
    cutaneous a.
    myalgic a.
    periodic a.

asthenic

asthenocoria

asthenope

asthenopia
    accommodative a.
    muscular a.
    nervous a.
    tarsal a.

asthenopic

asthenospermia

asthenoxia

asthmatiform

asthmogenic

astigmia

astigmic

astral

astroblast

astrocele

astrocinetic

astrocoele

astrocyte
    fibrillary a.
    fibrous a.

astrocyte (*continued*)
    gemistocytic a.
    plasmatofibrous a.
    protoplasmic a.

astrocytosis

astroglia

astrokinetic

astrophorous

astrosphere

astrostatic

asulfurosis

ASV
    antisnake venom

asyllabia

asymbolia

asymboly

asynapsis

asynchronism

asynchrony

asynclitism
    anterior a.
    posterior a.

asynergia

asynergic

asynergy

asynovia

asystole

asystolia

asystolic

ATA
    anti-*Toxoplasma* antibodies

atactic

atactiform

ataxia
    acute a.

ataxia (*continued*)
  acute cerebellar a.
  Bruns' frontal a.
  cerebellar a.
  cerebral a.
  Ferguson-Critchley ataxia
  Friedreich's a.
  frontal a.
  hereditary a.
  kinetic a.
  locomotor a.
  Menzel's a.
  motor a.
  ocular a.
  Sanger Brown a.
  sensory a.
  spinal a.
  spinocerebellar a.
  a.-telangiectasia
  thermal a.
  truncal a.

ataxiaphasia

ataxic

ataxy

ATCC
  American Type Culture
    Collection

ATD
  asphyxiating thoracic
    dystrophy

ATE
  adipose tissue extract

atelectasis

atelectatic

ATG
  antihyroglobulin

AT/GC ratio

atheroembolism

atheroembolus

atherogenesis

atherogenic

atheroma

atheromatosis

atheromatous

atherosclerosis obliterans

atherosis

athetoid

athetosic

athetosis

athetotic

athiaminosis

athrepsia

athrepsy

athreptic

athymia

athymism

athyrea

athyreosis

athyreotic

athyria

athyroidemia

athyroidism

athyroidosis

athyrosis

athyrotic

AT III, AT-III
  anithrombin III

ATL
  adult T-cell leukemia
  adult T-cell lyphoma

atmosphere
  a. absolute
  explosive a.

ATN
  acute tubular necrosis

atom
  asymmertric carbon a.

atomic
  a. absorption (AA)
  a. absorption
    spectrophotometer
  a. absorption
    spectrophotometry
    (AAS)
  a. mass
  a. mass unit
  a. number
  a. spectrum
  a. weight
  a. weight unit (awu)

atonia
  choreatic a.

atonic

atonicity

atony
  primary ureteral a.

atopognosia

atopognosis

ATP
  adenosine triphosphate
    ATP pyrophospho-
    hydrolase

ATPase
  adenosine triphosphatase
    calcium-activated A.
    magnesium-activated
    A.
    Padykula-Herman stain
    for myosin A.
    A. stain

ATPS
  ambient temperature and
    pressure, saturated

atransferrinemia

atrepsy

atreptic

atresia

atresic

atretic

atretoblepharia

atretogastria

atretopsia

atretorrhinia

atretostomia

atrichosis

atrichous

atriomegaly

atrioventricularis communis

atrophedema

atrophia
  a. bulborum hereditaria
  a. choroideae et retinae
  a. cutis
  a. cutis senilis
  a. dolorosa
  a. maculosa
  a. musculorum lipomatosa
  a. senilis
  a. testiculi

atrophie
  a. blanche
  a.e noire

atrophoderma
  a. biotripticum
  idiopathic a. of Pasini and
    Pierini
  a. maculatum
  a. neuriticum
  a. of Pasini and Pierini
  a. reticulatum
    symmetricum faciei
  a. senile
  a. vermicularis

atrophodermatosis

atrophodermia
  a. vermiculata

atrophy

- acute yellow a.
- Aran-Duchenne muscular a.
- arthritic a.
- black a.
- blue a.
- bone a.
- brown a.
- Charcot-Marie a.
- Charcot-Marie-Tooth a.
- circumscribed cerebral a.
- compensatory a.
- compression a.
- concentric a.
- corticostriatospinal a.
- Cruveilhier's a.
- degenerative a.
- Dejerine-Sottas a.
- Dejerine-Thomas a.
- denervated muscle a.
- dentatorubral a.
- a. of disuse
- Duchenne-Aran muscular a.
- eccentric a.
- Eichhorst's a.
- endocrine a.
- endometrial a.
- Erb's a.
- facial a.
- facioscapulohumeral muscular a.
- fatty a.
- Fazio-Londe a.
- gastric a.
- granular a. of kidney
- gray a.
- gyrate a. of choroid and retina
- healed yellow a.
- hemifacial a.
- hemilingual a.
- Hoffmann's a.
- Hunt's a.
- idiopathic muscular a.
- infantile a.
- inflammatory a.y
- interstitial a.
- essential a. of iris

atrophy (*continued*)

- ischemic muscular a.
- juvenile muscular a.
- lactation a.
- Landouzy-Dejerine a.
- leaping a.
- Leber's hereditary optic a.
- linear a.
- lobar a.
- macular a.
- multiple system a.
- muscular a.
- myelopathic muscular a.
- myopathic a.
- neural a.
- neuritic muscular a.
- neuropathic a.
- neurotrophic a.
- numeric a.
- olivopontocerebellar a.
- optic a.
- hereditary optic a.
- primary optic a.
- secondary optic a.
- pallidal a.
- Parrot's a. of the newborn
- pathologic a.
- periodontal a.
- peroneal a.
- peroneal muscular a.
- physiologic a.
- pigmentary a.
- postmenopausal a.
- post-traumatic a. of bone
- pressure a.
- progressive choroidal a.
- progressive hemifacial a.
- progressive muscular a.
- progressive neural muscular a.
- progressive neuromuscular a.
- pseudohypertrophic muscular a.
- red a.
- rheumatic a.
- segmental sensory dissociation with brachial muscular a.

atrophy (*continued*)
    senile a.
    senile a. of skin
    serous a.
    simple a.
    spinal muscular a.
    infantile spinal muscular a.
    progressive spinal muscular a.
    proximal spinal muscular a.
    Werdnig-Hoffmann spinal muscular a.
    subacute a. of liver
    subchronic a. of liver
    Sudeck's a.y
    Tooth's a.
    toxic a.
    trophoneurotic a.
    vascular a.
    Vulpian's a.
    white a.
    yellow a.
    Zimmerlin's a.

ATS
    antitetanic serum
    antihymocyte serum
    arteriosclerosis

attached cranial section

attachment
    a. plaque
    spindle a.

attack
    Adam-Stokes a. (ASA)
    a. rate
    transient ischemic a.

attenuant

attenuate

attenuated
    a. culture
    a. tuberculosis
    a. vaccine
    a. virus

attenuation

attenuator

attraction sphere

attribute

atypia
    cellular a.
    koilcytotic a.

atypical
    a. adenomatous hyperplasia (AAH)
    a. fibrous histiocytoma
    a. fibroxanthoma
    a. insulin
    a. lipoma
    a. lymphocyte
    a. measles
    a. melanocytic hyperplasia
    a. mycobacteria
    a. polypoid adenomyofibroma (APA)
    a. polypoid adenomyoma of low malignant potential (APA-LMP)
    a. polypoid adenomyoma (APA)
    a. primary pneumonia
    a. regeneration
    a. squamous cells of undetermined significance (ASCUS)
    a. verrucous endocarditis

atypism

AU
    antitoxin unit
    Australia antigen

Au Ag
    Australia antigen

audio amplifier

Auer
    A. body

D. rod

Auger
    A. effect

Auger (*continued*)
   A. electron

augmented histamine test
   (AHT)

Aujeszky
   A. disease
   A. disease virus

AUL
   acute undifferetiated
      leukemia

AUO
   amyloid of unknown origin

aural polyp

auramine
   a. O fluoroscent stain

auramine-rhodamine stain

aurantia

aurantiasis

aureolin

auricle
   cervical a.

aurid

aurin

aurochromoderma

Aus antigen

auscultatory gap

Australia antigen (AU, Au Ag)

Australian
   A. X disease
   A. X disease virus
   A. X encephalitis
   E. X encephalitis virus

autecic

autemesia

autoadsorption

autoagglutination

autoagglutinin
   anti-Pr cold a.
   cold a.

autoallergic hemolytic anemia

autoallergization

autoallergy

autoamputation

AutoAnalyzer

autoanalyzer
   sequential multichannel a.
      (SMA)

autobiotic

autocholecystectomy

autoclasis

autocytolysis

autocytolytic

autodigestion

autoecholalia

autoeczematization

autoerythrophagocytosis

autofluorescence

autogamous

autogamy

autohemagglutination

autohemagglutinin

autohemolysin

autohemolysis

autohemolytic

autolysate

autolysis
   postmortem a.

autolysosome

autolytic

autolyze

automaticity
    triggered a.

Automeris

automixis

autophagia

autophagolysosome

autophagosome

autophagy

autophony

autoproteolysis

autopsy

autoradiography

autosensitization
    erythrocyte a.

autosepticemia

autosomatognosis

autosomatognostic

autosome

autosplenectomy

autosynthesis

autotemnous

autotomy

autotopagnosia

autotrepanation

autovaccinia

auxochrome

auxochromous

A-V
    arteriovenous
    arterioventricular
    auriculoventricular
        A-V block

Av
    avoirdupois

avenolith

AV/AF
    anteverted/anteflexed

avalanche ionization

avascular
    a. necrosis

Avellis syndrome

average
    a. deviation (AD)
    a. gradient
    a. life
    Walsh a.
    weighted a.

AVF
    arteriovenous fistula

AVH
    acute viral hepatitis

avitaminosis

avitaminotic

AVM
    arteriovenous malformation

Avogadro number

avoirdupois (Av)

AVP
    arginine vasopressin

AVR
    aortic valve replacement

avulsed wound

avulsion

AW
    anterior wall

AWI
    anterior wall infarction

AWMI
    anterior wall myocardial
        infarction

awu
    atomic weight unit

Axenfeld syndrome

axenic

AXG
    adult-type
        xanthogranuloma

axial aneurysm

axilemma

axiopodium

axis
    cell a.
    renin-aldosterone a.
    a. of rotation
    a. of symmetry

axoaxonic

axodendritic

axolemma

axolysis

axon
    fusimotor a.
    myelinated a.
    naked a.
    unmyelinated a.

axonal
    a. degeneration
    a. demyelination

axonapraxia

axone

axoneme

axonopathy
    distal a.
    proximal a.

axonotmesis

axophage

axoplasm

axoplasmic

axopodium

axosomatic

axostyle

Ayerza
    A. disease
    A. syndrome

Ayoub-Shklar method

Ayre spatula

A-Z
    Achheim-Zondek
        A-Z test

azan stain

azar
    kala a.

azathioprine

azeotrope

azeotropic solution

azeotropy

azide

azidothymidine (AZT)

azin dye

azinphosmethyl

azo
    a. coupling reaction
    a. dye

azobenzene

azobilirubin

azocarmine
    a. B
    a. dye
    a. G

azoic
    a. dye

azoospermatism

azoospermia

azoprotein

azote

azotemia

azotemia (*continued*)
    chloropenic a.
    extrarenal a.
    hypochloremic a.
    nonrenal a.
    postrenal a.
    prerenal a.
    renal a.

azotemic

azotometer

azotorrhea

azoturia

azoturic

AZT
    Aschheim-Zondek test
    azidothymidine

azure
    a. I
    a. II
    a. A
    a. B
    a. C
    methylene a.

azure-eosin stain

azuresin

azurophil, azurophile
    a. granule

azurophilia

azurophilic granule

azymia

Azzopardi criteria

B

B
- bacillus
- Baumé scale
- Benoist scale
- whole blood
    - B cell
    - B cell antigen receptor
    - B lymphocyte
    - B virus
    - B virus hepatitis

b
- bis
- blood

4B

B5 fixative

B–5 sodium acetate-sublimate formalin

10B

B19 virus

B72.3
- B. antibody
- B. stain

BA
- bacterial agglutination
- blocking antibody
- bronchial asthma

Baastrup syndrome

Babcock tube

Babes-Ernst granule

Babesiidae

babesiosis
- b. serological test

Babès node

Babinski-Frölich syndrome

Babinski-Nageotte syndrome

Babinksi syndrome

Babinski-Vaquez syndrome

baby
- blue b.
- collodion b.
- giant b.

BAC
- blood alcohol concentration

Bachman-Pettit test

Bachman test

Bacillaceae

bacillary
- b. dysentery
- b. embolism
- b. emulsion (tuberculin) (BE)
- b. hemoglobinuria

Bacille
- F. bilié de Calmette-Guérin (BCG)

bacillemia

bacilli (*pl. of* bacillus)

bacilliform

bacillosis

bacilluria

bacitracin disk test

back
- adolescent round b.

backbone

backcross

background
- b. count
- flame b.
- b. interference
- pathoanatomic b.
- smear b.

backknee

backwash ileitis

Bactalert
    B. analyzer
    B. FAN culture medium
    B. system

BACTEC blood culture system

bacterascites
    monomicrobial non-
      neutrocytic b.
    polymicrobial b.

bacterid
    pustular b.

bacteriospermia

bacteriuria

bacteriuric

bacteruria

bagassosis

BAL
    bronchoalveolar lavage

Balamuth
    B. buffer solution
    B. culture medium

balance
    acid-base b.
    fluid b.
    water b.
    negative b.
    positive b.
    zero b.

balanitis
    amebic b.
    b. circinata
    b. circumscripta
      plasmacellularis
    b. diabetica
    erosive b.
    Follmann's b.
    b. gangraenosa
    gangrenous b.
    phagedenic b.
    plasma cell b.
    b. plasmacellularis
    b. xerotica obliterans

balanocele

balanoposthitis
    chronic circumscribed
      plasmocytic b.
    b. chronica circumscripta
      plasmocellularis
    specific gangrenous and
      ulcerative b.

balanoposthomycosis

balanorrhagia

balantidiasis

balantidiosis

balantidosis

Balbiani
    B. body
    B. chromosome
    B. ring

Balint syndrome

Balkan nephropathy

ball
    chondrin b.
    food b.
    fungus b.
    Marchi b.
    pleural fibrin b.

Baller-Gerold syndrome

Ballet disease

Ballingall disease

ballism

ballismus

balm
    b. of Gilead

Baló disease

balsam
    Canada b.
    b. of Gilead

Bamberger
    B. albuminuria
    B. disease

Bamberger-Marie
    B.-M. disease
    B.-M. syndrome

BamH1 enzyme

Bamle disease

Bancroft
    B. filarial worm
    B. filariasis

bancroftiasis

band
    A b.
    contraction b.
    H b.
    I b.
    Lane's b.
    M b.
    Soret b.
    Vicq d'Azyr's b.
    Z b.

Bandl ring

bandpass

Bannister disease

Banti
    B. disease
    B. spleen
    B. syndrome

BAO
    basal acid output

BAP
    blood agar plate

baragnosis

Barany caloric test

Barbados leg

barber's itch

barbiero

Barclay-Baron disease

Barcoo disease

Bardet-Beidl syndrome

Bard needle

bare lymphocyte syndrome

Bargen streptococcus

baritosis

barium test

Barlow
    B. disease
    B. syndrome

Barnett-Bourne acetic alcohol-
    silver nitrate method

baroagnosis

baro-otitis
    baro-otitis media

barosinusitis

barotitis
    b. media

barotrauma
    pulmonary b.
    otitic b.
    sinus b.

Barraquer disease

Barré-Guillain syndrome

barreling distortion

Barrett
    B. epithelium
    B. esophagus
    B. syndrome
    B. ulcer

barrier
    blood-air b.
    blood-brain b.
    blood-cerebral b.
    b. filter
    blood-gas b.
    blood-testis b.
    blood-thymus b.
    filtration b.

bartholinitis

Bartonella

Bartonella (*continued*)
    B. elizabethae
    B. vinsonii

bartonelliasis

bartonellosis

baruria

barytosis

basalis

bascule
    cecal b.

base
    buffer b.

basedoid

basedowiform

basicaryoplastin

basichromatin

basichromiole

basicytoparaplastin

basiparachromatin

basiparaplastin

basiphilic

basometachromophil

basophil
    beta b.
    Crooke-Russell ba.
    delta b.

basophile

basophilia
    diffuse b.
    punctate b.

basophilic

basophilism
    Cushing's b.
    pituitary b.

basophilopenia

basophilous

basoplasm

bathomorphic

bathrocephaly

bathyanesthesia

bathycardia

bathyhyperesthesia

bathyhypesthesia

batonet

BB
    blood bank
    blood buffer base
    blue bloater
    breakthrough bleeding
    breast biopsy
    buffer base
        orseillin BB

BBB
    blood-brain barrier
    bundle-branch block

BC
    bactericidal concentration

BCB
    brilliant cresyl blue

B-cell
    B.-c. differentiating factor
    B.-c. growth factor I, II
    B.-c. lymphoma (BCL)
    B.-c. malignancy
    B.-c. marker
    B.-c. stimulating factor

BCF .
    basophil chemotactic factor

BCG
    Bacille bilié de Calmette-
        Guérin
    bicolor guaiac (test)
    bromocresol green
        BCG vaccine

BCL
    B-cell lymphoma

bcl-2
   bcl-2 antibody
   bcl-2 gene arrangement
   bcl-2 oncogene
   bcl-2 protein
   bcl-2 proto-oncogene

bcl-1/PRAD1 gene
   rearrangement

BCNU
   bischloroethylnitrosourea
   bischloronitrosourea

BCP-D
   bromocresol purple
      desoxycholate

BD
   base deficit

BDG
   buffered desooxycholate
      glucose

BE
   bacillary emulsion
      (tuberculin)
   bacterial endocarditis
   base excess
   bovine enteritis

bead
   rachitic b.
   scorbutic b.

beading
   arteriolar b.

beaked pelvis

Be^a antigen

Beau
   B. disease
   B. line
   G. syndrome

Beauvais disease

Beaver direct smear method

Bechterew disease

Beck

Beck (*continued*)
   B. disease
   B. triad

Becker
   B. antigen
   B. disease
   B. distrophy
   B. nevus
   B. stain for spirochetes

Beckman
   B. Paragon SPE-II Gel
      Apparatus

Beckwith-Wiedemann
   syndrome

becquerel (Bq)

Becton-Dickinson needle

Bednar tumor

Begbie disease

Béguez César disease

Behçet
   B. disease
   B. syndrome

begma

Behnken unit (R)

Behr disease

BEI
   butanol-extractable iodine
      BEI test

Beigel disease

bejel

Bekhterev disease

Belgian Congo enemia

Belke-Kleihauer stain

Bell-Magendie law

Bence
   B. Jones (BJ)
   B. Jones albumin
   B. Jones albuminuria

Bence (*continued*)
    B. Jones cylinder
    B. Jones myeloma
    B. Jones protein
    B. Jones protein test
    B. Jones proteinuria
    Jones reaction

Benditt hypothesis

Benedict
    B. solution
    B. test for glucose

Benedict-Hopkins-Cole reagent

Bengston method

benzalin

1,2-benzenedicarboxylic acid

benzidine

benzopurpurine
    b. 4B

benzoylecgonine

benzoylglycine

Ber-EP4
    B.-E. antibody
    B.-E. immunoperoxidase
        stain

Berg
    B. chelate removal
        method
    B. stain

bergamot oil

Ber-H2 antibody

beriberi
    atrophic b.
    cerebral b.
    dry b.
    infantile b.
    paralytic b.
    wet b.

beriberic

Berkefeld filter

berylliosis
    acute b.
    chronic b.

beta-naphtholsulfonic acid

betanin

bezoar

Bezold abscess

BF
    blastogenic factor

B/F
    bound-free ratio

bf
    bouillon filtrate (tuberculin)

BFP
    biologic false-positive

BFR
    biologic false-positive
        reactor
    bone formation rate

BFT
    bentonite flocculation test

BFU-E
    burst-forming unit-erythroid

BGG
    bovine growth globulin

BGH
    bovine growth hormone

BGSA
    Blood granulocyte-specific
        activity

BGTT
    Borderline glucose
        tolerance test

BHBA
    β-hydroxybutyrate

BHC
    benzene hexachloride

BHI
    brain-heart infusion

BHS
 a-hemolytic strepococcus

BHTU microscope

BH/VH
 body hematocrit-venous
  hemacrit ratio

BI
 bacteriological index
 burn index

Bial
 B. reagent
 B. test

Bianchi syndrome

Bi antigen

biatriatum
 cor pseudotriloculare b.
 cor triloculare b.

bibulous

bicameral abscess

bicarbonate
 blood b.
 plasma b.
 standard b.

bicollis

BIDLB
 block in posteroinferior
  division of left branch

Biebrich
 B. scarlet
 B. scarlet-picroaniline blue
 B. scarlet red

Biedl disease

Bielschowsky
 B. disease
 B. method
 B. stain

Bielschowsky-Jansky disease

Biemond syndrome

Biermer

Biermer (*continued*)
 B. anemia
 B. disease

biferiens

biferious

bifid
 b. bacterium
 b. tongue
 b. ureter
 b. uterus

bifida
 spina b.

bigemina

bigeminal

bigeminy

BIH
 benign intracranial
  hypertension

bilateral
 b. left-sidedness
 b. otitis media (BOM)
 b. synnetrical, and equal
  (BSE)
 b. symmetry

bilayer

Bilderbeck disease

bilious

bilirachia

bilirubinemia

bilirubinuria

biliuria

biloma

binuclear

binucleate

binucleation

binucleolate

biomicroscope

biomicroscopy

bionecrosis

bioplasmic

biopyoculture

bisferiens

bisferious

bismuthia

bituminosis

bivalent

BJ
Bence Jones

Björnstad syndrome

BJP
Bence Jones protein

BK virus

BL
bleeding
blood loss
Burkitt lymphoma

black
fat b. HB
indulin b.
b. periodic acid method
b. peidra
b. plague
solvent b. 3
Sudan b. B

BLA 36 monoclonal antibody

Blancophor

blankophore

blastid

blastide

blastin

blastocyte

blastogenesis

blastogenetic

blastogenic

blastomere

blastomycosis
European b.
pulmonary b.

BLB
Bessey-Lowry Brock
Boothby, Lovelace,
Bulbulian
BLB mask
BLB unit

bleb
emphysematous b.

bleeding
dysfunctional uterine b.
implantation b.
occult b.

blennadenitis

blennemesis

blennorrhagia

blennorrhagic

blennorrhea
inclusion b.
b. neonatorum
Stoerk's b.

blennorrheal

blennothorax

blennuria

blepharadenitis

blepharelosis

blepharism

blepharitis
b. angularis
b. ciliaris
marginal b.
b. marginalis
nonulcerative b.
seborrheic b.
b. ulcerosa
squamous b.

blepharoadenitis

blepharochalasis

blepharochromidrosis

blepharoclonus

blepharoconjunctivitis

blepharodiastasis

blepharopachynsis

blepharophimosis

blepharoplegia

blepharoptosis

blepharopyorrhea

blepharospasm
essential b.
symptomatic b.

blepharostenosis

blepharosynechia

BLG
β-lactoglobulin

blindness
amnesic color b.
blue b.
blue-yellow b.
Bright's b.
color b.
complete color b.
concussion b.
cortical b.
cortical psychic b.
day b.
eclipse b.
electric-light b.
flight b.
functional b.
green b.
hysterical b.
legal b.
letter b.
music b.
night b.
object b.

blindness (*continued*)
psychic b.
red b.
red-green b.
river b.
snow b.
taste b.
text b.
total b.
total color b.
word b.
yellow b.

Bloch reaction

Bloch-Sulzberger
B.-S. disease
B.-S. syndrome

block
air b.
alveolar-capillary b.
anodal b.
anterior fascicular b.
atrioventricular b.
AV b.
2:1 AV b.
bifascicular b.
bilateral bundle branch b.
bundle branch b.
comparator b.
complete atrioventricular b.
complete heart b.
conduction b.
congenital complete heart
b.
depolarization b.
dynamic b.
entrance b.
exit b.
fascicular b.
first degree atrioventricular
b.
first degree heart b.
heart b.
high grade atrioventricular
b.
incomplete heart b.
interventricular b.

block (*continued*)
    intra-Hisian b.
    intrahisian b.
    intraventricular b.
    left anterior fascicular b.
    left bundle branch b.
    left posterior fascicular b.
    Mobitz type I b.
    Mobitz type II b.
    partial heart b.
    periinfarction b.
    posterior fascicular b.
    right bundle branch b.
    second degree
      atrioventricular b.
    second degree heart b.
    sinoatrial b.
    sinoatrial exit b.
    sinus b.
    spinal b.
    spinal subarachnoid b.
    third degree atrioventricular
      b.
    third degree heart b.
    trifascicular b.
    unifascicular b.
    ventricular b.
    Wenckebach b.
    sinus exit b.

blockade
    neuromuscular b.
    renal b.

blood
    occult b.
    sludged b.

BLT
    blood-clot lysis time

BLU
    Bessey-Lowry unit

blue
    alcian b.
    alizarin b.
    alkali b.
    aniline b.
    aniline b., W. S.
    anthracene b.

blue (*continued*)
    Berlin b.
    Borrel's b.
    brilliant b., C.
    brilliant cresyl b.
    bromchlorphenol b.
    bromphenol b.
    bromthymol b.
    china b.
    Congo b.e 3B
    cresyl b., 2 R. N. or B. B. S.
    cyanol b.
    Evans b.
    indigo b.
    soluble indigo b.
    isamine b.
    Kühne's methylene b.
    leukomethylene b.
    Löffler's methylene b.
    Luxol fast b. MBS
    marine b.
    methylene b.
    methylene b. O
    Niagara b. 3B
    Nile b., A.
    Nile b. sulfate
    polychrome methylene b.
    Prussian b.
    soluble b., 3 M.
    soluble b., 2 R.
    solvent b. 38
    spirit b.
    Swiss b.
    thymol b.
    toluidine b.
    toluidine b. O
    trypan b.
    Unna's alkaline methylene
      b.
    water b.

BLV
    bovine leukemia virus

B-lymphocyte stimulatory factor
    (BSF)

BM
    body mass

BMG
    benign monoclonal
      gammopathy

bmk
    birthmark

B-mode

BMR
    basal metabolic rate

BMT
    bone marrow
      transplantation

BN
    branchial neuritis

BNO
    bladder neck obstruction

BNS
    benign nephrosclerosis

B&O
    belladonna and opium

Boas-Oppler bacillus

bobbing
    ocular b.

Bodansky unit (BU)

Bodian
    B. copper-PROTARGOL
      stain
    B. method

body
    acetone b.
    Alder-Reilly b.
    Amato b.
    amylaceous b.
    amyloid b.
    apoptotic b.
    asbestos b.
    asbestosis b.
    Aschoff b.
    asteroid b.
    Babès-Ernst b.
    Bracht-Wächter b.
    brassy b.

body (*continued*)
    Cabot's ring b.
    cancer b.
    cell b.
    central b.
    chromophilous b.
    Civatte b.
    coccoid x b.
    colloid b.
    conchoid b.
    Councilman's b.
    Cowdry type I inclusion b.
    crystalloid b.
    cytoid b.
    demilune b.
    dense b.
    Döhle's b.
    Döhle's inclusion b.
    Dutcher b.
    elementary b.
    ferruginous b.
    fibrin b. of pleura
    fuchsin b.
    Gamna-Favre b.
    Golgi b.
    Guarnieri's b.
    Halberstaedter-Prowazek b.
    Harting b.
    Hassall's b.
    Hassall-Henle b.
    Heinz b.
    Heinz-Ehrlich b.
    hematoxylin b.
    Henderson-Paterson b.
    Hensen's b.
    Herring b.
    Hirano b.
    Howell's b.
    Howell-Jolly b.
    HX b.
    hyaline b.
    inclusion b.
    intermediate b. of
      Flemming
    Jaworski b.
    Jolly's b.
    ketone b.
    Lafora's b.

body (*continued*)
    Lallemand's b.
    Lallemand-Trousseau b.
    lamellar b.
    L.C.L. b.
    LE b.
    Levinthal-Coles-Lillie b.
    Lewy b.
    Lindner's initial b.
    Lipschütz b.
    Lostorfer's b.
    lyssa b.
    Mallory's b.
    Masson b.
    melon-seed b.
    metachromatic b.
    Michaelis-Gutmann b.
    molluscum b.
    Mooser b.
    Mott b.
    multilamellar b.
    multivesicular b.
    Negri b.
    nemaline b.
    Nissl b.
    Nothnagel's b.
    Odland b.
    oryzoid b.
    Pappenheimer b.
    paranuclear b.
    Paschen b.
    Pick b.
    Plimmer's b.
    polar b.
    polyglucosan b.
    postbranchial b.
    Prowazek's b.
    Prowazek-Greeff b.
    psammoma b.
    pyknotic b.
    Reilly b.
    Renaut's b.
    residual b.
    residual b. of Regnaud
    reticulate b.
    b. of Retzius
    rice b.
    Ross's b.

body (*continued*)
    Russell b.
    Schaumann's b.
    Schiller-Duval b.
    Schmorl b.
    sclerotic b.
    telobranchial b.
    tigroid b.
    Torres-Teixeira b.
    trachoma b.
    Trousseau-Lallemand b.
    ultimobranchial b.
    vermiform b.
    Winkler's b.
    zebra .

boil
    blind b.
    gum b.

bone
    Albers-Schönberg
      marble b.
    brittle b.
    cavalry b.
    chalky b.
    exercise b.
    ivory b.
    marble b.
    rider's b.

BOOP
    bronchiolitis obliterans
      with organizing
      pneumonia

Borchgrevink method

botryoid

botulism
    infant b.

bouton
    b. de passage
    b. en passant
    synaptic b.n
    b. terminal

bowl
    mastoid b.
    mastoidectomy b.

bowleg
    nonrachitic b.

BP
    blood pressure
    bypass

bp
    base pair
    boiling point

BPD
    bronchopulmonary
      dysplasia

BPH
    benign prostatic
      hypertrophy

Bq
    becquerel

bracelet
    Nageotte b.

brachialgia
    b. statica paresthetica

brachiocyllosis

brachiocyrtosis

Brachmann-de Lange syndrome

Bracht-Wachter lesion

brachybasia

brachycheilia

brachychily

brachydactyly

brachyesophagus

brachygnathia

brachygnathous

brachymetacarpalism

brachymetacarpia

brachymetapody

brachymetatarsia

brachyphalangia

brachyskelous

brachystasis

Bradshaw tst

bradyacusia

bradyarrhythmia

bradyarthria

bradyauxesis

bradycinesia

bradycrotic

bradydysrhythmia

bradyesthesia

bradyglossia

bradykinesia

bradylalia

bradylexia

bradylogia

bradyphagia

bradyphasia

bradyphrasia

bradyphrenia

bradypnea

bradypragia

bradyrhythmia

bradyspermatism

bradysphygmia

bradytachycardia

bradyteleocinesia

bradyteleokinesis

bradytocia

bradytrophia

bradytrophic

bradyuria

brain
    respirator b.
    wet b.

brancher enzyme deficiency

brash
    water b.

brazilin

BRM
    biuret-reactive material

breast
    caked b.
    chicken b.
    Cooper's irritable b.
    funnel b.
    pigeon b.
    proemial b.
    shoemakers' b.
    shotty b.
    thrush b.

breath
    liver b.

breathing
    Biot's b.
    Cheyne-Stokes b.
    mouth b.
    periodic b.
    pursed lip b.

brevicollis

breviradiate

bridge
    arteriolovenular b.
    cell b.
    cytoplasmic b.
    protoplasmic b.
    tarsal b.

bridging
    myocardial b.

bridou

brightic

brightism

bromoderma

bromomenorrhea

bromphenol

bronchadenitis

bronchiectasia

bronchiectasic

bronchiectasis
    capillary b.
    cylindrical b.
    cystic b.
    dry b.
    follicular b.
    fusiform b.
    saccular b.
    sacculated b.
    varicose br.

bronchiectatic

bronchiloquy

bronchiocele

bronchiolectasis

bronchiolitis
    constrictive b.
    b. exudativa
    exudative b.
    b. fibrosa obliterans
    b. obliterans
    b. obliterans with
      organizing pneumonia
    obliterative b.
    proliferative b.
    respiratory b.

bronchiospasm

bronchiostenosis

bronchismus

bronchitic

bronchitis
    arachidic b.
    asthmatic b.
    capillary b.
    Castellani's b.

bronchitis (*continued*)
　　chronic b.
　　exudative b.
　　fibrinous b.
　　hemorrhagic b.
　　laryngotracheal b.
　　membranous b.
　　b. obliterans
　　plastic b.
　　pseudomembranous b.
　　putrid b.
　　secondary b.
　　vanadium b.

bronchoadenitis

bronchoaspergillosis

bronchoblastomycosis

bronchocandidiasis

bronchocavernous

bronchocavitary

bronchocele

bronchodilatation

bronchoegophony

broncholith

broncholithiasis

bronchologic

bronchomalacia

bronchomycosis

bronchonocardiosis

bronchopancreatic

bronchopathy

bronchophony
　　whispered b.

bronchoplegia

bronchopleural

bronchopleuropneumonia

bronchopneumonia
　　postoperative b.

bronchopneumonic

bronchopneumonitis

bronchopneumopathy

bronchorrhagia

bronchorrhea

bronchosinusitis

bronchospasm

bronchospirochetosis

bronchostaxis

bronchostenosis

bronchus
　　tracheal b.

brown
　　aniline b.
　　Bismarck b. R
　　Bismarck b. Y
　　phenylene b.
　　Manchester b.

bruissement

brush
　　Ruffini's b.

Bruton
　　B. disease
　　B. type
　　　agammaglobulinemia

BSA
　　bismuth-sulfite agar
　　body surface area
　　bovine serum albumin

BSB
　　body surfaced burned

BSDLB
　　block in anterosuperior
　　　division of left branch

BSE
　　bilateral, symmetrical, and
　　　equal

BSF
　　B-lymphocyte stimulatory
　　　factor

BSFR
    basal secretory flow rate
        BSFR test
BSI
    bound serum iron

BSP excretion test

BSS
    balanced salt solution
    buffered saline solution

BSTFA
    bis-trimethylsilyltrifluoro-
        acetamide

BT
    bladder tumor
    bleeding time
    brain tumor

BTB
    breakthrough bleeding

BTPS
    body temperature, ambient
        pressure, saturated
            BTPS conditions of gas

bubonocele

bubonulus

buccoglossopharyngitis
    b. sicca

bud
    gustatory b.
    taste b.

buffer
    bicarbonate b.
    cacodylate b.
    phosphate b.
    protein b.
    veronal b.

bulb
    end b.
    end b. of Held
    end b. of Krause
    b. of Krause

bulb (*continued*)
    Krause's end b.
    onion b.
    terminal b. of Krause

bulbitis

bulbospiral

bulla
    emphysematous b.

bullate

bullation

bullosis
    diabetic bullosis

bullous

BUN
    blood urea nitrogen

BUN/creatinine ratio

bundle
    hair b.
    Kent's b.
    muscle b.
    papillomacular b.'s
    Weissmann's b.

buphthalmia

buphthalmos

buphthalmus

burbulence

burn
    brush b.
    chemical b.
    contact b.
    electric b.
    electrical b.
    flash b.
    friction b.
    radiation b.
    sun b.
    thermal b.
    x-ray b.

bursa
    adventitious b.
    supernumerary b.

bursitis
- Achilles .
- adhesive b.
- anserine b.
- calcific b.
- ischiogluteal b.
- olecranon b.
- omental b.
- pharyngeal b.
- popliteal b.
- prepatellar b.
- radiohumeral b.
- retrocalcaneal b.
- scapulohumeral b.
- septic b.
- subacromial b.
- subdeltoid b.
- superficial calcaneal b.
- Tornwaldt's (Thornwaldt's) b.

bursitis (*continued*)
- trochanteric b.

bursolith

bursopathy

burst
- spider b.

butyraceous

butyroid

butyrous

byssaceous

byssinosis
- acute b.
- chronic b.

byssinotic

byssoid

C

C
    calculus
    Celsius
    Celsius temperature scale
    centigrade temerpature scale
    curie
    large calorie
        C carbohydrate antigen
        C cell
        C group virus
        C lactose test
        C peptide
        C region
        C virus

C1q radioassay

C3
    C. proactivator
    C. proactivator convertase

CA
    carcinoma
    cardiac arrest
    chronological age
    common antigen
    cytosine arabinoside
        CA 19–9 assay
        CA virus

CA-125, CA125
    CA-125 assay

CABG
    coronary artery bypass graft

Cabot ring body

cacatory

Cacchi-Ricci syndrome

cachectic

cachexia
    cardiac c.
    hypophysial c.
    c. hypophysiopriva
    pituitary c.
    c. suprarenalis
    uremic c.

cachexy

cacogenesis

cacogeusia

cacosmia

cacotrophy

CAD
    coronary artery disease

cadmiosis

caffeine
    c. benzoate

CAG
    chronic atrophic gastritis

CAH
    chronic active hepatitis
    congenital adrenal
        hyperplasia

CAHD
    Coronary atherosclerotic
        heart disease

CAHM
    Complex atypical
        hyperplasia/metaplasia

caisson disease

Cajal
    C. astrocyte stain
    C. formol ammonium
        bromide solution
    C. gold sublimate
        method
    C. gold sublimate stain
    H. uranium silver method

Calabar swelling

C/alb/
    albumin clearance

calcaneitis

calcaneoapophysitis

calcaneocavus

calcaneodynia

calcaneovalgocavus

calcanodynia

calcareous

calcariuria

calcaroid

calcemia

calcibilia

calcicosilicosis

calcicosis

calcification
    dystrophic c.
    Mönckeberg's c.

calcineurin

calcinosis
    c. circumscripta
    c. cutis
    c. intervertebralis
    tumoral c.
    c. universalis

calciorrhachia

calcipenia

calcipenic

calciphilia

calciphylaxis
    systemic c.

calciprivia

calciprivic

calcipyelitis

calcium
    c. oxalate
    c. pyrophosphate

calciuria

calculogenesis

calculosis

calculous

calculus
    alternating c.
    apatite c.
    articular c.
    bile duct c.
    biliary c.
    bronchial c.
    brushite c.
    calcium oxalate c.
    cholesterol c.
    combination c.
    cystine c.
    decubitus c.
    dental c.
    encysted c.
    fibrin c.
    gastric c.
    gonecystic c.
    hemic c.
    hepatic c.
    intestinal c.
    joint c.
    lacrimal c.
    lacteal c.
    lung c.
    mammary c.
    matrix c.
    nasal c.
    nephritic c.
    oxalate c.
    pancreatic c.
    phosphate c.
    phosphatic c.
    pocketed c.
    preputial c.
    prostatic c.
    renal c.
    renal c., primary
    renal c., secondary
    salivary c.
    serumal c.
    shellac c.
    spermatic c.
    staghorn c.
    stomachic c.
    struvite c.

calculus (*continued*)
    subgingival c.
    supragingival c.
    tonsillar c.
    triple phosphate c.
    urate c.
    urethral c.
    uric acid c.
    urinary c.
    uterine c.
    vesical c.
    vesicoprostatic c.
    weddellite c.
    whewellite c.
    whitlockite c.
    xanthic c.
    xanthine c.

caldesmon

callositas

callosity

callus
    bony c.
    central c.
    definitive c.
    ensheathing c.
    external c.
    inner c.
    intermediate c.
    internal c.
    medullary c.
    myelogenous c.
    permanent c.
    provisional c.
    temporary c.

calmodulin

calotte

calpain

calvities

CAM
    contralateral axillary
      metastasis
        AE1 plus CAM
        CAM 5.2 antibody

C/am/
    amylase clearance

cambium

CAMP
    Christie-Atkins-Much-
      Petersen
        CAMP factor
        CAMP test

cAMP
    adenosime 3′,5′-cyclic
      phosphate (cyclic AMP)

Campanacci
    osteofibrous dysplasia of C.

campospasm

camptocormia

camptocormy

camptodactylia

camptodactylism

camptodactyly

camptomelia

camptomelic

camptospasm

canaliculitis

canaliculization

canaliculus
    apical c.
    bile c.
    bone c.
    c. dentales
    haversian c.
    intracellular c. of parietal
      cells
    pseudobile c.
    biliary c.

C-ANCA
    antineutrophil cytoplasmic
      antibody

cancrum
    c. nasi

cancrum (*continued*)
c. oris
c. pudendi

candidiasis
acute pseudomembranous
c.
atrophic c.
bronchopulmonary c.
cutaneous c.
endocardial c.
oral c.
pulmonary c.
vaginal c.
vulvovaginal c.

candidid

candiduria

canescent

canities

canthitis

C8/144 antibody

CAO
chronic airway obstruction

caoutchouc pelvis

capacity
total iron-binding c.

capillaritis

capillaropathy

capillary
bile c.
glomerular c.
peritubular c.

capistration

capotement

capriloquism

caprizant

capsitis

capsula
c. glomeruli

capsule
Bowman's c.
fibrous c. of graafian follicle
glomerular c.
c. of glomerulus
malpighian c.
müllerian c.
Müller c.

capsulitis
adhesive c.
hepatic c.

caput
c. distortum
c. medusae
c. natiforme
c. planum
c. quadratum
c. succedaneum

carbamoyl phosphate
synthetase deficiency

carbohydraturia

carbolfuchsin

carboluria

carbolxylene

carbonuria

carboxyhemoglobin

carboxyhemoglobinemia

carboxylase
multiple c. deficiency

carboxymyoglobin

carbuncle
renal c.

carbuncular

carbunculoid

carbunculosis

carcinoma
embryonal c.
infantile embryonal c.
juvenile embryonal c.

carcinoma (*continued*)
    Paget's c.
    yolk sac c.

cardialgia

cardiectasis

cardiocele

cardiochalasia

cardiocirrhosis

cardiocyte

cardiodynia

cardiohepatomegaly

cardiomalacia

cardiomegalia
    c. glycogenica diffusa

cardiomegaly

cardiomelanosis

cardiomyoliposis

cardiomyopathy

cardiopathic

cardiopathy
    infarctoid c.

cardiopericarditis

cardioptosia

cardioptosis

cardiorrhexis

cardiosclerosis

cardiothyrotoxicosis

cardiovalvulitis

Cardiovirus

carditis
    Lyme c.
    rheumatic c.
    streptococcal c.
    verrucous c.

Carey Ranvier technique

CA15-3 RIA test

caries
    backward c.
    cemental c.
    central c.
    dental c.
    dental caries, primary
    dental c., rampant
    dental c., secondary
    dentinal c.
    dry c.
    enamel c.
    internal c.
    lateral c.
    necrotic c.
    pit c.
    rampant c.
    c. sicca
    spinal c.

cariogenesis

cariogenic

cariogenicity

cariology

cariosity

carious

carmalum

carmine
    alizarin c.
    indigo c.
    lithium c.
    Schneider's c.

carminic acid

carminophil

carminum

carnification

carnitine palmityltransferase
    deficiency

carnosinase
    serum c. deficiency

carnosinemia

carnosinuria

carnosity

carotenemia

carotenosis

carotidynia

carotodynia

carphologia

carphology

carpoptosis

carpus
    c. curvus

caruncle
    urethral c.

caryochrome

caryophil

caseation

caseous

caseum

cast
    bacterial c.
    blood c.
    bronchial c.
    coma c.
    decidual c.
    epithelial c.
    false c.
    fatty c.
    fibrinous c.
    granular c.
    hair c.
    hemoglobin c.
    hyaline c.
    Külz's c.
    leukocyte c.
    mucous c.
    pus c.
    red cell c.
    renal c.
    spiral c.
    spurious c.

cast (*continued*)
    spurious tube c.
    tube c.
    urate c.
    urinary c.
    waxy c.

castroid

CAT
    chlormerodrin
      accumulation test

catabiosis

catabiotic

cataphoresis

cataphoretic

cataphoria

cataphoric

cataplectic

cataplexis

cataplexy

cataract
    after-c.
    aminoaciduria c.
    axial fusiform c.
    black c.
    blue c.
    blue dot c.
    brown c.
    brunescent c.
    calcareous c.
    capsular c.
    cerulean c.
    complete c.
    complicated c.
    congenital c.
    contusion c.
    coralliform c.
    coronary c.
    cortical c.
    cuneiform c.
    cupuliform c.
    dermatogenic c.
    developmental c.

cataract (*continued*)
 diabetic c.
 duplication c.
 electric c.
 embryonal nuclear c.
 embryopathic c.
 evolutionary c.
 galactosemic c.
 glassblowers' c.
 glaucomatous c.
 heat c.
 heterochromic c.
 hypermature c.
 hypocalcemic c.
 immature c.
 incipient c.
 intumescent c.
 juvenile c.
 lamellar c.
 mature c.
 membranous c.
 metabolic c.
 morgagnian c.
 nuclear c.
 nutritional deficiency c.
 overripe c.
 polar c.
 postinflammatory c.
 c. of prematurity
 presenile c.
 primary c.
 punctate c.
 pyramidal c.
 radiation c.
 ringform congenital c.
 ripe c.
 rubella c.
 secondary c.
 senile c.
 senile nuclear sclerotic c.
 snowflake c.
 snowstorm c.
 Soemmering's ring c.
 spindle c.
 subcapsular c.
 sunflower c.
 supranuclear c.
 sutural c.

cataract (*continued*)
 syndermatotic c.
 thermal c.
 total c.
 toxic c.
 traumatic c.
 zonular c.

cataracta
 c. brunescens
 c. caerulea
 c. centralis pulverulenta
 c. complicata
 c. nigra

cataractogenic

cataractous

catarrh
 postnasal c.
 sinus c.
 vernal c.

catarrhal

cathaeresis

catheresis

catheretic

cathetometer

caumesthesia

causalgia

CAV
 congenital absence of
  vagina
 congenital adrenal
  virilism

caveola

cavern
 Schnabel's c.

caverniloquy

cavernitis
 fibrous c.

cavernositis

cavitation

cavitis

cavosurface

cavovalgus

cavovarus

cavus

CB
 chocolate blood
 chronic bronchitis

CBA
 chronic bronchitis with
  asthma

C-banding
 C.-b. stain

CBC
 complete blood count

CBF
 cerebral blood flow
 coronary blood flow

CBG
 corticosteroid-binding
  globulin
 cortisol-binding globulin

CBS
 chronic brain syndrome

CBV
 central blood volume
 circulating blood volume
 corrected blood volume

CC
 cord compression
 creatinine clearance

CCA
 chick-cell agglutination

CCAT
 conglutinatin complement
  absorption test

CCC
 chronic calculous
  cholecystitis
 clear cell carcinoma

CCF
 cephalin-cholesterol
  flocculation
 compound comminuted
  fracture
 congestive cardiac failure

CC/MCL
 centrocytic/mantle-cell
  lymphoma

CCP
 ciliocytophthoria

C/cr/
 creatinine clearance

CCV
 conductivity cell volume

CD
 cadaver donor
 cardiac disease
 cardiovascular disease
 consanguineous donor
 curative dose

CD1 antigen

CD1a antibody

CD2

CD3
 cytoplasmic C.

CD4

CD4/CD8 count

CD15 antigen

CD20
 C. antibody
 C. antigen

CD_{50}
 median curative dose

CDA
 congenital
  dyserythropoietic anemia

CDH
 congenital dislocation of
  hip

cDNA
   complimentary DNA
      cDNA clone
      cDNA library

CDP
   continuous distending
      pressure

CDP-choline

CDP-diglyceride

CDP-ethanolamine

CDw75 antigen

CE
   California encephalitis
   cardiac enlargement

CEA
   carcinoembryonic
      antigen
   crystalline egg albumin
      CEA assay
      CEA immuno-
         peroxidase stain

CEA-M stain

ceanothus extract

CEA-P stain

ceasmic

cecitis

cecocele

cecum
   high c.
   mobile c.
   c. mobile

cedar
   red c.
   western red c.

CEEV
   Central European
      ecephalitis virus

CEF
   chick embryo fibroblast

celiomyositis

celiopathy

celitis

cell
   A c.
   absorptive c., intestinal
   acid c.
   acinar c.
   acinic c.
   acinous c.
   acoustic hair c.
   adventitial c.
   agger nasi c.
   algoid c.
   alpha c.
   alveolar c.
   alveolar c., great
   alveolar c., large
   alveolar c., small
   alveolar c., squamous
   alveolar c., type I
   alveolar c., type II
   alveolar epithelial c.
   Alzheimer c.
   amacrine c.
   ameboid c.
   amine precursor uptake
      and decarboxylation c.
   amphophilic c.
   Anichkov (Anitschkow) c.
   anterior horn c.
   antipodal c.
   apolar c.
   APUD c.
   argentaffin c.
   argyrophilic c.
   Arias-Stella c.
   Armanni-Ebstein c.
   Aschoff c.
   Askanazy c.
   auditory c.
   automatic c.
   B c.
   balloon c.
   basal c.
   basal granular c.

cell (*continued*)
    basket c.
    Beale's ganglion c.
    Bergmann c.
    berry c.
    beta c.
    Betz c.
    bipolar c.
    bipolar retinal c.
    bladder c.
    blast c.
    bone c.
    border c.
    Böttcher c.
    breviradiate c.
    bristle c.
    brood c.
    burr c.
    C c.
    Cajal c.
    cameloid c.
    capsule c.
    cartilage c.
    Caspersson type B c.
    castration c.
    caterpillar c.
    caudate c.
    caveolated c.
    cement c.
    central c.
    centroacinar c.
    chief c.
    chromaffin c.
    chromophobe c.
    chromophobic c.
    ciliated c.
    Clara c.
    Clarke c.
    Claudius c.
    cleavage c.
    clump c.
    commissural c.
    compound granule c.
    cone c.
    contractile fiber c.
    corneal c.
    c.of Corti
    corticotrope c.

cell (*continued*)
    corticotroph c.
    corticotroph-lipotroph c.
    corticotropic c.
    cribrate c.
    Crooke c.
    Custer c.
    cytotrophoblastic c.
    D c.
    daughter c.
    Davidoff (Davidov) c.
    decidual c.
    Deiters c.
    delta c.
    dendritic c.
    follicular dendritic c.
    dentin c.
    dome c.
    Downey c.
    dust c.
    elementary c.
    embryonic c.
    enamel c.
    endocrine c.of the gut
    endothelioid c.
    enterochromaffin c.
    enteroendocrine c.
    ependymal c.
    epidermic c.
    epithelioid c.
    eukaryotic c.
    F c.
    Fañanás c.
    fat-storing c.of liver
    fatty granule c.
    flagellate c.
    foam c.
    foot c.
    foreign body giant c.
    formative c.
    G c.
    gametoid c.
    gamma c.of hypophysis
    ganglion c.
    Gaucher c.
    Gegenbaur c.
    germ c.
    germ c., primordial

cell (*continued*)
    germinal c.
    ghost c.
    giant c.
    giant pyramidal c.
    Gierke c.
    gitter c.
    Gley c.
    glial c.
    glitter c.
    globoid c.
    glomerular c.
    glomus c.
    Golgi c.
    gonadotrope c.
    gonadotroph c.
    gonadotropic c.
    Goormaghtigh c.
    granular c.
    granule c.
    granulosa c.
    granulosa c., primitive
    granulosa c., primordial
    granulosa-lutein c.
    grape c.
    ground-glass c.
    gustatory c.
    H c.
    hair c.
    heart-disease c.
    heart-failure c.
    heart-lesion c.
    hecatomeral c.
    heckle c.
    Heidenhain c.
    HeLa c.
    helmet c.
    Hensen c.
    hepatic c.
    heteromeral c.
    heteromeric c.
    hilum c.
    Hofbauer c.
    horizontal c.
    horizontal c.of Cajal
    horizontal c.of retina
    horn c.
    Hortega c.

cell (*continued*)
    Hürthle c.
    hyperchromatic c.
    I-c.
    initial c.
    integrator c.
    intercalary c.
    intercalated c.
    intercapillary c.
    interdental c.
    interfollicular c.
    interstitial c.
    interstitial c.of Cajal
    interstitial c.of Leydig
    islet c.
    Ito c.
    juxtaglomerular c.
    karyochrome c.
    Kupffer c.
    L c.
    lacis c.
    lactotrope c.
    lactotroph c.
    lactotropic c.
    Langerhans c.
    Langhans c.
    Langhans giant c.
    large granule c.
    LE c.
    Leishman's chrome c.
    lepra c.
    Leydig c.
    light c.
    littoral c.
    liver c.
    luteal c.
    lutein c.
    M c.
    malpighian c.
    Marchand c.
    Martinotti c.
    matrix c.
    Mauthner c.
    Merkel c.
    Merkel-Ranvier c.
    Merkel tactile c.
    mesangial c.
    mesenchymal c.

cell (*continued*)

Mexican hat c.
Meynert c.
microglia c.
microglial c.
migratory c.
Mikulicz c.
mitral c.
morular c.
mossy c.
mother c.
motor c.
Mott c.
mucous neck c.
mulberry c.
c. of Müller
muriform c.
muscle c.
myeloma c.
myoepithelioid c.
myointimal c.
Nageotte c.
nerve c.
neuroendocrine c.
neuroepithelial c.
neuroglia c.
neuroglial c.
neurosecretory c.
neutrophilic c.
nevus c.
Niemann-Pick c.
nodal c.
nucleated c.
nurse c.
nursing c.
olfactory c.
olfactory receptor c.
osseous c.
osteoprogenitor c.
oxyntic c.
oxyphil c.
oxyphilic c.
P c.
pacemaker c.
Paget c.
pagetoid c.
Paneth c.
parafollicular c.

cell (*continued*)

paraluteal c.
paralutein c.
parenchymal hepatic c.
parenchymal liver c.
parent c.
parietal c.
pathologic c.
peg c.
peptic c.
pericapillary c.
periglomerular c.
perithelial c.
perivascular c.
pessary c.
phalangeal c.
pheochrome c.
photoreceptor c.
Pick c.
pillar c.
pineal c.
plasma c., flaming
PNH c.
polar c.
polyplastic c.
PP c.
prefollicle c.
pregnancy c.
prickle c.
primordial germ c.
principal c.
progenitor c.
prokaryotic c.
prolactin c.
pulmonary epithelial c.
pulpar c.
Purkinje c.
pus c.
pyramidal c.
radial c.of Müller
Renshaw c.
reserve c.
resting c.
rod c.
Rolando c.
root c.
Rouget c.
S c.

cell (*continued*)
- Sala c.
- sarcogenic c.
- satellite c.
- Schultze c.
- Schwann c.
- sclerotic c.
- seminal c.
- sensory c.
- septal c.
- Sertoli c.
- sex c.
- sexual c.
- shadow c.
- sickle c.
- skeletogenous c.
- small granule c.
- solitary c.of Meynert
- somatostatin c.
- somatotrope c.
- somatotroph c.
- somatotropic c.
- sperm c.
- spermatogenic c.
- spermatogonial c.
- spider c.
- spur c.
- stave c.
- stippled c.
- sympathicotrophic c.
- sympathochromaffin c.
- syncytiotrophoblastic c.
- synovial c.
- tactile c.
- target c.
- taste c.
- tautomeral c.
- teardrop c.
- tendon c.
- theca c.
- theca-lutein c.
- thyroidectomy c.
- thyrotrope c.
- thyrotroph c.
- thyrotropic c.
- touch c.
- Touton giant c.
- transitional c.

cell (*continued*)
- tufted c.
- Türk c.
- type I c.
- type II c.
- Tzanck c.
- ultimobranchial c.
- vacuolated c.
- vasofactive c.
- vasoformative c.
- ventricular c.
- Vignal c.
- Virchow c.
- visual c.
- von Hansemann c.
- von Kupffer c.
- wandering c.
- wandering c., primitive
- wandering c., primordial
- Warthin-Finkeldey c.
- wasserhelle c.
- water-clear c.
- Wedl c.
- wing c.
- xanthoma c.
- Zander c.
- zymogenic c.

celliferous

cellifugal

cellipetal

celloidin

cellula
- c. lentis

cellulicidal

cellulifugal

cellulipetal

cellulitis
- anaerobic c.
- clostridial anaerobic c.
- dissecting c.of scalp
- eosinophilic c.
- facial c.
- finger c.

cellulitis (*continued*)
    gangrenous c.
    indurated c.
    necrotizing c.
    nonclostridial anaerobic c.
    orbital c.
    pelvic c.
    periurethral c.
    phlegmonous c.
    preseptal c.

cellulofibrous

cellulotoxic

celophlebitis

CELO virus

cementicle
    adherent c.
    attached c.
    free c.
    interstitial c.

cementoblast

cementoclasia

cementoclast

cementocyte

cementoid

cementoma
    gigantiform c.

cementum
    acellular c.
    afibrillar c.
    cellular c.
    uncalcified c.

cenesthopathy

centrage

centraphose

centrifugate

centrifugation
    density gradient c.
    differential c.
    isopyknic c.

centrifuge
    microscope c.

centriole
    anterior c.
    distal c.
    posterior c.
    proximal c.
    ring c.

centrolecithal

centro-osteosclerosis

centrophose

centroplasm

centrosclerosis

centrosome

centrosphere

CEOT
    calcifying epithelial
      odontogenic tumor

CEP
    centromere enumeration
      probe
    congenital erythropoiectic
      porphyria

cephalalgia
    histamine c.
    pharyngotympanic c.
    quadrantal c.

cephaledema

cephalgia

cephalhematoma
    c. deformans

cephalhydrocele
    c. traumatica

cephalocele
    orbital c.

cephalodactyly
    Vogt's c.

cephalodynia

cephalohematoma

cephalomenia

cephalonia

cephalopathy

cephaloplegia

cephalostyle

ceraceous

ceramidase deficiency

ceramide trihexosidase
  deficiency

cercarienhullenreaktion

cerebellitis

cerebriform

cerebroid

cerebromalacia

cerebromeningitis

cerebropathia
  c. psychica toxemica

cerebropathy

cerebrosclerosis

cerebrosidosis

cerebrosis

cerumen
  impacted c.
  inspissated c.

ceruminoma

ceruminosis

cervicobrachialgia

cervicocolpitis
  c. emphysematosa

cervicodynia

cervicovaginitis

CES
  central excitatory state

CF
  carbol-fuchsin
  cardiac failure
  carrier-free
  chemotactic factor
  Chiari-Frommel-syndrome
  citrovorum factor
  complement fixation
  complement-fixing
  cystic fibrosis
    CF antibody
    CF antibody test
    CF test

CFF
  critical flicker fusion
    CFF test

c-fos oncogene

CFP
  chronic false-positive
  cystic fibrosis of pancreas

CFT
  complement-fixation test

CFU-C
  Colony-forming unit-culture

CFU-E
  colony-forming unit-
    erythroid

CFU/mL
  colony-forming units/mL

CFWM
  cancer-free white mouse

CG
  Cardio-Green
  chorionic gonadotropin
  chronic glomerulonephritis
  colloidal gold
  phosgene (choking gas)
    chrome violet CG

CGD
  chronic granulomatous
    disease

CGL

CGL (*continued*)
    chronic granulocytic
      leukemia

C-glycoholic acid breath test

CGN
    chronic glomerulonephritis

CG/OQ
    cerebral glucose oxygen
      quotient

CGP
    chorionic growth hormone
      prolactin
    circulating granulocyte pool

CGRP
    calcitonin gene-related
      peptide

CGS, cgs
    centimeter-gram-second
        CGS system
        CGS unit

CGT
    chorionic gonadotropin

CGTT
    cortisone-glucose tolerance
      test

CH
    cholesterol
    crown-heel

CHA
    congenital hypoplastic
      anemia

Chabert disease

Chaetoconidium

Chagas
    C. disease
    C. disease serological
      test

chalasia

chalazia

chalazion

chalazodermia

chalcitis

chalcosis
    c. corneae

chalicosis

chalkitis

chamber
    diffusion c.

change
    Armanni-Ebstein c.
    Crooke's c.
    Crooke-Russell c.
    fatty c.
    harlequin color c.
    hyaline c.
    hydropic c.

channel
    acetylcholine c.
    blood c.
    calcium c.
    calcium-sodium c.
    fast c.
    gated c.
    ligand-gated c.
    potassium c.
    protein c.
    slow c.
    sodium c.
    voltage-gated c.
    water c.

chasmatoplasson

chaude-pisse

CHB
    complete heart block

CHD
    congestive heart disease
    coronary heart diseas

ChE
    cholesterol ester
    cholinesterase

Cheadle disease

check
   alert c.
   c. bit
   Δ c.
   δ c.
   c. digit
   limit c.
   parity c.
   previous value c.

cheilectropion

cheilitis
   actinic c.
   angular c.
   apostematous c.
   commissural c.
   c. exfoliativa
   c. glandularis
   c. glandularis
     apostematosa
   c. granulomatosa
   granulomatous c.
   impetiginous c.
   Miescher's granulomatous
     c.
   migrating c.
   solar c.
   c. venenata

cheilognathopalatoschisis

cheilognathoprosoposchisis

cheilognathoschisis

cheilognathouranoschisis

cheiloschisis

cheilosis
   angular c.

cheiragra

cheiralgia
   c. paresthetica

cheirarthritis

cheiromegaly

cheiropodalgia

cheiropompholyx

cheirospasm

Chelex DNA amplification

chelicera

cheloid

cheloma

chemical
   c. adsorption
   c. asphyxiant
   c. bond
   c. equation
   c. equilibrium
   c. incompatibility
   incompatible c.
   c. inhibition isoamylase test
   c. interference
   c. mediator
   c. peritonitis
   c. pneumonia
   c. pneumonitis
   c. prophylaxis
   c. reaction
   c. shift
   c. styptic
   c. waste

chemically pure

chemiluminescence

chemiosmotic
   a. hypothesis

chemiosorption

chemiotaxis

chemistry
   analytical c.
   clinical c.
   inorganic c.
   organic c.
   physical c.
   physiologic c.
   c. profile

chemoattractant

chemoceptor

chemokine

chemokinesis

chemokinetic

chemoreception

chemoreceptor

chemosis

chemotactic

chemotaxin

chemotaxis

chemotic

cherubism

chest
    alar c.
    barrel c.
    blast c.
    cobbler's c.
    flail c.
    flat c.
    foveated c.
    funnel c.
    keeled c.
    paralytic c.
    pigeon c.
    pterygoid c.
    tetrahedron c.

cheyletiellosis

CHF
    congestive heart failure

CHH
    cartilage-hair hypoplasia

Chiari
    C. disease
    C. II syndrome
    C. net

Chiari-Arnold syndrome

Chiari-Budd syndrome

Chiari-Frommel syndrome (CF)

chiasma

chick-cell agglutination (CCA)

chick embryo fibroblast (CEF)

chilblain

CHILD
    congenital hemidysplasia
    with ichthyosiform
    erythroderma and limb
    defects
        CHILD test

Child
    C. hepatic risk criteria

childbed fever

childhood
    c. hemolytic uremic
        syndrome
    c. type tuberculosis

chilitis

chilomastigiasis

chilopod

Chilopoda

chilopodiasis

chimera
    blood group c.
    dispermic c.
    heterologous c.
    homologous c.
    isologous c.
    radiation c.

chimeric
    c. antibody

chimerism
    hematolymhoid c.

chimney sweep's cancer

chin
    galoche c.

Chinese
    C. liver fluke
    C. restaurant syndrome
        (CCA)

chionablepsia

chiral
    c. center
    c. crystal

chiromegaly

chiropodalgia

chirospasm

chloasma

chloracne

chloremia

chlorhydria

chloridimeter

chloridimetry

chloridometer

chloridorrhea
    familial c.

chloriduria

chloronaphthalene

chloropia

chloroprivic

chloropsia

chlorosis

chloruresis

chloruretic

chloruria

CHN
    central hemorrhagic
      necrosis

CHO
    carbohydrate

choanocyte

cholangeitis

cholangiectasis

cholangiohepatitis
    Oriental c.

cholangiolar

cholangiole

cholangiolitis

cholangitis
    chronic nonsuppurative
      destructive c.
    c. lenta
    Oriental c.
    primary sclerosing c.
    progressive nonsuppurative
      c.
    recurrent pyogenic c.
    sclerosing c.

cholecystalgia

cholecystatony

cholecystectasia

cholecystitis
    acute c.
    chronic c.
    cholecystitis c.
    emphysematous c.
    follicular c.
    gaseous c.
    c. glandularis proliferans

cholecystolithiasis

cholecystopathy

cholecystoptosis

cholecystosis
    hyperplastic c.

choledochitis

choledochocele

choledocholith

choledocholithiasis

cholelith

cholelithiasis

cholelithic

cholemesis

cholemia
    familial c.
    Gilbert c.

cholemic

cholemimetry

choleperitoneum

choleperitonitis

cholera
    c. morbus
    pancreatic c.
    summer c.

cholestasia

cholestasis

cholestatic

cholesteatoma
    congenital c.
    c. tympani

cholesteatomatous

cholesteatosis

cholesterohydrothorax

cholesterol desmolase
    deficiency

cholesterolemia

cholesterolestersturz

cholesterolosis

cholesteroluria

cholesterosis
    extracellular c.

choleuria

cholohemothorax

chololith

chololithiasis

chololithic

cholothorax

choluria

choluric

chondralgia

chondralloplasia

chondriome

chondriosome

chondritis
    costal c.
    c. intervertebralis calcanea

chondroblast

chondrocalcinosis

chondroclast

chondrocyte
    isogenous c.

chondrodermatitis
    c. nodularis chronica
    helicis

chondrodynia

chondrodysplasia
    metaphyseal c.
    c. punctata

chondrodystrophia
    c. calcificans congenita
    c. congenita punctata
    c. fetalis calcificans

chondrodystrophy
    hyperplastic c.
    hypoplastic c.
    hypoplastic fetal c.

chondroepiphysitis

chondroid

chondroitinuria

chondroma
    joint c.
    synovial c.

chondromalacia
    c. patellae

chondrometaplasia
    synovial c.

chondrometaplasia (*continued*)
    tenosynovial c.

chondromitome

chondromucin

chondromucoid

chondromucoprotein

chondronecrosis

chondropathia
    c. tuberosa

chondropathology

chondropathy

chondrophyte

chondroplasia
    c. punctata

chondroplast

chonechondrosternon

CHOP
    cyclophosphamide,
      doxorubicon
      hydrochloride, vincristine
      (Oncovin), prednisone

chordee

chorditis
    c. fibrinosa
    c. nodosa
    c. tuberosa
    c. vocalis
    c. vocalis inferior

chordoblastoma

chordoma
    chondroid c.

chorea
    acute c.
    chronic c.
    chronic progressive
      hereditary c.
    chronic progressive
      nonhereditary c.

chorea (*continued*)
    c. cordis
    dancing c.
    degenerative c.
    c. dimidiata
    Dubini's c.
    electric c.
    fibrillary c.
    c. gravidarum
    hemilateral c.
    hereditary c.
    Huntington's c.
    juvenile c.
    methodic c.
    mimetic c.
    c. minor
    c. nocturna
    c. nutans
    one-sided c.
    paralytic c.
    posthemiplegic c.
    saltatory c.
    senile c.
    simple c.
    Sydenham's c.

choreal

choreic

choreiform

choreoacanthocytosis

choreoathetoid

choreoathetosis
    familial paroxysmal c.
    paroxysmal c.
    paroxysmal kinesigenic c.

choreoid

chorioamnionitis

chorioblastosis

choriocele

choriomeningitis
    lymphocytic c.

chorioretinitis
    c. sclopetaria

chorioretinitis (*continued*)
    toxoplasmic c.

chorioretinopathy

choristoblastoma

choristoma

choroideremia

choroiditis
    acute diffuse serous c.
    anterior c.
    areolar c.
    areolar central c.
    central c.
    diffuse c.
    disseminated c.
    Doyne's familial
        honeycombed c.
    exudative c.
    focal c.
    Förster's c.
    c. guttata senilis
    juxtapapillary c.
    macular c.
    metastatic c.
    senile macular
        exudative c.
    c. serosa
    suppurative c.
    Tay's c.

choroidocyclitis

choroidoiritis

choroidopathy

choroidoretinitis

Chotzen syndrome

chr
    chronic

ChrA
    chromogranin A
        ChrA immuno-
            peroxidase stain

Chr⁹ antigen

Christeller reaction

Christensen urea agar

Christian
    C. disease
    C. syndrome

Christian-Hand-Schuller disease

Christian-Weber disease

Christie-Atkins-Munch-Petersen
    (CAMP)
    C.-A.-M.-P. factor

Christison formula

Christman disease

Christmas
    C. disease
    C. factor

Christopherson nuclear grading
    system

Christ-Siemens syndrome

Christ-Siemens-Touraine
    syndrome

chromaffin
    c. body
    c. cell
    Gomori method of c.
    c. hormone
    c. paraganglioma
    c. reaction
    c. reaction time
    c. tumor

chromaffinity

chromaffinopathy

chromaphil

chromargentaffin

chromatin

chromatism

chromatoblast

chromatocinesis

chromatogram

chromatograph

chromatographic

chromatography
    adsorption c.
    affinity c.
    column c.
    gas c.
    gas-liquid c.
    gas-solid c.
    gel-filtration c.
    gel-permeation c.
    high-performance liquid c.
    high-pressure liquid c.
    ion exchange c.
    liquid-liquid c.
    molecular exclusion c.
    molecular sieve c.
    paper c.
    partition c.
    thin-layer c.

chromatoid

chromatokinesis

chromatolysis

chromatophagus

chromatophil

chromatophile

chromatophilia

chromatophilic

chromatophilous

chromatophorotropic

chromatoplasm

chromatopsia

chromatoscopy
    gastric c.

chromatotaxis

chromaturia

chromhidrosis

chromidrosis

chromoblast

chromoblastomycosis

chromocholoscopy

chromodacryorrhea

chromodiagnosis

chromogranin

chromometer

chromomycosis

chromophage

chromophil

chromophile

chromophilic

chromophilous

chromophobe

chromophobia

chromophore

chromophoric

chromophorous

chromophose

chromoplast

chromoplastid

chromopsia

chromorhinorrhea

chromoscopy

chromospermism

chromotoxic

chronotaraxis

chrotoplast

CHR reaction

chrysiasis

chrysoderma

CHS
        Chédiak-Higashi syndrome

chylaqueous

chylemia

chylomediastinum

chylomicrograph

chylomicronemia

chylopericarditis

chylopericardium

chyloperitoneum

chylopleura

chylopneumothorax

chylorrhea

chylothorax
    congenital c.
    traumatic c.

chyluria

CI
    cerebral infarction
    chemoimmunotherapy
    chemotherapeutic index
    color index
    Colour index
    coronary insufficiency
        CI number

Ciaccio
    C. fluid
    C. method
    C. stain

Ciaccio-positive lipid

Ciarrocchi disease

cicatrical
    c. horn
    c. pemphigoid

cicatrix, pl. cicatrices
    brain c.
    meningocerebral c.

cicatrizant

cicatrization

cicatrizing enterolitis

cicutoxin

CID
    cytomegalic inclusion
        disease

CIDS
    cellular immunity
        deficiency syndrome

CIE
    countercurrent
        immunoelectrophoresis

CIEP
    Counterimmunoelectrophor
        esis

CIF
    clone-inhibiting factor

cigarette-paper scar

ciguatera

ciguatoxin

Ci-hr
    curie-hour

cilia

ciliary dysentery

Ciliata

ciliate dysentery

ciliates

ciliocytophothoria (CCP)

ciliogenesis

Ciliophora

ciliorum

cilium
    olfactory c.

cillosis

cimbia

cimicosis

CIN
cervical intraepithelial
neoplasia
chronic interstitial nephritis

C/in/
insulin clearance

cinclisis

cinemicrography
time-lapse c.

cinesalgia

cinoplasm

circuit
macroreentrant c.
microreentrant c.
reentrant c.
reentry c.

circulation
collateral c.
compensatory c.
persistent fetal c.
portoumbilical c.

circumcrescent

circumgemmal

circumnuclear

cirrhogenous

cirrhonosus

cirrhosis
acholangic biliary c.
acute juvenile c.
alcoholic c.
atrophic c.
bacterial c.
biliary c.
biliary c. of children
calculus c.
cardiac c.
Charcot's c.
congestive c.
Cruveilhier-Baumgarten c.
decompensated c.
fatty c.

cirrhosis (*continued*)
Laënnec's c.
c. of liver
macronodular c.
malarial c.
metabolic c.
multilobular c.
periportal c.
pigment c.
pigmentary c.
pipestem c.
portal c.
posthepatitic c.
postnecrotic c.
primary biliary c.
secondary biliary c.
stasis c.
syphilitic c.
Todd's c.
toxic c.
unilobular c.
vascular c.

cirrhotic

cirsocele

cirsoid

cirsomphalos

cirsophthalmia

CIS
carcinoma in situ
central inhibitory state

cistern
terminal c.

cisterna
cylindrical confronting c.
perinuclear c.
subsarcolemmal c.

cis/trans test

citrullinemia

citrullinuria

CJD
Creutzfeldt-Jakob disease

CK
    creatine kinase

c-Ki-*ras* gene

CLA
    Certified Laboratory
        Assistant
    cyclic lysine anhydride

cladosporiosis
    c. epidermica

Clark
    C. level
    C. mailgnant melanome
        staging
    C. oxygen elctrode
    C. rule
    C. test

Clarke fluid

Clarke-Hadfield syndrome

CLAS
    congenital localized
        absence of skin

clasmatocyte

clasmatocytosis

clasmatosis

classification
    American Urological
        System cancer staging c.
    Ann Arbor staging c.
    Ann Arbor tumor c.
    Arneth c.
    Astler-Coller modification of
        Dukes c.
    Bergey c.
    Bessman anemia c.
    Black c.
    Borrmann c.
    Broders c.
    Caldwell-Moloy c.
    Denver c.
    Dukes c.
    Eggel tumor c.
    Enzinger tumor c.

classification (*continued*)
    FAB leukemia c.
    Frankel c.
    Fredrickson and Lees c.
    Fredrickson
        dyslipoproteinemia c.
    Gell and Coombs c.
    Horie tumor c.
    Keith-Wagener c.
    Keith-Wagener-Barker c.
    Keil c.
    Lancefield c.
    Lennert c.
    Levine-Rosai c.
    Lukes-Butler con-Hodgkin
        lymphoma c.
    Lukes-Collins c.
    Lund-Browder c.
    McNeer c.
    Moss c.
    New York Heart Association
        (NYHA) c.
    Paris c.
    Portmann c.
    Rappaport c.
    Runyon c.
    Rye c.
    Seattle c.
    Skinner c.

clastothrix

clathrate

Clauberg
    C. test
    C. unit

Claude
    C. Bernard-Horner
        syndrome
    C. syndrome

claudicant

claudication
    intermittent c.
    jaw c.
    neurogenic c.
    venous c.

claudicatory

clausura

claviculus

clavus
c. durus
c. mollis
c. syphiliticus

CLBBB
complete left bundle-branch block

CLD
chronic liver disease
chronic lung disease

clearance
p-aminohippurate c.
blood-urea c.
creatinine c.
free water c.
inulin c.
osmolal c.
renal c.
total body c.
total c.
urea c.
whole body c.

cleft
facial c.
facial c., lateral
facial c., oblique
facial c., transverse
Lanterman's c.
Maurer's c.
primary synaptic c.
Schmidt-Lanterman c.
secondary synaptic c.
subneural c.
synaptic c.

cleidagra

cleidarthritis

cleisagra

CLH
chronic lobular hepatitis

CLH (*continued*)
cutaneous lymphoid hyperplasia

click
Ortolani's c.

climacteric
delayed c.

climacterium
c. praecox

clinarthrosis

Clinistix

Clinitest

clinodactylism

clinodactyly

clitoridauxe

clitoriditis

clitorimegaly

clitorism

clitoritis

clitoromegaly

CLL
chronic lymphatic leukemia
chronic lymphocytic leukemia

cloaca

cloacal

cloacogenic
c. carcinoma
c. polyp

clomiphene test

Clonad monoclonal antibody

clone-inhibiting factor

clonicity

clonicotonic

clonidine suppression test

clonism

clonismus

clonorchiasis

clonorchiosis

clonospasm

clonus

Cloquet canal remnant

clot
   agonal c.
   agony c.
   antemortem c.
   blood c.
   chicken fat c.
   sentinel c.
   currant jelly c.
   distal c.
   external c.
   heart c.
   internal c.
   laminated c.
   marantic c.
   passive c.
   plastic c.
   postmortem c.
   proximal c.
   spider-web c.
   stratified c.
   washed c.
   white c.

CLOtest test

Cloudman melanoma

cloudy
   c. swelling
   c. swelling degeneration
   c. urine

Clough-Ricter syndrome

Clouston syndrome

cloverleaf skull

cloxacillin sodium

CLS

CLS (*continued*)
   Certified Laboratory
      Scientist

CLSL
   chronic lymphosarcoma
      leukemia

CLSM
   confocal laser scan
      microscopy

CLT
   clot lysis time

cluster of differentiation
   b. o. d. 2, 3, 4, 8

Clutton joint

CMB
   carbolic methylene blue

CMC
   critical micelle
      concentration

CM-cellulose
   carboxymethyl cellulose

CMF
   chondromyxoid fibroma

CMGN
   chronic membranous index
   cell-mediated immunity

CMI
   carbohydrate metabolism
      glomerulonephritis

CMID
   cytomegalic inclusion
      disease

c/min
   cycles per minute

CML
   chronic myeloctic leukemia
   chronic myelogenous
      leukemia

CMM
   cutaneous malignant
      melanoma

cmm
   cubic millimeter

CMN
   cystic medial necrosis

CMN-AA
   cystic medial necrosis of
      ascending aorta

CMO
   calculated mean organism

cMo
   centimorgan

CMoL
   chronic monoblastic
      leukemia
   chronic monocytic
      leukemia

CMOS logic

CMP
   cardiomyopathy

CMP-*N*-acetyl-D-neuraminate

CMR
   cerebral metabolic rate
   crude mortality ratio

CMRG
   cerebral metabolic rate of
      glucose

CMRO
   cerebral metabolic rate of
      oxygen

CMRR
   common mode rejection
      ratio

CMV
   cytomegalovirus
      CMV culture
      CMV isolation

cnemitis

cnemoscoliosis

CNHD
   congenital nonspherocytic
      hemolytic disease

Cnidospora

Cnidosporia

CO
   corneal opacity

coacervate

coacervation

coag
   coagulation

Coag-a-mate prothrombin
   device

coagglutinin

coagulable

coagulant

coagulase
   c. test

coagulation
   diffuse intravascular c.
   disseminated intravascular
      c.
   exogenous
      anticoagulant c.
   c. factor transfusion
   massive c.

coagulopathy
   consumption c.

coagulum

coalition
   calcaneocuboid c.
   calcaneonavicular c.
   cubonavicular c.
   naviculocuneiform c.
   talocalcaneal c.
   talonavicular c.
   tarsal c.

coarctate

coarctation
   c. of aorta
   c. of aorta, adult type
   c. of aorta, infantile type
   reversed c.

coat
   extraneous c.
   proper c. of corium
   proper c. of dermis

cobalamin

cobalt assay

cobaltinitrite method

cobaltosis

cobaltous chloride

Cobas
   C. Fara H centrifugal
      analyzer
   C. Helios differential
      analyzer

Coblentz test method

COBS
   cesarean-obtained barrier-
      sustained

cocaethylene

cocaine
   c. hydrochloride
   c. metabolic assay
   tetracaine, epinephrine,
      and c. (TAC)

cocarboxylase

cocacinogen

coccerin

coccidioidoma

coccidioidomycosis
   primary c.

coccinella

coccinellin

coccode

coccyalgia

coccydynia

coccygalgia

coccygodynia

coccyodynia

cochineal

cochlea
   Mondini's c.

cochleitis

cochlitis

coctoprecipitin

cocultivation

cocurrent

codeine assay

CODE-ON Immunoslide Stainer

codocyte

coefficient
   creatinine c.
   cryoscopic c.
   c. of demineralization

coenuriasis

coenurosis

coeur
   c. en sabot

COF
   cemento-ossifying fibroma

cofactor
   cobra venom c.
   heparin c.
   platelet c.
   platelet c. I, II, V
   ristocetin c.
   c. of thromboplastin

Coffin-Lowry syndrome

Coffin-Siris syndrome

Cogan syndrome

COGTT
   cortisone-primed oral
      glucose tolerance test

COHB
   Carboxyhemoglobin

coherent smallpox

cohesive termini

Cohnheim theory

coin lesion

Colcemid

Colcher-Sussman method

colchicine

COLD
   chronic obstructive lung
      disease

cold-knife conization

cold-reacting antibody

cold-reactive antibody

cold-sensitive mutation

colectasia

Cole hematoxylin

Coleman-Schiff reagent

Coleoptera

coleoptosis

colestipol hydrochloride

Coley toxin

coli-aerogenes group

colibacillemia

colibacillosis
   c. gravidarum

colibacilluria

colic
   appendicular c.
   biliary c.
   bilious c.
   endemic c.
   flatulent c.
   gallstone c.
   gastric c.
   hepatic c.
   infantile c.

colic (*continued*)
   intestinal c.
   menstrual c.
   nephric c.
   ovarian c.
   pancreatic c.
   renal c.
   stercoral c.
   tubal c.
   ureteral c.
   uterine c.
   vermicular c.
   verminous c.
   worm c.

colicystitis

colicystopyelitis

colitides

colitis
   amebic c.
   antibiotic-associated c.
   balantidial c.
   cathartic c.
   chemical c.
   collagenous c.
   Crohn's c.
   c. cystica profunda
   c. cystica superficialis
   diversion c.
   granulomatous c.
   c. gravis
   hemorrhagic c.
   infectious c.
   irradiation c.
   ischemic c.
   lymphocytic c.
   microscopic c.
   mucous c.
   necrotizing amebic c.
   c. polyposa
   pseudomembranous c.
   radiation c.
   regional c.
   segmental c.
   soap c.
   transmural c.
   c. ulcerativa

colitis (*continued*)
    ulcerative c.
    uremic c.

coliuria

collacin

collagenoblast

collagenocyte

collar
    Casal's c.
    circumaortic venous c.
    c. of pearls
    Spanish c.
    c. of Stokes
    venereal c.
    c. of Venus

collarette
    Biett's c.

collastin

collateral
    Schaffer c.

colliculitis

collimation

colliquative

colloidin

collum
    c. distortum
    c. valgum

coloboma
    atypical c.
    bridge c.
    c. of choroid
    c. of ciliary body
    complete c.
    Fuchs' c.
    c. of fundus
    c. iridis
    c. of iris
    c. of lens
    c. lentis
    c. lobuli
    c. of optic disk

coloboma (*continued*)
    c. of optic nerve
    c. at optic nerve entrance
    c. palpebrale
    peripapillary c.
    c. of retina
    c. retinae
    retinochoroidal c.
    typical c.
    c. of vitreous

colodyspepsia

coloenteritis

colonalgia

colonorrhagia

colopathy

colophony

coloproctitis

coloptosis

color
    confusion c.
    pseudoisochromatic c.

colorimeter
    Duboscq's c.
    titration c.

colorrhea

colpalgia

colpatresia

colpectasia

colpectasis

colpismus

colpitis
    c. emphysematosa
    emphysematous c.
    c. macularis
    c. mycotica

colpocele

colpocephaly

colpocystitis

colpocystocele

colpocytology

colpodynia

colpohyperplasia
    c. cystica
    c. emphysematosa

colpoptosis

colporrhagia

colporrhexis

colpospasm

colpostenosis

colpoxerosis

column
    enamel c.
    c. of Kölliker
    muscle c.
    c. of Sertoli

colypeptic

comedo
    closed c.
    open c.

comedogenic

comedomastitis

comminution

commotio
    c. cerebri
    c. retinae
    c. spinalis

comorbid

comorbidity

comparascope

comparator

compartmentalization

compartmentation

complex
    AIDS dementia c.

complex (*continued*)
    atrial premature c.
    atrioventricular (AV)
      junctional escape c.
    atrioventricular (AV)
      junctional premature c.
    basal c. of choroid
    Carney's c.
    EAHF c.
    Eisenmenger's c.
    Ghon c.
    Golgi c.
    interpolated ventricular
      premature c.
    jumped process c.
    junctional premature c.
    juvenile nephronophthisis-
      medullary cystic disease
      c.
    juxtaglomerular c.
    Lutembacher's c.
    Meyenburg's c.
    pore c.
    primary c.
    Ranke c.
    sicca c.
    sling ring c.
    supraventricular c.
    synaptonemal c.
    ventricular premature c.

compression
    c. of the brain
    cerebral c.
    nerve c.
    spinal c.
    spinal cord c.

compressorium

concha
    c. bullosa

conchiolinosteomyelitis

conchitis

conclination

concrement

concretio

concretio (*continued*)
    c. cordis
    c. pericardii

concretion
    calculous c.
    preputial c.
    prostatic c.
    tophic c.

concussion
    abdominal c., hydraulic
    air c.
    c. of the brain
    c. of the labyrinth
    pulmonary c.
    c. of the retina
    c. of the spinal cord

condenser
    Abbe's c.
    cardioid c.
    darkfield c.
    paraboloid c.

conduction
    aberrant c.
    anomalous c.
    concealed c.
    concealed retrograde c.
    decremental c.
    delayed c.
    retrograde c.
    ventriculoatrial c.

condyloma
    c. acuminatum
    flat c.
    c. latum
    pointed c.

condylomata

condylomatoid

condylomatosis

condylomatous

cone
    acrosomal c.
    antipodal c.
    attraction c.

cone (*continued*)
    bifurcation c.
    cerebellar pressure c.
    ectoplacental c.
    fertilization c.
    growth c.
    implantation c.
    pressure c.
    retinal c.
    sarcoplasmic c.
    twin c.

confertus

congelation

conglutinatio
    c. orificii externi

conglutination

congophilic

coniofibrosis

coniolymphstasis

coniosis

coniosporosis

coniotoxicosis

conjunctivitis
    actinic c.
    acute contagious c.
    acute epidemic c.
    acute hemorrhagic c.
    angular c.
    arc-flash c.
    atopic c.
    atropine c.
    blennorrheal c.
    calcareous c.
    catarrhal c., acute
    catarrhal c., chronic
    chemical c.
    croupous c.
    diphtheritic c.
    diplobacillary c.
    eczematous c.
    Egyptian c.
    epidemic c.

conjunctivitis (*continued*)
follicular c.
gonococcal c.
gonorrheal c.
granular c.
inclusion c.
infantile purulent c.
Koch-Weeks c.
larval c.
lithiasis c.
c. medicamentosa
membranous c.
meningococcus c.
molluscum c.
Morax-Axenfeld c.
mucopurulent c.
necrotic infectious c.
neonatal c.
c. nodosa
nodular c.
Parinaud's c.
Pascheff's c.
c. petrificans
phlyctenular c.
pseudomembranous c.
purulent c.
scrofular c.
shipyard c.
simple c.
simple acute c.
spring c.
swimming pool c.
trachomatous c.
tularemic c.
uratic c.
vaccinial c.
vernal c.
welder's c.
Widmark's c.

conjunctivoma

conoid
Sturm's c.

conophthalmus

conotruncal

constipation

constipation (*continued*)
atonic c.
gastrojejunal c.
proctogenous c.
spastic c.

contraction
atrial premature c.
atrioventricular (AV)
junctional premature c.
automatic ventricular c.
carpopedal c.
clonic c.
Dupuytren's c.
escaped ventricular c.
fibrillary c.
hourglass c.
junctional premature c.
palmar c.
premature c.
supraventricular premature
c.
ventricular premature c.

contracture
Dupuytren's c.
ischemic c.
organic c.
postpoliomyelitic c.
Volkmann's c.

contrafissure

contrasexual

contrecoup

contund

contuse

contusion
brain c.
contrecoup c.
myocardial c.
c.of spinal cord

conus
distraction c.
myopic c.
supertraction c.

convergence

convergence (*continued*)
    negative c.

convexobasia

convulsibility

convulsion
    central c.
    clonic c.
    essential c.
    febrile c.
    local c.
    mimetic c.
    mimic c.
    puerperal c.
    salaam c.
    tetanic c.
    tonic c.
    uremic c.

convulsivant

COP
    colloidal osmotic pressure

COPD
    chronic obstructive
        pulmonary disease

Cope method of bronchography

copepod

Copepoda

copiopia

copracrasia

copremesis

coprolith

coprology

coproma

coproporphyria
    erythropoietic c.
    hereditary c.

coproporphyrinuria

coprostasis

coprosterol

coprozoa

coprozoic
    c. emeba

CoQ
    coenzyme Q

cor
    c. adiposum
    c. biloculare
    c. bovinum
    c. pulmonale, acute
    c. pulmonale, chronic
    c. taurinum
    c. triatriatum
    c. triloculare
    c. triloculare biatriatum
    c. triloculare biventriculare

coracoiditis

corallin
    yellow c.

Corbin technique

Corbus disease

cord
    c. blood
    c. blood serum
    c. compression (CC)
    c. factor
    marginal insertion of
        umblical c.
    prolapsed umbilical c.
    ruptured umbilical c.
    sex c.'s

cordis

core
    air c.
    c. antigen
    hyaline c.
    magnetic c.
    c. memory
    c. pneumonia

corectasis

corectopia

corediastasis

corestenoma
    c. congenitum

cornea
    conical c.
    c. farinata
    flat cornea
    c. globosa
    c. guttata
    c. plana
    c. verticillata

corneitis

corneoblepharon

corneocyte

corneoiritis

corodiastasis

corona
    c. radiata
    c. veneris

corps
    c. ronds

corpse

corpulency

corpus
    c. amylacea
    c. atretica
    c. lutea atretica
    c. oryzoidea
    c. versicolorata

corpuscle
    amylaceous c.
    amyloid c.
    articular c.
    axile c.
    axis c.
    bone c.
    bridge c.
    bulboid c.
    cartilage c.
    chorea c.
    chromophil c.

corpuscle (*continued*)
    chyle c.
    colloid c.
    compound granular c.
    concentric c.
    corneal c.
    Dogiel's c.
    genital c.
    Gierke c.
    Gluge's c.
    Golgi's c.
    Golgi-Mazzoni c.
    Guarnieri's c.
    Hassall's c.
    Jaworski's c.
    Krause's c.
    lamellar c.
    lamellated c.
    Leber's c.
    lingual c.
    Lostorfer's c.
    lymph c.
    lymphoid c.
    malpighian c. of kidney
    Mazzoni's c.
    meconium c.
    Meissner's c.
    Merkel's c.
    Norris' c.
    Pacini's c.
    pacinian c.
    paciniform c.
    Paschen's c.
    pessary c.
    pus c.
    renal c.
    Ruffini's c.
    salivary c.
    Schwalbe's c.
    tactile c.
    taste c.
    tendon c.
    terminal nerve c.
    thymus c.
    Timofeew's c.
    touch c.
    Toynbee's c.

corpuscle (*continued*)
Tröltsch's c.
typhic c.
Valentin's c.
Vater's c.
Vater-Pacini c.
Virchow's c.

corpusculum
c. articulare
c. bulboideum
c. genitale
c. lamellosum
c. nervosum terminale
c. renis
c. tactus

correspondence
anomalous retinal c.

corticocancellous

corticolipotrope

corticopleuritis

corticosterone methyl oxidase
deficiency

corticotrope

corticotroph

corticotroph-lipotroph

coruscation

corymbiform

corymbose

Corynebacterium
C. acnes

coryza
c. foetida

costalgia

costogenic

cotransport

cough
aneurysmal c.
Balme's c.
barking c.

cough (*continued*)
brassy c.
dry c.
ear c.
habit c.
hacking c.
privet c.
productive c.
psychogenic c.
trigeminal c.
wet c.
whooping c.
winter c.

counterbalance
renal c.

counterstain

countertransport

coup
c. de fouet
c. de sabre
en c. de sabre
c. de soleil

coupling
fixed c.
variable c.

couvercle

coverglass

cowage

cowperitis

coxa
c. adducta
c. flexa
c. magna
c. plana
c. valga
c. vara
c. vara luxans

coxalgia

coxarthria

coxarthritis

coxarthrocace

coxarthropathy

coxarthrosis

coxitis
    c. fugax
    senile c.

coxodynia

coxotuberculosis

CP
    cerebral palsy
    chemically pure
    coproporphyrin
    cystosarcoma phyllodes

C/P
    cholesterol-phospholipid
        ratio

C/pah/
    p-aminohippurate
        clearance

CPB
    cardiopulmonary bypass
    competitive protein-binding
        CPB assay

CPC
    chronic passive congestion
    clinicopathologic
        conference

CPD
    cephalopelvic disproportion

CPD-adenine

CPE
    chronic pulmonary
        emphysema
    coronary prognostic index

C-peptide
    C-p. test

CPI
    chronic pneumonitis of
        infancy
    coronary prognostic index

CPN
    chronic pyelonephritis

CPPD
    calcium pyrophosphate
        deposition disease

CPR
    cerebral cortex perfusion
        rate
    cortisol production rate

C_3 proactivator

CQ
    circadian quotient

C_1 immune complex detection

CR
    crown rump

craniocele

craniomalacia

craniomeningocele

craniopathy
    metabolic c.

craniosclerosis

craniostenosis

craniostosis

craniosynostosis

craniotabes

crapulent

CRBBB
    complete right bundle-
        branch block

CRD
    chronic renal disease
    complete reaction of
        degeneration

C-reactive
    C.-r. protein (CRP)
    C.-r. protein assay
    C.-r. protein test

creatine
    c. kinase
    c. kinase assay

creatine (*continued*)
    c. kinase isoenzyme
    c. kinase isoenzyme
      electrophoresis
    c. kinase test
    c. phosphate
    c. phosphokinase

creatinemia

creatinine

creatinuria

creatorrhea

crenate

crenated

crenation

crenocyte

crenocytosis

crenulation

crepitant

crepitation

crepitus
    articular c.
    bony c.
    false c.
    c. indux
    joint c.
    c. redux
    silken c.

crepuscular

crescent
    epithelial c.
    glomerular c.
    myopic c.

cresolphthalein

CREST
    calcinosis, Raynaud
      phenomenon, esophageal
      motility disorders,
      sclerodactyl, and
      telangiectasia
    CREST syndrome

crest
    mitochondrial c.

cretin

cretinism
    athyreotic c.
    athyrotic c.
    endemic c.
    myxedematous c.
    neurologic c.
    spontaneous c.
    sporadic c.
    sporadic goitrous c.
    sporadic nongoitrous c.

cretinistic

cretinoid

cretinous

CRF
    chronic renal failure
    corticotropin-releasing
      factor

cricoidynia

crinophagy

crisis
    addisonian c.
    adrenal c.
    aplastic c.
    bronchial c.
    cardiac c.
    celiac c.
    clitoris c.
    deglobulinization c.
    Dietl's c.
    febrile c.
    gastric c.
    genital c. of newborn
    glaucomatocyclitic c.
    hemolytic c.
    hepatic c.
    hypertensive c.
    intestinal c.
    laryngeal c.
    megaloblastic c.
    myasthenic c.

crisis (*continued*)
    nephralgic c.
    ocular c.
    oculogyric c.
    parkinsonian c.
    pharyngeal c.
    rectal c.
    renal c.
    salt-depletion c.
    salt-losing c.
    sickle cell c.
    tabetic c.
    thoracic c.
    thyroid c.
    thyrotoxic c.
    vaso-occlusive c.
    vesical c.
    visceral c.

crispation

crista
    mitochondrial c.
    c. mitochondriales

criterion
    Ranson's c.

CRM
    cross-reacting material

cRNA
    chromosomal RNA

crocein

crocidismus

cross
    Ranvier's c.
    silver c.

croupous

croupy

CRP
    C-reactive protein

^{51}Cr red cell survival

CRS
    Chinese restaurant
      syndrome

CRST
    calcinosis cutis, Raynaud
      phenomenon,
      sclerodactyl, and
      telangiectasia
    CRST syndrome

CRT
    cathode ray tube
      CRT terminal

cruor

crusta
    c. lactea

crustae

crustosus

cryalgesia

cryanesthesia

cryesthesia

crymodynia

cryofibrinogen

cryofibrinogenemia

cryogammaglobulin

cryoglobulin
    type I c.
    type II c.
    type III c.

cryoglobulinemia
    essential mixed c.

cryopathy

cryostat

CRYO-VAC-A cryostat vacuum
  system

cryptitis
    anal c.

cryptococcosis
    cutaneous c.
    pulmonary c.

cryptoempyema

cryptoglandular

cryptolith

cryptomenorrhea

cryptomere

cryptomerorachischisis

cryptopodia

cryptopyic

cryptorchid

cryptorchidism

cryptorchidy

cryptorchism

crystal
- asthma c.
- blood c.
- calcium pyrophosphate dihydrate (CPPD) c.
- Charcot-Leyden c.
- coffin lid c.
- CPPD c.
- dumbbell c.
- ear c.
- hedgehog c.
- hydroxyapatite c.
- knife rest c.
- Lubarsch's c.
- c. of Reinke
- thorn apple c.
- Virchow's c.
- whetstone c.

crystalloid
- Charcot-Böttcher c.
- c. of Reinke

crystalluria

CS
- chorionic somatomammotropin

C&S
- culture and sensitivity
  - C & S test

CSA
- colony-stimulating activity
- compressed spectral assay

CSF
- cerebrospinal fluid
- colony-stimulating factor
- CSF glutamine test

CSH
- capsular synovial-like hyperplasia
- chronic subdural hematoma
- cortical stromal hyperplasia

Csillag disease

CSM
- cerebrospinal meningitis

CSR
- corrected sedimentation rate
- cortisol secretion rate

cSt
- centistoke

CT
- cerebral thrombosis
- circulation time
- clotting time
- coagulation time
- Coombs test
- coronary thrombosis
- corrected transposition
- cytotechnologist
  - CT number

CTCL
- Cutaneous T-cell lymphoma

CTD
- carpal tunnel syndrome
- congenital thymic dysplasia

C-terminal

ctetosome

CT-guided sterotactic biopsy

CTL
- cytologic T lymphocyte

CTP
    cytidine triphosphate
    cytosine triphosphate

C/u/
    urea clearance

Cuban itch

CUC
    chronic ulcerative colitis

cubitus
    c. valgus
    c. varus

cucurbitol

cuirass
    tabetic c.

culture medium

cumulus
    ovarian c.
    c. ovaricus

cuniculi

cuniculus

cup
    glaucomatous c.

cupping
    pathologic c.

cupremia

cupriuria

cupruresis

cupulolithiasis

curse
    Ondine's c.

curvature
    Pott's c.
    spinal c.
    penile c.

curve
    Harrison's c.
    Wunderlich's c.

cushingoid

cushion
    intimal c.

cuticle
    dental c.
    enamel c.
    primary c.
    c. of root sheath
    secondary c.

cutis
    c. hyperelastica
    c. laxa
    c. rhomboidalis nuchae
    c. verticis gyrata

cuvet
    c. oximeter

CV
    cell volume
    coefficient of variation
    cresyl violet

CVA
    cardiovascular accident
    cerebrovascular accident

CVD
    cardiovascular disease

CVH
    combined ventricular
      hypertrophy
    common variable
      hypogammaglobulinemia

CVOD
    cerebrovascular obstructive
      disease

CVP
    cell volume profile

CVR
    cardiovascular-renal
    cerebrovascular resistance

CVRD
    cardiovascular renal
      disease

CVS
    chorionic villus sampling

CWDF
cell wall-deficient bacterial forms

CWP
coal workers' pneumoconiosis

cyanocrystallin

cyanophil

cyanophilous

cyanophose

cyanopsia

cyanosis
autotoxic c.
enterogenous c.
false c.
hereditary methemoglobinemic c.
c. lienis
pulmonary c.
c. retinae
shunt c.
tardive c.

cyanotic

cyanuria

cyanurin

cycle
aberrant c.
anovulatory c.
asexual c.
cell c.
citrate-pyruvate c.
forced c.

cyclitis
heterochromic c.
plastic c.
pure c.
purulent c.
serous c.

cycloceratitis

cyclochoroiditis

cyclodamia

cyclokeratitis

cyclomastopathy

cyclophoria
accommodative c.
minus c.
plus c.

cycloplegia

cycloplegic

cyclosis

cyclospasm

cyclotropia

cyestein

cyesthein

cylinder
axis c.
Bence Jones c.
Külz's c.
Leydig's c.
Ruffini's c.
terminal c.
urinary c.

cylindroid

cylindruria

cyllosis

cymbocephalia

cymbocephalic

cymbocephalous

cymbocephaly

cyrtosis

Cys
cysteine

cyst
adventitious c.
allantoic c.
alveolar c.
amnionic c.

cyst (*continued*)
  apical c.
  arachnoid c.
  atheromatous c.
  Baker's c.
  Bartholin's c.
  Blessig's c.
  blue dome c.
  Boyer's c.
  branchial c.
  branchial cleft c.
  branchiogenetic c.
  branchiogenous c.
  bronchial c.
  bronchogenic c.
  bronchopulmonary c.
  bursal c.
  calcifying odontogenic c.
  cervical c.
  cervical lymphoepithelial c.
  chocolate c.
  choledochal c.
  choledochus c.
  chyle c.
  colloid c.
  corpus luteum c.
  dental c.
  dentigerous c.
  dermoid c.
  dilatation c.
  distention c.
  endometrial c.
  endometriotic c.
  endothelial c.
  enteric c.
  enterogenous c.
  ependymal c.
  epidermal c.
  epidermal inclusion c.
  epidermoid c.
  epithelial c.
  eruption c.
  esophageal duplication c.
  extravasation c.
  exudation c.
  false c.
  fissural c.
  follicular c.

cyst (*continued*)
  ganglionic c.
  Gartner's c.
  Gartner's duct c.
  gartnerian c.
  gas c.
  gingival c.
  globulomaxillary c.
  Gorlin's c.
  hemorrhagic c.
  heterotopic oral
    gastrointestinal c.
  implantation c.
  incisive canal c.
  inclusion c.
  intraepithelial c.
  intraluminal c.
  involution c.
  Iwanoff's (Iwanow's) c.
  keratinizing c.
  keratinous c.
  Klestadt's c.
  lacteal c.
  lateral periodontal c.
  leptomeningeal c.
  lutein c.
  lymphoepithelial c.
  median anterior maxillary c.
  median mandibular c.
  median palatal c.
  meibomian c.
  mesenteric c.
  milk c.
  mucous c.
  mucus retention c.
  myxoid c.
  Naboth's c.
  nabothian c.
  nasoalveolar c.
  nasolabial c.
  nasopalatine duct c.
  necrotic c.
  neural c.
  neurenteric c.
  nevoid c.
  odontogenic c.
  oil c.
  omental c.

cyst (*continued*)
oophoritic c.
pancreatic c.
paranephric c.
parapyelitic c.
parovarian c.
pearl c.
periapical c.
pericardial c.
perineurial c.
periodontal c.
pilar c.
piliferous c.
pilonidal c.
placental c.
porencephalic c.
congenital preauricular c.
primordial c.
pyelogenic renal c.
radicular c.
Rathke's cleft c.
residual c.
retention c.
Sampson's c.
sebaceous c.
secretory c.
seminal c.
serous c.
simple bone c.
soapsuds c.
solitary bone c.
springwater c.
subchondral c.
sublingual c.
subsynovial c.
synovial c.
Tarlov c.
tarry c.
tarsal c.
thecal c.
theca-lutein c.
thymic c.
thyroglossal c.
thyrolingual c.
traumatic bone c.
trichilemmal c.
true c.
tubular c.

cyst (*continued*)
umbilical c.
unicameral bone c.
urachal c.
urinary c.
vitellointestinal c.
wolffian c.

cystalgia

cystathionine β-synthase
  deficiency

cystathioninuria

cystatrophia

cystelcosis

cysterethism

cysthypersarcosis

cystiferous

cystiform

cystigerous

cystinemia

cystinosis
adolescent nephropathic c.
adult nephropathic c.
benign c.
early onset c.
infantile nephropathic c.
late onset juvenile c.

cystinuria

cystinuric

cystirrhagia

cystirrhea

cystis

cystistaxis

cystitis
allergic c.
bacterial c.
catarrhal c., acute
c. colli
croupous c.

cystitis (*continued*)
    cystic c.
    c. cystica
    diphtheritic c.
    c. emphysematosa
    eosinophilic c.
    exfoliative c.
    c. follicularis
    c. glandularis
    hemorrhagic c.
    incrusted c.
    interstitial c.
    mechanical c.
    panmural c.
    c. papillomatosa
    c. senilis feminarum
    submucous c.

cystoblast

cystocele

cystodynia

cystoenterocele

cystoepiplocele

cystogenesis

cystoid

cystolith

cystolithiasis

cystolithic

cystoma
    c. serosum simplex

cystonephrosis

cystoneuralgia

cystoparalysis

cystoparesis

cytopathological

cystophorous

cystophthisis

cystoplegia

cystoptosis

cystopyelitis

cystopyelonephritis

cystorrhagia

cystorrhea

cystoschisis

cystosclerosis

cystose

cystospasm

cystospermitis

cystostaxis

cystoureteritis

cystoureteropyelitis

cystoureteropyelonephritis

cystourethritis

cystourethrocele

cystous

cytaster

cytoanalyzer

cytobiology

cytocentrum

cytochalasin
    c. B

cytochemism

cytochemistry

cytochrome-c oxidase
   deficiency

cytochylema

cytocidal

cytocide

cytocinesis

cytoclasis

cytoclastic

cytode

cytodendrite

cytodieresis

cytodistal

cytofluorimeter

cytogenesis

cytogenic

cytogenous

cytogeny

cytoglucopenia

cytoglycopenia

cytohistogenesis

cytohormone

cytohyaloplasm

cytokalipenia

cytokeratin

cytokinesis

cytologic

cytologist

cytology
    aspiration biopsy c.
    exfoliative c.

cytolymph

cytolysate

cytolysis

cytolysosome

cytolytic

cytomegalic

cytomegaloviruria

cytometaplasia

cytometer
    flow c.

cytometry
    flow c.
    image c.

cytomitome

cytomorphology

cytomorphosis

cyton

cytonecrosis

cytopathic

cytopathogenesis

cytopathogenetic

cytopathogenic

cytopathogenicity

cytopathologic

cytopathologist

cytopathology

cytopenia

cytophotometer

cytophotometric

cytophotometry

cytophylactic

cytophylaxis

cytophyletic

cytophysics

cytophysiology

cytopigment

cytopipette

cytoplasm

cytoplasmic

cytoplast

cytoproximal

cytoreticulum

Cyto-Rich cervical cytology
    monolayer system

cytorrhyctes

cytoscopy

cytosiderin

cytoskeletal

cytoskeleton

cytosol

cytosolic

cytosome

cytospin
  c. analysis
  c. cup
  c. slide centrifuge Gram-
    stained smear

cytospongium

cytost

cytostasis

cytostatic

cytostromatic

cytotactic

cytotaxigen

cytotaxin

cytotaxis

cytothesis

cytotoxic

cytotoxicity

cytotrophoblast

cytotrophoblastic

cytotropic

cytotropism

cyturia

Cytyc
  C. CytoLyl preservative
    solution
  C. Preservcyt preservative
    solution

Czapek-Dox
  C.-D. agar
  C.-D. medium

Czapek solution agar

Czerny disease

D

Δ (*var. of* Delta)

δ (*var. of* delta)
    δ agent
    δ antigen
    δ cell islet
    δ check
    δ hepatitis
    δ ray
    δ staphylolysin
    δ virus

D
    D antigen
    D colony
    D line
    D value

D_{CO}
    diffusing capacity for carbon monoxide

D10 antigen

D-3-hydroxyacyl coenzyme A

DA
    degenerative arthritis
    direct agglutination
    disaggregated
        DA pregnancy test

Daae disease

Daae-Finsen disease

DAB
    diaminobenzidine
        DAB reaction

Dabska tumor

DAC
    diazacholesterol
    digital-to-analog converter

D/A converter

DaCosta
    D. disease
    D. syndrome

dacroyte

dacryadenalgia

dacryadenitis

dacrycystalgia

dacrycystitis

dacryelcosis

dacryoadenalgia

dacryoadenitis

dacryoblennorrhea

dacryocanaliculitis

dacryocele

dacryocystalgia

dacryocystectasia

dacryocystitis

dacryocystoblennorrhea

dacryocystocele

dacryocystoptosis

dacryocystorhinostenosis

dacryocystostenosis

dacryocyte

dacryohelcosis

dacryohemorrhea

dacryolith

dacryolithiasis

dacryoma

dacryops

dacryopyorrhea

dacryopyosis

dacryorrhea

dacryosinusitis

dacryosolenitis

dacryostenosis

dactyledema

dactylion

dactylitis

dactylocampsodynia

dactylogryposis

dactylomegaly

dactylospasm

Dade Hepzyme heparinase

Da Fano stain

DAGT
  direct anitglubulin test

DAH
  disordered action of heart

dahlia

DAKO
  D. Envision System
    Peroxidase
  D. target retrieval solution

dalapon

Dale-Laidlaw clotting time
  method

Dalen-Fuchs nodule

daltonism

Dalton law

damage
  irradiation d.
  minimal brain d. (MBD)
  myocardial d. (MD)
  radiation d.

D-amino acid oxidase

dAMP
  deoxyadenosine
    monophosphate

dammar

Danbolt-Close syndrome

dance
  brachial d.
  hilar d.
  hilus d.
  St. Anthony's d.
  St. Guy's d.
  St. John's d.
  St. Vitus' d.

dander

dandruff

Dandy-Walker syndrome

Dane
  D. and Herman keratin
    stain
  D. method
  D. particle

Danielssen-Boeck disease

Danielssen disease

Danlos syndrome

DANS
  1-dimethylamino
    aphthalene-5 sulfonic acid

dansyl chloride

Danubian endemic familial
  nephropathy

Danysz phenomenon

DAP
  direct agglutination
    pregnancy

DAPI
  4′6-diamidino-2-
    phenylindole-2 HC1
      DAPI solution

DAPT
  direct agglutination
    pregnancy test

D-arabitol dehydrogenase

Darier disease

dark
  d. current
  d. reaction
  d. reactivation

dark-field
  d.-f. condenser
  d.-f. examination
  fluorescent antibody d.-f.
    (FADF)
  d.-f. microscope

Darling disease

Darlington amplifier

Darrow
    D. red
    D. red stain

d'Arsonval meter

dartoic

dartoid

DAT
    differential agglutination tier
    diphtheria antitoxin
    direct agglutination test

Datril

daunomycin

daunorubicin
    d., cytarabine,
        6-mercatopurine,
        prednisone (DCMP)

Davaineidae

Davenport graph

David disease

Davidson differential absorption
    test

Davies disease

Dawson encephalitis

Day test

DB
    dextran blue

DBC
    dye-binding capacity

DBCL
    dilute blood clot lysis
        (method)

DBI
    development-at-birth index

DCA
    deoxycholate-citrate agar

DCF
    direct centrifugal flotation

DCIS
    ductal carcinoma in situ

DCMP
    daunorubicin, cytarabine, 6-
        mercaptopurine,
        prednisone

DDD
    dense-deposit disease
    dihydroxydinaphthyl
        disulfide

D-dimer
    D-d. assay
    D-d. test

DDS
    dystrophy-dystocia
        syndrome

DEA
    dehydroepiandrosterone

deacylase
    acylsphingosine d.

deacylate

dead
    d. of disease (DOD)
    d. fetus in utero (DFU)
    d. finger
    d. on arrival (DOA)
    d. time

dead-end host

deadly agaric

DEAE-cellulose
    diethylaminoethyl cellulose

deafferentation

deafness
    acoustic trauma d.
    Alexander's d.
    bass d.
    boilermakers' d.
    central d.
    conduction d.
    conductive d.
    cortical d.

deafness (*continued*)
    functional d.
    hysterical d.
    labyrinthine d.
    Michel's d.
    midbrain d.
    Mondini's d.
    music d.
    nerve d.
    neural d.
    organic d.
    pagetoid d.
    paradoxic d.
    perceptive d.
    postlingual d.
    prelingual d.
    Scheibe's d.
    sensorineural d.
    tone d.
    toxic d.
    vascular d.
    word d.

dearterialization

death
    activation-induced cell d.
    brain d.
    cause of d.
    cell d.
    cerebral d.
    cognitive d.
    cot d.
    crib d.
    fetal d.
    fetal d., early
    fetal d., intermediate
    fetal d., late
    functional d.
    genetic d.
    indirect maternal d.
    infant d.
    intrauterine d.
    late neonatal d.
    liver d.
    local d.
    maternal d.
    molecular d.
    natural d.

death (*continued*)
    perinatal d.
    programmed cell d.
    somatic d.
    sudden cardiac d.
    sudden coronary d.
    sudden unexpected d.
    sudden unexpected,
      unexplained d.
    sudden unexplained d.
    sudden unexplained infant d.

DeBakey aortic assay

debrancher deficiency limit
   dextrinosis

debranching enzyme

Debré phenomenon

Debré-Semelaigne syndrome

déridement, debridement

debris

decalcification

decameter

decanoic acid

decantation

decarboxylase
    branched-chain alpha
      ketoacid d.
    branched-chain α-ketoacid d.
    d. broth
    glutamate d.
    glutamic acid d. (GAD)
    histidine d.
    methylmalonyl-CoA d.
    ornithine d.
    orotidine d.
    orotidine-5′-phosphate d.
    orotidylate d.
    oxaloacetate d.
    uroprophyrigen d.

decarboxylation
    amine precursor uptake
      and d. (APUD)

decay
    α-d.
    alpha d.
    d. antibody-accelerating
      factor
    β-d.
    beta d.
    branching d.
    d. coefficient
    d. constant
    exponential d.
    d. mode
    positron beta d.
    d. product
    radioactive d.
    d. rate
    d. scheme

deceration

decerebrate
    d. rigidity

decerebellation

decidua
    d. tuberosa papulosa

deciduitis

deciduomatosis

deciduosis

decompensation

decomposition
    d. of movement

decubital

decubitus
    Andral's d.
    d. calculus
    d. ulcer

decussate

decussation

dedifferentiated liposarcoma

dedifferentiation

de-efferentiation

deep agar

Deetjen body

defatigation

defecation
    fragmentary d.

defect
    acquired d.
    aortic septal d.
    aorticopulmonary septal d.
    atrial septal d.
    atrioseptal d.
    birth d.
    congenital d.
    cortical d.
    congenital ectodermal d.
    endocardial cushion d.
    genetic d.
    intercalary d. of pollical ray
    neural tube d.
    ostium primum d.
    ostium secundum d.
    polytopic field d.
    retention d.
    salt-losing d.
    septal d.
    ventricular septal d.

defective
    d. bacteriophage
    d. interfering particle
    d. phage
    d. probacteriophage
    d. prophage
    d. virus

defense
    host d.'s
    mechanism d.
    muscular d.

defensis

deferentitis

deferoxamine
    d. mesylate
    d. mesylate infusion test

deficiency
- adenosine deaminase d.
- ADH d.
- alpha-1 antitrypsin d.
- d. anemia
- antidiuretic hormone deficiency d.
- antitrypsin d.
- brancher d.
- caramoyl phosphate synthetase I d.
- 20,22-desmolase d.
- debrancher d.
- dihydropteridine reductase d.
- disaccharidase d.
- duplication d.
- d. factor (DF)
- d. factors I, II, VII, VIII, IX, X, XI
- familial apolipoprotein C-II (apo C-II) d.
- familial high-density lipoprotein (HDL) d.
- familial lipoprotein d.
- galactokinase d.
- glucose-6-phosphate dehydrogenase d.
- glucosesephosphate isomerase d.
- gluthathione synthetase d.
- growth hormone d. (GHD)
- hereditary plasmathromboplastin component d.
- immunity d.
- immunological d.
- iron d.
- iron d., latent
- iron d., prelatent
- lactase d.
- LCAT d.
- lecithin-cholesterol acyltransferase d.
- leukocyte adhesion d.
- lipoprotein lipase d.
- molybdenum cofactor d.

deficiency (*continued*)
- multiple acyl CoA dehydrogenation d.
- oxygen d.
- plasma thromboplastin antecedent d.
- PTA d.
- sucrase-α-dextrinase d., intestinal
- sucrase-isomaltase d., congenital
- vitamin d.
- color vision d.

deficit
- oxygen d.
- pulse d.
- reversible ischemic neurologic d.

defluvium
- postpartum d.
- d. unguium

defluxion

deformity
- Arnold-Chiari d.
- boutonnière d.
- buttonhole d.
- Chiari's d.
- crossbar d.
- Dandy-Walker d.
- gun stock d.
- Ilfeld-Holder d.
- Madelung's d.
- Mondini's d.
- recurvatum d.
- rocker-bottom d.
- rolled edge d.
- seal-fin d.
- silver fork d.
- Sprengel's d.
- swan neck d.
- thumb-in-palm d.
- ulnar drift d.
- Velpeau's d.
- Volkmann's d.

deg
   degeneration
   degree

degeneratio
   d. micans

degeneration
   adipose d.
   adiposogenital d.
   Alzheimer's neurofibrillary
      d.
   angiolithic d.
   Armanni-Ebstein d.
   ascending d.
   atheromatous d.
   axonal d.
   ballooning d.
   calcareous d.
   caseous d.
   cerebellar d., primary
      progressive
   cerebromacular d.
   cerebroretinal d.
   cheesy d.
   colloid d.
   colloid d. of choroid
   comma d.
   corticostriatal-spinal d.
   Crooke's hyaline d.
   cystic d.
   cystoid d.
   descending d.
   Doyne's familial colloid d.
   Doyne's honeycomb d.
   dystrophic d.
   earthy d.
   elastoid d.
   familial colloid d.
   fascicular d.
   fatty d.
   fibrinous d.
   fibroid d.
   fibrous d.
   gelatiniform d.
   glassy d.
   glistening d.
   glycogenic d.
   Gombault's d.

degeneration (*continued*)
   granulovascular d.
   gray d.
   hepatolenticular d.
   Holmes' d.
   Horn's d.
   hyaline d.
   hydropic d.
   lattice d. of retina
   lipoidal d.
   macular d.
   macular d., congenital
   macular d., disciform
   macular d., senile
      exudative
   macular d., Stargardt's
   macular d., vitelliform
   macular d., vitelline
   macular disciform d.
   Mönckeberg's d.
   mucinoid d.
   mucinous d.
   mucoid d.
   mucous d.
   myelinic d.
   myofibrillar d.
   myxomatous d.
   Nissl d.
   olivopontocerebellar d.
   pallidal d.
   pigmental d.
   pigmentary d.
   red d.
   retrograde d.
   rim d.
   Rosenthal's d.
   sclerotic d.
   secondary d.
   senile d.
   senile disciform d.
   spongy d. of central
      nervous system
   spongy d. of white matter
   striatonigral d.
   subacute combined d. of
      spinal cord
   tapetoretinal d.
   transneuronal d.

degeneration (*continued*)
    traumatic d.
    Türck's d.
    uratic d.
    vacuolar d.
    vitelliform d. of Best
    vitreous d.
    wallerian d.
    Wilson's d.
    Zenker's d.

Degos
    D. disease
    D. syndrome

degranulation

degree (deg)
    d.'s of freedom
    second d.

dehiscence

dehydrase
    aminolevulinic acid d.
      (ALAD)

dehydratase
    carbonate d.

dehydrated alcohol

dehydration
    absolute d.
    hypernatremic d.
    relative d.
    voluntary d.

dehydroascorbic acid

dehydrobilirubin

dehydroepiandrosterone (DEA, DHA, DHEA)

dehydroepiandrosterone sulfate (DHEAS, DS)

dehydrogenase
    acyl-CoA d.
    alcohol d.
    aldehyde d.
    branched-chain alpha
      ketoacid d.

dehydrogenase (*continued*)
    D-arabitol d.
    glucose-6-phosphate d.
    glutamate d.
    glyceraldehyde phosphate
      d. (GAPD, GAPDH)
    heat-stable lactic d. (HLDH)
    hexosephosphate d.
    3-hydroxybutyrate d.
    iditol d.
    isocitrate d.
    isocitric d.
    isovaleyrl-CoA d.
    lactate d. (LD, LDH)
    lactic d. (LD)
    L-arabinose d.
    L-arabitol d.
    lysine d.
    malate d.
    malic d. (MD)
    oxoglutarate d.
    2-oxoisovalerate d.
    phosphogluconate d.
    polyol d.
    proline d.
    1-pyrroline-5-carboxylate d.
    saccharopine d.
    sarcosine d.
    serum hydroxybutyrate d.
      (SHBD)
    serum isocitric d. (SICD)
    sorbitol d.
    tetrahydrofolate d.
    triosephosphate d.
    xylitol d.
    L-xylulose d.

dehyrdogenate

dehydrogenation

dehydroisoandrosterone (DHIA)

deiminase
    arginine d.

Dejerine
    D. disease
    D. syndrome

Dejerine-Klumpke syndrome

Dejerine-Roussy syndrome

Dejerine-Sottas
    D.-S. disease
    D.-S. syndrome

dekanem (DK)

delacrimation

Delafield
    D. fixative solution
    D. hematoxylin
    D. hemotoxyling stain

Delaney clause

delayed
    d. adrenarche
    d. allergy
    d. climacteric
    d. hemolytic transfusion
      reaction
    d. hypersensitivity
    d. hypersensitivity reaction
    d. menopause
    d. primary closure (DPC)
    d. puberty

delayed-type hypersensitivity
  (DTH)

deletion
    antigenic d.
    chromosomal d.
    intercalary d.
    interstitial d.
    d. mutation
    terminal d.
    d. theory

deliquescence

deliquescent

delirium
    febrile d.
    senile d.

delirium tremens (DT)

delle

delphian node

delta, δ
    d. agent
    d. aminolevulinic acid
    d. antigen
    d. base
    d. cell
    d. cell islet
    d. check
    d. hepatitis
    d. ray
    d. staphylolysin

demarcation
    line of d.
    surface d.

Dematiaceae

dematiaceous
    d. fungi

demeclocycline

dementia
    Alzheimer's d.
    d. of the Alzheimer type
    arteriosclerotic d.
    Binswanger's d.
    boxer's d.
    dialysis d.
    epileptic d.
    multi-infarct d.
    myoclonic d.
    d. myoclonica
    paralytic d.
    d. paralytica
    posttraumatic d.
    presenile d.
    d. pugilistica
    senile d.
    subcortical d.
    vascular d.

demilune
    d. body

demineralization

demonstration
    calcium deposit d.
    copper deposit d.
    degenerating myelin d.

demonstration (*continued*)
  iron-positive d.

demyelinate

demyelinated myelitis

demyelinating
  d. diseases
  d. encephalopathy

demyelination
  axonal d.
  segmental d.

demyelinization

denaturation
  protein d.

denaturing
  d. gels
  d. gradient gel
    electrophoresis

dendrite
  apical d.

dendritic

dendrocyte
  dermal d.

dendrodendritic

dendron

dendrophagocytosis

dengue
  hemorrhagic d.
  d. hemorrhagic fever
  d. shock syndrome
  d. virus
  d. virus, types 1, 2, 3, 4

denitrifying bacterium

Dennie-Marfan syndrome

Dennis technique

dens
  d. in dente
  d. invaginatus

dense-core neurosecretory
  granule

dense deposit disease

densimeter

densitometer
  gas d.

densitometry

density
  arciform d.
  buoyant d.
  character d.
  count information d.
  fiber d.
  d. function
  d. gradient centrifugation
  luminous flux d.
  optical d. (OD)
  scan information d.
  subplasmalemmal d.
  total body d. (TBD)

density-dependent repair

dental
  d. calculus
  d. caries
  d. fluorosis
  d. follicular cyst
  d. granuloma
  d. lymph
  d. pathology
  d. plaque

dentalgia

dentate nucleus

denticulated

dentigerous
  d. cyst
  d. mixed tumor

dentin
  calcified d.
  crystal d.
  dysplasia .d
  hereditary opalescent d.
  mantle d.
  opalescent d.
  sclerotic d.
  transparent d.

dentinoblast

dentinogenesis
    d. imperfecta

denucleated

denudation

Denver classification

Denys-Leclef phenomenon

deorsumvergence

deossification

deoxyadenosine
    monophosphate (dAMP)

deoxyadenosine-'5-phosphate

deoxyadenylic acid

6-deoxy-beta-L-galactose

deoxygenated hemoglobin

deoxyguanosine
    d. monophosphate
        (dGMP)
    d. phosphate

deoxyguanonsine-5'-phosphate

2-deoxyguanosine-5'-
    triphosphate (dGTP)

deoxyguanylic acid

deoxyhemoglobin

6-deoxy-β-L-mannose

deoxynucleotidyl transferase

deoxyribonuclease (DNase,
    DNAse)
    d. agar
    d. digestion
    d. I
    d. II
    d. test

deoxyribonucleic
    d. acid
    d. acid stain
    d. acid staining

deoxyribonucleic acid (DNA)
    competitor DNA

deoxyribonucleoprotein

deoxyribonucleoside

deoxyriboncleotide

deoxyribose

deoxysugar

deoxythymidine triphosphate
    (dTTP)

deoxyuridine
    d. monophosphate (dUMP)
    d. phosphate
    d. suppresion test

deoxyuridine-5'-phosphate

deoxyuridylic acid

deoxyvirus

deparaffinization

dependence
    anchorage d.
    drug d.

depigmentation

deplasmolysis

deplasmolyze

deposition
    bilharzial pigment d.
    calcium d.
    cholesterol d.
    collagen d.
    fatty d.
    ferrocalcinotic d.
    hemosiderin d.
    Kupffer cell iron d.
    malarial pigment d.
    particule crystalline
        material d.
    xanthomatous d.

depolarization
    atrial premature d.
    ventricular premature d.

depot
    fat d.
    d. reaction

depramine assay

depressed
    d. adenoma
    d. fracture

depression
    congenital chondrosternal
      d.

deprivation
    d. disease

deproteinization

depth
    d. dose
    d. of field
    d. of focus
    relative sagittal d. (RSD)

depulization

DeR
    reaction of degeneration

der
    derivative chromosome

deradelphus

derangement
    chromosomal d.
    Hey's internal d.

Dercum disease

derepressed gene

derepression
    transient d.

derivation

derivative
    d. chromosome (der)
    purified protein d. (PPD)

derivative-standard
    purified protein d. (PPD-S)

derived
    d. albumin
    d. protein

dermal
    d. bone
    d. dendritic cell
    d. dendrocyte
    d. duct tumor
    d. eccrine cylindroma
    d. epidermal necus
    d. nevus
    d. papilla
    d. sinus
    d. tuberculosis

dermal-epidermal nevus

dermamyiasis

dermatan sulfate

dermatitides

dermatitis
    actinic d.
    allergic d.
    allergic contact d.
    ammonia d.
    d. artefacta
    ashy d.
    atopic d.
    berlock d.
    berloque d.
    brown-tail moth d.
    d. bullosa striata pratensis
    d. calorica
    caterpillar d.
    cercarial d.
    contact-type d.
    contagious pustular d.
    cosmetic d.
    dhobie mark d.
    diaper d.
    eczematous d.
    d. exfoliativa
    d. exfoliativa neonatorum
    exfoliative d.
    exudative discoid and
      lichenoid d.
    factitial d.
    d. gangrenosa infantum
    d. herpetiformis
    d. hiemalis

dermatitis (*continued*)
  industrial d.
  infectious eczematoid d.
  insect d.
  irritant d.
  Jacquet d.
  lichenoid d.
  livedoid d.
  marine d.
  meadow d.
  meadow-grass d.
  d. medicamentosa
  moth d.
  napkin d.
  nickel d.
  nummular eczematous d.
  occupational d.
  onion mite d.
  d. papillaris capillitii
  Pelodera d.
  perfume d.
  periocular d.
  perioral d.
  photoallergic contact d.
  photocontact d.
  phototoxic d.
  phytophototoxic d.
  pigmented purpuric
    lichenoid d.
  poison ivy d.
  poison oak d.
  poison sumac d.
  primary irritant d.
  radiation d.
  rat-mite d.
  d. repens
  rhabditic d.
  rhus d.
  roentgen-ray d.
  sabra d.
  Schamberg d.
  schistosome d.
  seborrheic d.
  d. seborrheica
  stasis d.
  d. striata pratensis bullosa
  swimmers' d.
  uncinarial d.

dermatitis (*continued*)
  d. vegetans
  d. venenata
  verrucose d.
  verrucous d.
  vesicular d.

dermatoarthritis

dermatochalasis

dermatochalazia

dermatoconjunctivitis

dermatodysplasia

dermatofibrosis
  d. lenticularis disseminata

dermatographic

dermatographism
  black d.
  white d.

dermatolysis
  d. palpebrarum

dermatomegaly

dermatomycosis
  d. furfuracea

dermatomyiasis

dermatomyositis

dermato-ophthalmitis

dermatopathic

dermatopathology

dermatopathy

dermatophiliasis

dermatophilosis

dermatophyte

dermatophytid

dermatophytosis

dermatopolyneuritis

dermatorrhagia

dermatorrhexis

dermatosclerosis

dermatosis
    acute febrile neutrophilic d.
    ashy d. of Ramirez
    d. cenicienta
    chronic bullous d. of
      childhood
    dermatolytic bullous d.
    industrial d.
    lichenoid d.
    linear IgA d. of adulthood
    linear IgA d. of childhood
    d. papulosa nigra
    progressive pigmentary d.
    Schamberg's d.
    Schamberg's progressive
      pigmented purpuric d.
    subcorneal pustular d.
    transient acantholytic d.

dermatosome

dermatotropic

dermatozoiasis

dermatozoonosis

dermographism

dermolipoma

dermopathic

dermopathy
    diabetic d.
    infiltrative d.

dermosynovitis

dermotropic

DES
    diethylstilbestrol

desalivation

desalt

desaturation

descemetitis

descemetocele

descending
    d. degeneration

descensus
    d. uteri

desetope

desferrioxamine

deshydremia

desiccant

desiccate

desiccation

desiccative

desiccator

designated blood donation

desipramine assay

desmalgia

Desmarres dacryolith

desmectasia

desmectasis

desmin
    d. antibody

desmitis

desmodynia

desmoid
    extra-abdominal d.
    d. tumor

desmolase
    17,20-d.
    20,22-d.
    20,22-d. deficiency

desmopathy

desmoplasia

desmoplastic
    d. cerebral astrocytoma
    d. fibroma
    d. infantile ganglioglioma
    d. medulloblastoma

desmoplastic (*continued*)
  d. melanoma
  d. small round-cell tumor (DSRCT)
  d. stroma
  d. trichoblastoma
  d. trichoepithelioma

desmorrhexis

desmosine

desmosis

desmosome
  half d.

desmosterol

desolvation

desoxycholate
  bromocresol purple d. (BCP-D)

11-desoxycorticosterone

despeciate

despeciation

desquamate

desquamation
  furfuraceous d.
  lamellar d. of the newborn

desquamative
  d. inflammatory vaginitis
  d. interstitial pneumonia (DIP)
  d. interstitial pneumonitis (DIP)
  d. interstitial poisoning

desquamatory

destructive
  d. distillation
  d. interference

desynchronization

detached cranial section

detachment
  d. of retina
  retinal d.

detection
  antibody d.
  cardiac shunt d.
  C_1q immune complex d.

detector
  alpha-particle d.
  cadmium telluride d.
  combustible gas d.
  EC d.
  electron capture d.
  error d.
  flame ionization d.
  lithium-drifted d.
  paralyzable d.
  surface-barrier d.
  TC d.
  thermal conductivity d.
  thermoluminescent d.
  d. transfer function (DTF)

detergent
  anionic d.
  nonionic d.

determinant
  allotypic d.
  antigenic d.
  genetic d.
  d. group
  idiotypic antigenic d.
  immunogenic d.
  isoallotypic d.
  R d.
  resistance d. (RD)
  rough d.

determination
  activity d.
  lactate dehydrogenase isoenzymes d.
  lecithin-sphingomyelin ratio d.
  sex d.
  Shimadzu hemoglobin d.

detersice

detoxicate

detoxification
  metabolic d.

detritic synovitis

detrition

detritus

detumescence

deutan

deuteranomal

deuteranomalous

deuteranomaly

deuteranope

deuteranopia

deuteranopic

deuteranopsia

deuteropathic

deuteropathy

deuterosome

deuthyalosome

DEV
    duck embryo vaccine

devascularization

developmental
    d. arrest
    d. jaw cyst
    d. mixoploid
    d. synchronism

development-at-birth index
    (DBI)

Devergie disease

deviation
    average d.
    immune d.
    d. to the left
    mean d.
    mean square d.
    no significant d. (NSD)
    relative standard d. (RSD)
    d. to the right
    right axis d. (RAD)
    standard d.
    sum of square d.'s (SSD)

Devic disease

device
    Boyden chamber assay d.
    Coag-a-mate prothrombin
        d.
    Coumatrak prothrombin
        time d.
    I/O d.
    OraSure HIV-1 Oral
        Specimen Collection D.
    Riechert-Mundiger
        stereotactic d.
    semiconductor d.

devil's grip

devolution

Dewar flask

dexamethasone (DXM)
    d. suppression test (DST)

dexiocardia

dextran
    d. blue (DB)
    low molecular weight d.
        (LMD, LMDX)

dextrin
    limit d.

dextrinosis
    debrancher deficiency limit
        d.
    limit d.

dextrinuria

dextrocardia
    corrected d.
    false d.
    isolated d.
    mirror-image d.
    secondary d.
    type 1, 2, 3, 4 d.
    d. with situs inversus

dextroclination

dextrocycloduction

dextrogastria

dextroposition
    d. of the heart

dextrorotatory

dextrose
    d. solution mixture (DSM)
    d. test

dextrose-nitrogen ratio

dextrose-saline

dextrose in water (percent)
    (D/W)

Dextrostix

dextrosuria

dextrothyroxine sodium

dextrotorsion

dextroversion
    d. of the heart

DF
    deficiency factor
    disseminated foci

df
    degrees of freedom

DFA
    direct fluorescent antibody
    direct fluorescent assay

DFA-TP
    direct fluorescent antibody-
      Treponema pallidum test
    DFA-TP test

DFB
    diffuse panbronchiolitis

DFSP
    dermatofibrosarcoma
      protuberans

DFU
    dead fetus in utero
    dideoxyfluorouridine

DGGE
    denaturing gradient gel
      electrophoresis
        DGGE technique

dGMP
    deoxyguanosine
      monophosphate

dGTP
    2-deoxyguanosine-5′-
      triphosphate

DHA
    dehydroepiandrosterone

Dharmendra antigen

DHE
    dihydroergotamine

DHEA
    dehydroepiandrosterone
      DHEA test

DHEAS
    dehydroepiandrosterone
      sulfate

d'Herelle phenomenon

DHFR
    dihydrofolate reductase

DHIA
    dehydroisoandrosterone

DHL
    diffuse histocytic
      lymphoma

DHMA
    dihydroxymandelic acid

dhobie itch

DHT
    dihydrotachysterol
    dihydrotestosterone
    DHT test

DI
    diabetes insipidus

Di
    D. antigen
    D. Guglielmo disease
    D. Guglielmo syndrome

diabetes
    adult-onset d.

diabetes (*continued*)
    alimentary d.
    alloxan d.
    brittle d.
    bronze d.
    bronzed d.
    calcinuric d.
    chemical d.
    gestational d.
    d. innocens
    d. insipidus
    d. insipidus, central
    d. insipidus, nephrogenic
    d. insipidus, pituitary
    insulin-dependent d.
      mellitus (IDDM)
    juvenile-onset d.
    latent d.
    lipoatrophic d.
    maturity-onset d.
    d. mellitus
    d. mellitus, adult-onset
    d. mellitus, gestational
    d. mellitus, growth-onset
    d. mellitus, insulin-
      dependent
    d. mellitus, juvenile
    d. mellitus, juvenile-onset
    d. mellitus, ketosis-prone
    d. mellitus, ketosis-resistant
    d. mellitus, malnutrition-
      related
    d. mellitus, maturity-onset
    d. mellitus, non-insulin-
      dependent
    d. mellitus, tropical
    d. mellitus, tropical
      pancreatic
    d. mellitus, type 1
    d. mellitus, Type I
    d. mellitus, type 2
    d. mellitus, Type II
    non-insulin-dependent d.
      mellitus (NIDDM)
    phloridzin d.
    posttransplant d.
    preclinical d.
    puncture d.

diabetes (*continued*)
    renal d.
    steroid d.
    steroidogenic d.
    subclinical d.
    thiazide d.

diabetic
    d. acidosis
    d. amyotrophy
    d. angiopathy
    d. coma
    d. dermopathy
    d. gangrene
    d. glomerulosclerosis
    hyperosmolar d. coma
    d. ketoacidosis
    d. lipemia
    d. microangiopathy
    d. myelopathy
    d. nephropathy
    d. neuropathy
    d. retinopathy (DR)
    d. ulcer
    d. urine

diabeticorum
    bullosis d.

diabetogenic hormone

diabetogenous

diabrosis

diacetate

diacetemia

diacetic acid

diacetonuria

diaceturia

diacylglycerol

Diagnex
    D. Blue
    D. Blue test

diagnosis
    biological d.
    clinical d.

diagnosis (*continued*)
    cytohistologic d.
    cytologic d.
    direct d.
    laboratory d.
    pathologic d.
    physical d.
    prenatal d.
    provocative d.
    serum d.

diagram
    acid-base d.
    block d.
    scatter d.
    Venn d.

diakinesis

dial
    d. unit
    vernier d.

dialysance

dialysate

dialysis
    equilibrium d.
    extracorporeal d.
    peritoneal d.

dialyzer

diamagnetic

diameter
    Mantoux d. (MD)
    mean cell d. (MCD)
    mean corpuscular d.
      (MCD)
    outside d. (OD)

4′6-diamidino-2-phenylindole-2
  HCl (DAPI)

diaminobenzidine (DAB)
    d. reaction
    d. stain
    3-3′-d. tetrahydrochloride

ρ-diaminodiphenyl

diaminuria

Diamond-Blackfan
    D.-B. anemia
    D.-B. syndrome

diamond fuchsin

Diamyl

diapedesis

Diaphane
    D. solution

diaphanometer

diaphanometry

diaphanoscope

diaphragm
    antral d.
    eventration d.
    pyloric d.
    splinted d.
    slit d.

diaphragmalgia

diaphragmatic
    d. hernia
    d. peritonitis
    d. pleurisy

diaphragmatitis

diaphragmatocele

diaphragmitis

diaphysial, diaphyseal
    d. aclasis
    d. dyplasia
    d. juxtaepiphysial exostosis

diaphysitis
    tuberculous d.

diapyesis

diapyetic

diarrhea
    Brainerd d.
    cachectic d.
    choleraic d.
    d. chylosa
    congenital chloride d.

diarrhea (*continued*)
    dientameba d.
    dysenteric d.
    enteral d.
    epidemic d. of newborn
    familial chloride d.
    fermental d.
    fermentative d.
    flagellate d.
    gastrogenic d.
    hill d.
    infantile d.
    inflammatory d.
    irritative d.
    lienteric d.
    mechanical d.
    morning d.
    mucous d.
    neonatal d.
    osmotic d.
    d. pancreatica
    pancreatogenous fatty d.
    paradoxical d.
    parenteral d.
    putrefactive d.
    secretory d.
    serous d.
    stercoral d.
    summer d.
    toxigenic d.
    traveler's d.
    tropical d.
    virus d.
    watery d.
    weanling d.
    white d.

diarrheagenic *E. coli*

diarrheal

diarrheic

diarrheogenic

diaschisis

diaspironecrobiosis

diaspironecrosis

diastasic

diastasis
    iris d.
    d. recti abdominis

diastasuria

diastatic

diastematocrania

diastematomyelia

diastereoisomer

diastereoisomerism

diastereomer

Diastix

diastolic hypertension

diastrophic

diataxia
    cerebral d.
    d. cerebralis infantilis

diathesis
    d. of connective tissue
    gouty d.
    hemorrhagic d.

diathetic

diatom

diatomaceous earth

diauxic

diauxie

diaxon

diazacholesterol (DAC)

diazepam
    d. assay
    d. breath test

diazinon

diazo
    d. reaction
    d. reagent
    d. stain for argentaffin
      granules
    d. staining method

diazobenzenesulfonic acid

diazomethane generator

diazonal

diazone

diazonium salt

diazosulfobenzol

diazotize

dibasic
    d. acid
    d. potassium phosphate

debenzopyridine

diborane

dibothriocephaliasis

dibrachius
    monocephalus tetrapus d.
    monocephalus tripus d.

1,2-dibromethane

dibromide
    ethylene d.

dibucaine number (DN)

DIC
    diffuse intravascular
        coagulation
    disseminated intravascular
        coagulation

dicarbamylamine

dicarboxylic acid

dicarboxylicaciduria

dicentric

dicephalus
    d. dipus dibrachius
    d. dipus tetrabrachius
    d. dipus trirachius
    d. dipygus
    d. tripus tribrachius

dicheirus

dichlobenil

dichloride
    ethylene d.
    ethylidene d.

dichlorodiethyl sulfide

dichlorodiphenyl-
    trichloroethane

1,1-dichloroethane

1,2-dichloroethane

sym-dichloroethylene

2,6-dichlorophenol-indophenol

(2,4-dichlorophenoxy)acetic
    acid

dichloropropene-
    dichloropropene mixture

dichlorvos
    dimethyldichlorovinyl
        phosphate

dichorionic
    d. diamniotic placenta
    d. placenta twins

dichotomous variable

dichotomy

dichroic filter system

dichroism
    circular d.

dichromacy

dichromate
    potassium d.

dichromatic

dichromatism

dichromatopsia

dichromophil, dichromophile

dichromophilism

Dick
    D. method
    D. test
    D. test toxin

dicloxacillin

dicofol

dicrocoeliosis

dictyokinesis

dictyosome

dictyotene

didelphia

didelphic

didymalgia

didymitis

didymodynia

Diego antigen

dieldrin

dielectric
   d. constant
   d. strength

diet
   elimination d.

dietary protein

Dieterie
   D. method

dietetic albuminuria

diethylamide
   lysergic acid d. (LDS)

diethylamine

diethyldithiocarbamate

diethylenetriaminepentaacetic
   acid

diethylstilbestrol (DES)

diethyl sulfate

Difco EST testing system

difference
   alveolar-arterial carbon
      dioxide d.
   alveolar-arterial oxygen d.

difference (*continued*)
   arteriovenous carbon
      dioxide d.
   arteriovenous oxygen d.
   cation-anion d.
   electric potential d.
   d. limen (DL)
   mean of consecutive d.'s
      (MCD)
   no significant d. (NSD)

differential
   d. agglutination titer (DAT)
   d. diagnosis
   d. leukocyte count (DLC)
   d. leukocyte count
      automation
   d. renal function test
   d. thermometer
   d. ureteral catheterization
      test
   d. white blood count

differentiation
   amphicrine d.
   biphenotypic d.
   endothelial d.
   epithelial d.
   meissnerian d.
   mesenchymal d.
   myofibroblastic d.
   neuroendocrine d.
   rhabdomyoblastic d.

differentiator

Diff-Quik smear

diffraction
   x-ray d.

diffraction grating

diffuse
   d. acute inflammation
   d. acute peritonitis
   d. amyloidosis
   d. angiokeratoma
   d. arterial ectasia
   d. bronchopneumonia
   d. chronic inflammation

diffuse (*continued*)
    d. emphysema
    d. esophageal spasm
    d. ganglion
    d. glomerulonephritis
    d. goiter
    d. histocytic lymphoma
      (DHL)
    d. hyperplasia
    d. hypertrophy
    d. infantile familial sclerosis
    d. infiltrative lung disease
      (DILD)
    d. interstitial pneumonia
    d. interstitial pulmonary
      disease
    d. intravascular coagulation
      (DIC)
    d. lymphatic tissue
    d. meningiomatosis
    d. mesangial proliferation
    d. necrosis
    d. neuroendocrine system
    d. nontoxic goiter
    d. panbronchiolitis (DFB)
    d. peritonitis
    d. phlegmon
    d. poorly differentiated
      lymphoma (DPDL)
    d. pulmonary disease
    d. pyelonephritis
    d. reflection
    d. septal cirrhosis
    d. small cleaved cell
      lymphoma
    d. ulceration
    d. waxy spleen

diffusible

diffusing
    d. capacity for carbon
      monoxide

diffusion
    d. coefficent
    d. constant
    d. current
    facilitated d.

diffusion (*continued*)
    gel d.
    d. potential
    d. shell

diffusivity

Digenea

DiGeorge syndrome

digestion
    deoxyribonuclease d.
    lipolytic d.
    neuraminidase d.
    stalidase d.
    d. vacuole

digitonin

digitus
    d. hippocraticus
    d. malleus
    d. mortuus
    d. valgus
    d. varus

dihydrobiopterin synthetase
   deficiency

2,8-dihydroxyadenine

dihydroxyfluorane

dihysteria

dikaryote

dilaceration

dilatancy

dilatant

dilatation
    gastric d.
    d. of the heart
    idiopathic d.
    poststenotic d.
    prognathic d.
    prognathion d.
    d. of the stomach

DILD
    diffuse infiltrative lung
      disease

dilute blood clot lysis (method) (DBCL)

diluted whoel blood clot lysis

dilution
 doubling d.
 serial d.

dilution-filtration technique

DIM
 divalent ion metabolism

3,4-dimethoxyphenylethylamine

p-dimethylaminoazobenzene

dimethylbenzene

dimethyl ketone

dimethylnitrosamine

dimethyl-p-phenylenediamine

dimorphic
 d. anemia
 d. pathogenic fungi

dimorphous

dinitrate
 ethylene glycol d.

dinitrobenzene

dinitrochlorobenzene

dinitrogen tetroxide

dinitro-orthocresol

diphenylamino-azo-benzene

diphenyldiimide

diphtheria
 cutaneous d.
 faucial d.
 laryngeal d.
 laryngotracheal d.
 nasal d.
 pharyngeal d.

diphtherial

diphtheric

diphtheritic

diphtheroid

diphtherotoxin

diphyllobothriasis

dipicolinic acid

diplacusia

diplacusis
 binaural d.
 disharmonic d.
 echo d.
 monaural d.
 d. monauralis

diplegia
 atonic-astatic d.
 facial d.
 facial d., congenital
 Förster's d.
 infantile d.
 masticatory d.
 spastic d.

diploalbuminuria

dipobacterium

diploblastic

diplochromosome

diplococcemia

diplococcin

diplococcus
 Gram-negative intracellular
  diplococci (GNID)
 d. of Morax-Axenfeld
 d. of Neisser
 Weichselbaum d.

diploid

diploidy

diplomelituria

diplomyelia

diplont

diplopia
    binocular d.
    crossed d.
    direct d.
    heteronymous d.
    homonymous d.
    horizontal d.
    monocular d.
    paradoxical d.
    torsional d.
    uncrossed d.
    vertical d.

diplopod

diplosome

diplotene

dipolar

dipole moment

Diptera

dipsosis

dipygus
    d. parasiticus

dipylidiasis

direct
    d. agglunation (DA)
    d. antiglobulin test
    d. bilirubin
    d. centrifugal flotation
        (DCF)
    d. Coombs test
    d. fluorescent antibody
        (DFA)
    d. maternal death
    d. reacting bilirubin
    d. vision spectroscope

direct-reading potentiometer

dirofilariasis

disaccharidase deficiency

disaccharide
    d. tolerance test

disappearing bone disease

disarray
    lobular d.

discharge
    double d.
    epileptiform d.
    d. frequency
    urethral d.

discitis

discogenetic

discogenic

discopathy
    traumatic d.

discocyte

discoid lupus erythematous
    (DLE)

discoria

discontinuous
    d. sterilization

discordant lymphoma

discrete
    d. subaortic stenosis

discus
    d. oophorus
    d. ovigerus
    d. proligerus

discutient

disdiaclast

disdiadochokinesia

disease
    Acosta's d.
    Addison's d.
    adult celiac d.
    Akureyri d.
    Åland eye d.
    Albers-Schönberg d.
    Alexander's d.
    Alpers' d.
    alpha chain d.
    altitude d.
    Alzheimer's d.

disease (*continued*)
Anders' d.
Andersen's d.
Andes d.
anti-glomerular basement
    membrane antibody d.
apatite deposition d.
Apert-Crouzon d.
Aran-Duchenne d.
arc welder's d.
Armstrong's d.
arteriosclerotic
    cardiovascular d.
arteriosclerotic heart d.
atopic d.
Australian X d.
autoimmune d.
aviators' d.
Ayerza's d.
Azorean d.
Baastrup's d.
Baelz' d.
Baló's d.
Bamberger's d.
Bamberger-Marie d.
Bannister's d.
Banti's d.
Barcoo d.
Barlow's d.
Barraquer's d.
Basedow's d.
Batten d.
Batten-Mayou d.
bauxite workers' d.
Bayle's d.
Bazin's d.
Beck's d.
Béguez César d.
Behr's d.
Beigel's d.
Bekhterev's (Bechterew's) d.
Benson's d.
Berger's d.
Berlin's d.
Bernhardt's d.
Bernhardt-Roth d.
Besnier-Boeck d.
Best's d.

disease (*continued*)
Biedl's d.
Bielschowsky-Jansky d.
Bilderbeck's d.
Billroth's d.
Binswanger's d.
Blocq's d.
Blount d.
Boeck's d.
Bornholm d.
Bouchard's d.
Bouchet-Gsell d.
Bourneville's d.
Bradley's disease
Breisky's d.
Bright's d.
brittle bone d.
broad beta d.
Brodie's d.
bronzed d.
Brown-Symmers d.
Bruck's d.
Bruton's d.
Buerger's d.
Buhl's d.
Busquet's d.
Cacchi-Ricci d.
Caffey's disease
caisson disease
calcium hydroxyapatite
    deposition d.
calcium pyrophosphate
    deposition d.
caloric d.
Calvé-Perthes d.
Camurati-Engelmann d.
Canavan's d.
Canavan-van Bogaert-
    Bertrand d.
Caroli's d.
Carrión's d.
Castellani's d.
Castleman's d.
Cavare's d.
celiac d.
central core d.
Charcot's d.
Charcot-Marie-Tooth d.

disease (*continued*)
    cheese handler's d.
    cheese washer's d.
    Chester's d.
    Chiari-Frommel d.
    cholesteryl ester storage d.
    Christensen-Krabbe d.
    Christian's d.
    Christian-Weber d.
    Christmas d.
    chronic granulomatous d.
    chronic granulomatous d.
     of childhood
    chronic obstructive lung d.
    chronic obstructive
     pulmonary d.
    climatic d.
    Coats' d.
    collagen d.
    combined
     immunodeficiency d.
    combined system d.
    complicating d.
    compressed-air d.
    Concato's d.
    Conradi's d.
    constitutional d.
    Cooley's d.
    Corbus' d.
    Cori's d.
    cork handler's d.
    coronary artery d.
    coronary heart d.
    Corrigan's d.
    Corvisart's d.
    Cotugno's d.
    Cowden d.
    CPPD d.
    creeping d.
    Creutzfeldt-Jakob d.
    Creutzfeldt-Jakob d., new
     variant
    Crigler-Najjar d.
    Crohn's d.
    Crouzon's d.
    Cruveilhier's d.
    Cushing's d.
    cystic d. of breast

disease (*continued*)
    cystic d. of lung
    cystine d.
    cystine storage d.
    cytomegalic inclusion d.
    Czerny's d.
    Daae's d.
    Dalrymple's d.
    Darier's d.
    Darier-White d.
    David's d.
    deficiency d.
    degenerative joint d.
    Dejerine's d.
    Dejerine-Sottas d.
    demyelinating d.
    dense deposit d.
    Dent's d.
    deprivation d.
    de Quervain's d.
    Dercum's d.
    Deutschländer's d.
    Devic's d.
    disappearing bone d.
    diverticular d.
    Döhle d.
    Dubini's d.
    Dubois' d.
    Duchenne's d.
    Duchenne-Aran d.
    Duchenne-Griesinger d.
    Duhring's d.
    Dukes' d.
    Duncan's d.
    Durante's d.
    Duroziez's d.
    Eales d.
    Ebstein's d.
    Economo's d.
    Edsall's d.
    elevator d.
    end-stage renal d.
    Engelmann's d.
    Engel-Recklinghausen d.
    eosinophilic
     endomyocardial d.
    Epstein's d.
    Erb's d.

disease (*continued*)
   Erb-Charcot d.
   Erb-Goldflam d.
   Erdheim's d.
   Eulenburg's d.
   extrapyramidal d.
   Fabry's d.
   Fahr-Volhard d.
   Farber's d.
   fat-deficiency d.
   fatty liver d.
   Fazio-Londe d.
   Feer's d.
   Fenwick's d.
   fibrocystic d.
   fibrocystic d. of breast
   fibrocystic d. of the
      pancreas
   Filatov-Dukes d.
   fish eye d.
   Flajani's d.
   Flatau-Schilder d.
   flax-dresser's d.
   Flegel's d.
   Fleischner's d.
   flint d.
   floating beta d.
   focal d.
   Fölling d.
   foot process d.
   Forbes' d.
   Fordyce's d.
   Forestier d.
   Förster's d.
   Fournier's d.
   fourth d.
   fourth venereal d.
   Fox-Fordyce d.
   Freiberg's d.
   Friedländer's d.
   Friedreich's d.
   Frommel's d.
   functional d.
   Gaisböck's d.
   gamma chain d.
   Gamna's d.
   Gamstorp's d.
   Gandy-Nanta d.

disease (*continued*)
   Garré's d.
   gastroesophageal reflux d.
   Gaucher's d.
   Gee's d.
   Gee-Herter d.
   Gee-Herter-Heubner d.
   Gee-Thaysen d.
   genetic d.
   Gerhardt's d.
   Gerlier's d.
   Gibney's d.
   Gilbert's d.
   Gilles de la Tourette's d.
   Glanzmann's d.
   glycogen storage d.
   Goldflam's d.
   Goldflam-Erb d.
   Goldstein's d.
   Gorham's d.
   graft-versus-host d.
   grass d.
   Graves' d.
   Greenfield's d.
   grinder's d.
   Gross d.
   Guinon's d.
   Gull's d.
   Günther's d.
   GVH d.
   H d.
   Habermann's d.
   Haglund's d.
   Hagner's d.
   Hailey-Hailey d.
   Hallervorden-Spatz d.
   Haltia-Santavuori d.
   Hamman's d.
   Hammond's d.
   Hand's d.
   hand-foot-and-mouth d.
   Hand-Schüller-Christian d.
   Hansen's d.
   d. of the Hapsburgs
   Harada's d.
   hard metal d.
   Hartnup d.
   Hashimoto's d.

disease (*continued*)

heart d.
heavy chain d.
Heberden's d.
Hebra's d.
Heckathorn's d.
Heerfordt's d.
Heine-Medin d.
Heller-Döhle d.
hemoglobin d.
hemoglobin C d.
hemoglobin C-thalassemia d.
hemoglobin D d.
hemoglobin E d.
hemoglobin E-thalassemia d.
hemoglobin H d.
hemoglobin SC d.
hemoglobin SD d.
hemolytic d. of the newborn
hemorrhagic d. of the newborn
Henderson-Jones d.
hepatic veno-occlusive d.
hepatolenticular d.
hepatorenal glycogen storage d.
hereditary d.
heredodegenerative d.
Herlitz' d.
Hers' d.
Herter's d.
Herter-Heubner d.
Heubner's d.
Heubner-Herter d.
hip-joint d.
Hippel's d.
Hippel-Lindau d.
Hirschsprung's d.
Hodgson's d.
Hoffa's d.
Horton's d.
Huchard's d.
hunger d.
hungry d.
Hunt's d.
Huntington's d.
Hurler's d.

disease (*continued*)

Hurst d.
Hutchinson's d.
Hutinel's d.
hyaline membrane d.
hydrocephaloid d.
hypophosphatemic bone d.
hypopigmentation-immunodeficiency d.
Iceland d.
I-cell d.
idiopathic d.
immune complex d.
immunoproliferative small intestine d.
inborn lysosomal d.
inclusion d.
infantile celiac d.
inflammatory bowel d.
inherited d.
intercurrent d.
interstitial d.
interstitial lung d.
iron storage d.
ischemic bowel d.
ischemic heart d.
Jaffe-Lichtenstein d.
Jakob's d.
Jakob-Creutzfeldt d.
Jansen's d.
Jansky-Bielschowsky d.
Jensen's d.
Johnson-Stevens d.
Joseph d.
jumping d.
Kashin-Bek (Kaschin-Beck) d.
Kawasaki d.
Keshan d.
Kienböck's d.
Kikuchi's d.
Kikuchi-Fujimoto d.
kinky hair d.
Kinnier Wilson d.
Klebs' d.
knight's d.
Köhler's bone d.
Köhler's second d.

disease (*continued*)

Köhler-Pellegrini-Stieda d.
Koshevnikoff's
   (Koschewnikow's,
   Kozhevnikov's) d.
Krabbe's d.
Kufs' d.
Kuhnt-Junius d.
Kümmell's d.
Kümmell-Verneuil d.
Kussmaul's d.
Kussmaul-Maier d.
Kyrle's d.
Laënnec's d.
Lafora's d.
Landing d.
Lane's d.
Larsen's d.
Larsen-Johansson d.
Lauber's d.
laughing d.
Leber's d.
Legg's d.
Legg-Calvé d.
Legg-Calvé-Perthes d.
Legg-Calvé-Waldenström d.
legionnaires' d.
Leigh d.
Leiner's d.
Lenègre's d.
Leriche's d.
Letterer-Siwe d.
Lev's d.
Leyden's d.
Libman-Sacks d.
Lichtheim's d.
Lindau's d.
Lindau-von Hippel d.
lipid storage d.
Lipschütz's d.
Little's d.
Lobstein's d.
local d.
Lorain's d.
Lou Gehrig d.
Lowe's d.
L-S d.
Luft's d.

disease (*continued*)

lung fluke d.
Lyell's d.
lymphoproliferative d.
lymphoreticular d.
lysosomal storage d.
McArdle's d.
Machado-Joseph d.
MacLean-Maxwell d.
Madelung's d.
Majocchi's d.
Malassez's d.
Malibu d.
maple bark d.
maple bark stripper's d.
maple syrup urine d.
marble bone d.
Marchiafava-Bignami d.
margarine d.
Marie-Bamberger d.
Marie-Strümpell d.
Marie-Tooth d.
Marion's d.
Marsh's d.
Medin's d.
Mediterranean d.
medullary cystic d.
medullary cystic kidney d.
Meige's d.
Meleda d.
Ménétrier's d.
Meniere's d.
Merzbacher-Pelizaeus d.
metabolic d.
Meyer's d.
Meyer-Betz d.
microdrepanocytic d.
Mikulicz's d.
Miller's d.
Milroy's d.
Milton's d.
minimal change d.
Minor's d.
Mitchell's d.
mixed connective tissue d.
Möbius' d.
Moeller-Barlow d.
molecular d.

disease (*continued*)
    Mondor's d.
    Monge's d.
    monoclonal
        immunoglobulin
        deposition d.
    Morquio's d.
    Morquio-Ullrich d.
    Morton's d.
    Moschcowitz's d.
    motor neuron d.
    motor system d.
    mountain d.
    moyamoya d.
    Mozer's d.
    Mucha's d.
    Mucha-Habermann d.
    mu chain d.
    Münchmeyer's d.
    Murray Valley d.
    mushroom picker's d.
    mushroom worker's d.
    myeloproliferative d.
    Niemann's disease
    Niemann-Pick d.
    nil d.
    Nonne-Milroy d.
    Norrie's d.
    Norum-Gjone d.
    oasthouse urine d.
    obstructive small airways d.
    occupational d.
    Oguchi's d.
    oid-oid d.
    Opitz' d.
    Ormond's d.
    Osgood-Schlatter d.
    Osler's d.
    Osler-Vaquez d.
    Osler-Weber-Rendu
        disease
    Otto's d.
    Owren's d.
    ox-warble d.
    Paas's d.
    Paget's d.
    Paget d., juvenile
    Paget's d. of bone

disease (*continued*)
    Panner's d.
    parenchymatous d.
    Parkinson's d.
    Parrot's d.
    parrot d.
    Parry's d.
    Patella's d.
    Payr's d.
    Pel-Ebstein d.
    Pelizaeus-Merzbacher d.
    Pellegrini's d.
    Pellegrini-Stieda d.
    pelvic inflammatory d.
    periodic d.
    Perrin-Ferraton d.
    Perthes' d.
    Peyronie's d.
    phytanic acid storage d.
    Pick's d.
    pink d.
    plaster-of-Paris d.
    Plummer's d.
    pneumatic hammer d.
    policeman's d.
    polycystic kidney d.
    polycystic d. of kidneys
    polycystic liver d.
    polycystic ovary d.
    polycystic renal d.
    polyendocrine autoimmune
        d.
    polyglandular autoimmune
        d.
    Pompe's d.
    Poncet's d.
    Portuguese-Azorean d.
    Pott's d.
    Preiser's d.
    primary electrical d.
    Pringle's d.
    prion d.
    pulmonary veno-occlusive
        d.
    pulseless d.
    Purtscher's d.
    Pyle's d.
    Quervain's d.

disease (*continued*)

Quincke's d.
Raynaud's d.
Recklinghausen's d.
Recklinghausen-
    Applebaum d.
Recklinghausen's d. of
    bone
Refsum's d.
remnant removal d.
respiratory bronchiolitis-
    associated interstitial lung
    d.
restrictive lung d.
rheumatoid d.
Rh hemolytic d.
rice d.
Riedel's d.
Riga-Fede d.
Ritter's d.
Roger's d.
Romberg's d.
Rosai-Dorfman d.
Rossbach's d.
Roth's (Rot's) d.
Roth-Bernhardt (Rot-
    Bernhardt) d.
Rougnon-Heberden d.
Rust's d.
Ruysch's d.
saccharine d.
Sachs' d.
sacroiliac d.
salivary gland d.
Salla d.
Sanders' d.
Sandhoff's d.
sandworm d.
Santavuori d.
Santavuori-Haltia d.
Saunders' d.
Schamberg's d.
Schanz's d.
Schaumann's d.
Scheuermann's d.
Schilder's d.
Schimmelbusch's d.
Schlatter's d.

disease (*continued*)

Schlatter-Osgood d.
Schmorl's d.
Scholz' d.
Schönlein's d.
Schroeder's d.
Schüller's d.
Schüller-Christian d.
Schwediauer's d.
Seitelberger's d.
self-limited d.
Selter's d.
septic d.
serum d.
Sever's d.
severe combined
    immunodeficiency d.
Shaver's d.
sickle cell d.
sickle cell-hemoglobin C d.
sickle cell-hemoglobin D d.
sickle cell-thalassemia d.
silo filler's d.
Simmonds' d.
Simons' d.
Sinding-Larsen d.
Sinding-Larsen-Johansson d.
sixth d.
small airways d.
Smith-Strang d.
Sneddon-Wilkinson d.
specific d.
specific heart muscle d.
Spencer's d.
Spielmeyer-Vogt d.
Stargardt's d.
startle d.
Steinert's d.
Stieda's d.
Still's d.
stone d.
storage d.
storage pool d.
structural disease
Strümpell's d.
Strümpell-Leichtenstern d.
Strümpell-Marie d.
Sudeck's d.

disease (*continued*)

Sutton's d.
Swediaur's (Schwediauer's) d.
Swift's d.
Swift-Feer d.
swineherd's d.
Sylvest's d.
systemic d.
Takahara's d.
Takayasu's d.
Talma's d.
Tangier d.
Tarui's d.
Tay's d.
Tay-Sachs d.
thalassemia-sickle cell d.
Thaysen d.
Thiemann d.
Thomsen d.
Thomson d.
Thornwaldt d.
thyrocardiac d.
thyrotoxic heart d.
Tietze d.
Tillaux d.
Tooth d.
Tornwaldt (Thornwaldt) d.
transmissible neurodegenerative d.
Trevor d.
tuberculosis-respiratory d.
tubotympanic d.
tungsten carbide d.
Tyzzer d.
Underwood d.
Unna-Thost d.
Unverricht d.
Univerricht-Lundborg d.
Urbach-Wiethe d.
uremic bone d.
vagabonds' d.
vagrants' d.
van Buren d.
van den Bergh d.
Vaquez d.
Vaquez-Osler d.
veno-occlusive d. of the liver

disease (*continued*)

Verneuil d.
Verse d.
vibration d.
Vogt-Spielmeyer d.
Volkmann d.
Voltolini d.
von Economo d.
von Gierke d.
von Hippel-Lindau d.
von Recklinghausen d.
von Willebrand d.
Vrolik d.
Waldenström d.
Wartenberg d.
wasting d.
Weber d.
Weber-Christian d.
Weber-Rendu-Osler d.
Wegner d.
Weir Mitchell d.
Werdnig-Hoffmann d.
Werlhof d.
Werner Schultz d.
Wernicke d.
Weston Hurst d.
Westphal-Strümpell d.
wheat weevil d.
Whipple d.
white spot d.
Whytt d.
Wilson d.
Winckel d.
Winiwarter-Buerger d.
Winkler d.
Witkop d.
Witkop-Von Sallmann d.
Wolman d.
woolsorter d.
X-linked lymphoproliferative d.
Zahorsky d.
Ziehen-Oppenheim d.

disequilibrium

disesthesia

disgerminoma

disintegration constant

disjunction
    craniofacial d.

disjunctive absorption

disk
    Amici's d.
    anangioid d.
    anisotropic d.
    anisotropous d.
    Bowman's d.
    choked d.
    contained d.
    cupped d.
    Engelmann's d.
    extruded d.
    Hensen's d.
    herniated d.
    intercalated d.
    intermediate d.
    isotropic d.
    Merkel's d.
    micrometer d.
    noncontained d.
    protruded d.
    Ranvier's tactile d.
    ruptured d.
    sequestered d.
    tactile d.
    thin d.
    transverse d.

dislocatio
    d. erecta

dislocation
    Bell-Dally d.
    complete d.
    complicated d.
    compound d.
    congenital d.
    congenital d. of the hip
    consecutive d.
    divergent d.
    fracture d.
    habitual d.
    incomplete d.
    intrauterine d.
    Kienböck's d.

dislocation (*continued*)
    d. of the lens
    Lisfranc's d.
    Monteggia's d.
    Nélaton's d.
    partial d.
    pathologic d.
    primitive d.
    recent d.
    simple d.
    Smith's d.
    subastragalar d.
    subcoracoid d.
    subglenoid d.
    subspinous d.
    traumatic d.

disomy
    uniparental d.

disorder
    breathing-related sleep d.
    collagen d.
    d. of consciousness
    developmental d.
    factitious d. by proxy
    functional d.
    genetic d.
    LDL-receptor d.
    lymphoproliferative d.
    lymphoreticular d.
    mendelian d.
    monogenic d.
    multifactorial d.
    myeloproliferative d.
    phagocytic dysfunction d.
    plasma cell d.
    postconcussional d.
    rapid eye movement sleep
        behavior d.
    REM sleep behavior d.
    single-gene d.
    sleep d. d.

disordered action of the heart
    (DAH)

dispermic chimera

disperse phase

dispersion
    collodial d.
    molecular d.
    optical rotary d. (ORD)

dispersive medium

dispira

dispireme

displacement
    fish-hook d.
    gallbladder d.
    tissue d.

disproportion
    cephalopelvic d.

dissecting aneurysm

disseminata
    dermatofibrosis lenticularis
        d.

disseminate coccidiodomycosis

disseminated
    d. acute lupus
        erythematosus
    d. asperigillosis
    d. lipogranulomatosis
    d. superficial actinic
        porokeratosis (DSAP)

disseminatum
    xanthoma d. (XD)

disseminatus
    lupus erythemaosus d.
        (LED)

dissociation
    albuminocytologic d.
    atrial d.
    atrioventricular (AV) d.
    electromechanical d.
    interference atrioventricular
        d.
    isorhythmic atrioventricular
        d.
    syringomyelic d.
    tabetic d.

distance
    interelectrode d.
    skin to tumor d.
    working d.

distention, distension

distichia

distichiasis

distillation
    destructive d.
    fractional d.
    molecular d.

distome

distomiasis
    pulmonary d.

distress
    idiopathic respiratory d. of
        newborn

distribution
    anomalous vascular d.
    cumulative d.
    probability d.

districhiasis

distrix

disulfide
    dihydroxydinaphthyl d.
        (DDD)

disulfiram assay

DIT
    diiodotyrosine
    drug-induced
        thrombocytopenia

dithionite test

dithiothreitol

Dittrich
    D. plug
    D. stenosis

diuria

divarication

divergence
    negative vertical d.
    positive vertical d.

diverticula

diverticular

diverticularization

diverticulitis

diverticulosis

diverticulum
    acquired d.
    caliceal d.
    calyceal d.
    cervical d.
    d. of colon
    colonic d.
    false d.
    ganglion d.
    Ganser's d.
    giant d.
    Graser's d.
    d. ilei verum
    intestinal d.
    Kirchner's d.
    laryngeal d.
    Meckel's d.
    Pertik's d.
    pharyngoesophageal d.
    pressure d.
    pulsion d.
    Rokitansky's d.
    supradiaphragmatic d.
    synovial d.
    d. of trachea
    tracheal d.
    traction d.
    vesical d.
    Zenker's d.

divicine

division
    cell d.
    cell d., direct
    cell d., indirect
    equational d.
    maturation d.
    reduction d.

DJD
    degenerative joint disease

DK
    diseased kidney

DL
    difference limen
    Donath-Landsteiner

D-L Ab
    Donath-Landsteiner
      antibody

DLC
    differential leukocyte count

DLE
    discoid lupus
      erythematosus
    disseminated lup
      erythematosus

DMD
    Duchenne muscular
      dystrophy

DN
    dextrose-nitrogen ratio
    dibucaine number

DNA
    deoxyribonucleic acid
      DNA aneuploidy
      DNA complexity
      DNA flow cytometry
      DNA homology
      DNA
        nucleotidylexotransfe
        rase
      ribosomal DNA (rDNA)

DNAase

DNA-DNA hybridization

DNA-RNA hybridization

DNCB
    dinitrochlorobenzene

DNOC
    dinitro-orthocresol

DNP
    deoxyribonucleoprotein

DOC
   deoxycorticosterone

DOCA
   deoxycorticosterone
      acetate

docimasia
   auricular d.
   hepatic d.
   pulmonary d.

DOCS
   deoxycorticoids

Döderlein bacillus

Döhle
   D. disease
   D. inclusion

Döhle-Heller aortitis

doigt
   d. mort

dolichocolon

dolichostenomelia

dolor
   d. capitis
   d. coxae

dolorific

dolorogenic

DOMA
   dihydroxymandelic acid

domiciliated

Donnan potential

Donohue syndrome

DOPA
   dihydroxyphenylalamine
      DOPA test

Doriden

Dorner stain

dorsalgia

dorsodynia

dosimeter

dosimetry

dot
   Maurer d.
   Mittendorf d.
   Schüffner d.
   Trantas d.

double
   d. antibody sandwich assay
   d. (gel) diffusion preciptin
      test in one dimension
   d. (gel) diffusion preciptin
      test in two dimensions

double masked experiment

double-precision variable

doublet
   Wollaston d.

douglascele

douglasitis

doxepin
   d. hydrochloride assay

DPN
   diphosphopyridine
      nucleotide

Drabkin reagent

dracontiasis

dracunculiasis

dracunculosis

Dragendorff
   D. solution
   D. test

drepanocyte

drepanocytic

drepanocytosis

drop
   enamel d.
   foot d.
   d. phalangette

drop (*continued*)
    wrist d.

dropsical

dropsy
    abdominal d.
    d. of amnion
    articular d.
    d. of belly
    d. of chest
    cutaneous d.
    peritoneal d.
    salpingian d.
    wet d.

drug
    d. abuse screen
    d. screening assay

drusen

DTM
    dermatophyte test medium

DTN
    diphtheria toxin normal

Ducrey
    D. bacillus
    D. test

duct
    Bellini's d.
    collecting d.
    collecting d., cortical
    collecting d., medullary
    müllerian d., persistent
    papillary d.
    Rokitansky-Aschoff d.
    sudoriferous d.
    sweat d.

ductopenia

ductus
    d. papillaris
    patent d. arteriosus

dumbbell
    d. ganglioneuroma
    d. of Schäfer

Dunnet multiple component test

duodenitis

duodenocholangeitis

Duran-Reynals permeability
    factor

duroarachnitis

DVT

dwarf
    achondroplastic d.
    Amsterdam d.
    asexual d.
    ateliotic d.
    bird-headed d.
    Brissaud's d.
    cretin d.
    diastrophic d.
    geleophysic d.
    hypophysial d.
    hypothyroid d.
    infantile d.
    Laron d.
    Lévi-Lorain d.
    Lorain-Lévi d.
    micromelic d.
    nanocephalic d.
    normal d.
    phocomelic d.
    physiologic d.
    pituitary d.
    primordial d.
    pure d.
    rachitic d.
    renal d.
    rhizomelic d.
    Russell d.
    Seckel's bird-headed d.
    sexual d.
    Silver d.
    true d.

dwarfism
    bird-headed d.
    camptomelic d.
    hypophysial d.
    Laron d.
    Lévi-Lorain d.
    Lorain-Lévi d.

dwarfism (*continued*)
    pituitary d.
    renal d.
    Robinow d.
    Russell d.
    Russell-Silver d.
    Silver-Russell d.
    Seckel d.
    symptomatic d.
    Walt Disney d.

DXM
    dexamethasone

dyad

dyaster

dye
    acid d.
    acidic d.
    amphoteric d.
    anionic d.
    azo d.
    basic d.
    cationic d.
    metachromatic d.
    orthochromatic d.
    vital d.

dyed starch method

dynamopathic

dynein

dysacousia

dysacousis

dysacousma

dysacusis

dysadaptation

dysadrenalism

dysallilognathia

dysanagnosia

dysantigraphia

dysaphia

dysaptation

dysarteriotony

dysarthria
    ataxic d.

dysarthric

dysarthrosis

dysautonomia
    familial d.

dysbarism

dysbasia
    d. lordotica progressiva

dysbetalipoproteinemia
    familial d.

dysbolism

dyscalculia

dyscephaly
    mandibulo-oculofacial d.

dyschesia

dyschezia

dyschiasia

dyschiria

dyscholia

dyschondrosteosis

dyschromasia

dyschromatopsia

dyschromia

dyschylia

dyscinesia

dyscoria

dyscorticism

dyscrasia
    blood d.
    plasma cell d.

dyscrasic

dyscratic

dysdiadochocinesia

dysdiadochokinesia

dysdiadochokinetic

dysdipsia

dysecoia

dysencephalia splanchnocystica

dysenteric

dysenteriform

dysentery
    amebic d.
    bacillary d.
    balantidial d.
    bilharzial d.
    catarrhal d.
    ciliary d.
    ciliate d.
    epidemic d.
    flagellate d.
    Flexner's d.
    fulminant d.
    institutional d.
    Japanese d.
    malarial d.
    malignant d.
    protozoal d.
    schistosomal d.
    scorbutic d.
    Sonne d.
    spirillar d.
    sporadic d.
    viral d.

dysequilibrium
    dialysis d.

dysergia

dyserythropoiesis

dysesthesia
    auditory d.

dysesthetic

dysfibrinogenemia

dysfunction
    constitutional hepatic d.
    erectile d.
    familial autonomic d.
    myofascial pain d.
    d. of uterus

dysgalactia

dysgammaglobulinemia
    hyper-IgM d.

dysgenesis
    epiphyseal d.
    gonadal d.
    gonadal d., mixed
    gonadal d., pure
    gonadal d., 46,XY
    reticular d.
    seminiferous tubule d.

dysgenitalism

dysgeusia

dysglobulinemia

dysglycemia

dysgnathia

dysgnathic

dysgonesis

dysgrammatism

dysgraphia

dyshematopoiesis

dyshematopoietic

dyshemopoiesis

dyshemopoietic

dyshepatia
    lipogenic d.

dyshesion

dyshidrosis

dyshydrosis

dysidrosis

dyskaryosis

dyskaryotic

dyskeratosis
 d. congenita
 congenital d.
 hereditary benign
  intraepithelial d.

dyskeratotic

dyskinesia
 biliary d.
 d. intermittens
 orofacial d.
 primary ciliary d.
 tardive d.
 withdrawal-emergent d.

dyskinetic

dyslipidemia
 familial combined d.
 mixed d.

dyslipidosis

dyslipoidosis

dyslipoproteinemia

dyslochia

dysmature

dysmaturity
 pulmonary d.

dysmegalopsia

dysmenorrhea
 acquired d.
 congestive d.
 essential d.
 inflammatory d.
 d. intermenstrualis
 mechanical d.
 membranous d.
 obstructive d.
 ovarian d.
 primary d.
 secondary d.
 spasmodic d.
 tubal d.
 uterine d.

dysmetria
 ocular d.

dysmetropsia

dysmnesia

dysmnesic

dysmorphic

dysmorphism

dysmorphopsia

dysmorphosis

dysmyelination

dysmyelopoiesis

dysmyotonia

dysnomia

dysodontiasis

dysopia
 d. algera

dysopsia

dysorexia

dysosmia

dysosteogenesis

dysostosis
 cleidocranial d.
 craniofacial d.
 d. enchondralis epiphysaria
 mandibulofacial d.
 mandibulofacial d. with
  epibulbar dermoids
 metaphyseal d.
 d. multiplex
 Nager's acrofacial d.
 orodigitofacial d.
 postaxial acrofacial d.

dyspareunia

dyspepsia
 acid d.
 appendicular d.
 appendix d.
 catarrhal d.

dyspepsia (*continued*)
    cholelithic d.
    colon d.
    fermentative d.
    flatulent d.
    gastric d.
    intestinal d.
    nonulcer d.

dyspeptic

dysperistalsis

dysphagia
    contractile ring d.
    esophageal d.
    d. inflammatoria
    d. lusoria
    d. nervosa
    oropharyngeal d.
    dysphagia d.
    sideropenic d.
    d. spastica
    vallecular d.

dysphagy

dysphasia

dysphonia
    d. clericorum
    dysplastic d.
    d. plicae ventricularis
    d. puberum
    spasmodic d.
    spastic d.
    d. spastica

dysphrasia

dyspigmentation

dysplasia
    anhidrotic ectodermal d.
    arrhythmogenic right
      ventricular d.
    arteriohepatic d.
    bronchopulmonary d.
    chondroectodermal d.
    cleidocranial d.
    cortical d.

dysplasia (*continued*)
    craniocarpotarsal d.
    craniodiaphyseal d.
    craniometaphyseal d.
    cretinoid d.
    cystic renal d.
    dentinal d.
    developmental d.
      of the hip
    diaphyseal d.
    ectodermal d.
    encephalo-ophthalmic d.
    epiphyseal d.
    d. epiphysealis hemimelica
    d. epiphysealis multiplex
    d. epiphysealis punctata
    faciogenital d.
    familial white folded
      mucosal d.
    fibromuscular d.
    fibrous d., monostotic
    fibrous d., polyostotic
    fibrous d. of bone
    fibrous d. of jaw
    florid osseous d.
    frontonasal d.
    hereditary bone d.
    hidrotic ectodermal d.
    hypohidrotic ectodermal d.
    d. linguofacialis
    metaphyseal d.
    multicystic renal d.
    multiple epiphyseal d.
    neuronal colonic d.
    neuronal intestinal d.
    oculoauricular d.
    oculoauriculovertebral
      (OAV) d.
    oculodentodigital (ODD) d.
    oculodento-osseous d.
    ophthalmomandibulomelic
      d.
    periapical cemental d.
    primary adrenocortical
      nodular d.
    progressive diaphyseal d.

diaphyseal d. (*continued*)
    renal d.
    renal-retinal d.
    retinal d.
    septo-optic d.
    spondyloepiphyseal d.
    spondylothoracic d.
    Streeter's d.
    thymic d.
    ureteral neuromuscular d.

dysplastic

dyspnea
    cardiac d.
    exertional d.
    expiratory d.
    inspiratory d.
    nocturnal d.
    nonexpansional d.
    orthostatic d.
    paroxysmal nocturnal d.
    renal d.

dyspneic

dyspoiesis

dysponderal

dysponesis

dyspragia
    d. intermittens
      angiosclerotica intestinalis

dyspraxia

dysproteinemia

dysraphia

dysraphism

dysreflexia
    autonomic d.

dysrhaphism

dysrhythmia
    esophageal d.

dyssebacea

dyssebacia

dyssomnia

dysspermia

dysstasia

dysstatic

dyssymbolia

dyssymboly

dyssynergia
    biliary d.
    d. cerebellaris myoclonica
    d. cerebellaris progressiva
    detrusor-external sphincter
      d.
    detrusor-sphincter d.
    detrusor-striated sphincter
      d.
    vesico-sphincter d.

dystasia
    hereditary areflexic d.
    Roussy-Lévy hereditary
      areflexic d.

dystaxia

dysthyreosis

dysthyroid

dysthyroidal

dysthyroidism

dystithia

dystocia
    cervical d.
    constriction ring d.
    contraction ring d.
    fetal d.
    maternal d.
    placental d.

dystonia
    d. deformans progressiva
    d. lenticularis
    d. musculorum deformans
    oromandibular d.
    tardive d.
    torsion d.

dystrophia
- d. adiposa corneae
- d. adiposogenitalis
- d. brevicollis
- d. endothelialis corneae
- d. epithelialis corneae
- d. mediana canaliformis
- d. mesodermalis congenita hyperplastica
- d. myotonica
- d. unguis mediana canaliformis
- d. unguium

dystrophin

dystrophoneurosis

dystrophy
- adiposogenital d.
- Albright's d.
- asphyxiating thoracic d.
- Becker's muscular d.
- Becker type muscular d.
- Best's macular d.
- Biber-Haab-Dimmer d.
- corneal d.
- craniocarpotarsal d.
- Dejerine-Landouzy d.
- distal muscular d.
- Duchenne's d.
- Duchenne's muscular d.
- Duchenne type muscular d.
- Duchenne-Landouzy d.
- Emery-Dreifuss muscular d.
- Erb's d.
- Erb's muscular d.
- facioscapulohumeral muscular d.
- familial osseous d.
- Fuchs' d.
- Fukuyama type congenital muscular d.
- Gowers' muscular d.
- agranular corneal d.
- Groenouw's type I corneal d.
- Groenouw's type II corneal d.

dystrophy (*continued*)
- hereditary vitelliform d.
- infantile neuroaxonal d.
- Landouzy d.
- Landouzy-Dejerine d.
- Landouzy-Dejerine muscular d.
- lattice d. (of cornea)
- Leyden-Möbius muscular d.
- limb-girdle muscular d.
- macular corneal d.
- muscular d.
- amyotonic d.
- neuraxonal d.
- neuroaxonal d.
- oculocerebrorenal d.
- oculopharyngeal d.
- oculopharyngeal muscular d.
- pelvifemoral muscular d.
- progressive muscular d.
- progressive tapetochoroidal d.
- pseudohypertrophic muscular d.
- reflex sympathetic d.
- Salzmann's nodular corneal d.
- scapulohumeral muscular d.
- scapuloperoneal muscular d.
- Simmerlin's d.
- tapetochoroidal d.
- thoracic-pelvic-phalangeal d.
- wound d.

dystrypsia

dysuresia

dysuria

dysuriac

dysuric

dysvascular

dyszoospermia

E

Eadie-Hofstee equation

EAE
    experimental allergic
        encephalomyelitis

ear
    aviator's e.
    Aztec e.
    bat e.
    beach e.
    Blainville e.
    Cagot e.
    cat's e.
    cauliflower e.
    cup e.
    Darwin's e.
    diabetic e.
    glue e.
    hairy e.
    Hong Kong e.
    hot weather e.
    lop e.
    Morel e.
    Mozart e.
    prizefighter e.
    satyr e.
    scroll e.
    Singapore e.
    swimmer's e.
    tank e.
    tropical e.
    Wildermuth's e.

EBER1 riboprobe

EBNA
    Epstein-Barr nuclear
        antigen

eburnation
    e. of dentin

eburnitis

EC
    enterochromaffin-cell
        hyperplasia

ECBV
    effective circulating blood
        volume

eccentrochondroplasia

eccentro-osteochondrodysplasia

ecchymoma

ecchymosed

ecchymoses

ecchymosis
    cadaveric e.

ecchymotic

eccyesis

ECFV
    extracellular fluid
        volume

echinocyte

echinophthalmia

echinosis

echo
    amphoric e.

echoacousia

echographia

echophony

ECIS
    endometrial carcinoma in
        situ

ECL
    emitter-coupled logic
    enterochromaffin-like

eclampsia
    puerperal e.
    uremic e.

eclamptic

eclamptogenic

ECLT
    euglobulin clot lysis time

ecsomatics

ecstrophy

ECT
    ectomesenchymal
        chondromyoxid tumor
    euglobulin clot test

ectacolia

ectasia
    alveolar e.
    annuloaortic e.
    corneal e.
    diffuse arterial e.
    hypostatic e.
    mammary duct e.
    papillary e.
    scleral e.
    tubular e.

ectasis

ectatic

ecthyma
    contagious e.
    e. gangrenosum

ecthymiform

ectobiology

ectoblast

ectocervical smear

ectocolon

ectocytic

ectodermosis
    e. erosiva pluriorificialis

ectolysis

ectomesenchyme

ectonuclear

ectoperitonitis

ectopia
    e. cloacae

ectopia (*continued*)
    crossed renal e.
    e. lentis
    e. pupillae congenita
    renal e.
    e. renis
    e. testis
    e. vesicae

ectoplasm

ectoplasmatic

ectoplast

ectoplastic

ectosphere

ectotoxin

ectropion
    atonic e.
    cervical e.
    cicatricial e.
    flaccid e.
    e. luxurians
    aparalytic e.
    e. of pigment layer
    e. sarcomatosum
    senile e.
    aspastic e.
    e. uveae

ectropionize

ectropium

ECV
    extracellular volume

ECW
    extracellular water

eczema
    allergic e.
    asteatotic e.
    atopic e.
    e. craquelé
    dyshidrotic e.
    flexural e.
    e. herpeticum
    infantile e.
    e. intertrigo

eczema (*continued*)
    e. marginatum
    nummular e.
    seborrheic e.
    e. vaccinatum
    xerotic e.

eczematization

eczematogenic

eczematoid

eczematous

edema
    alimentary e.
    alveolar e.
    angioneurotic e.
    Berlin's e.
    brain e.
    brown e.
    e. bullosum vesicae
    e. calidum
    acardiac e.
    acerebral e.
    circumscribed e.
    cytotoxic e.
    dependent e.
    famine e.
    e. frigidum
    e. fugax
    gaseous e.
    giant e.
    hepatic e.
    hereditary angioneurotic e.
    hunger e.
    hydremic e.
    idiopathic e.
    inflammatory e.
    interstitial e.
    invisible e.
    e. of lung
    lymphatic e.
    Milroy's e.
    Milton's e.
    mucous e.
    e. neonatorum
    nephrotic e.
    noninflammatory e.
    nonpitting e.

    nutritional e.
    passive e.
    aperiodic e.
    periretinal e.
    pitting e.
    aplacental e.
    prehepatic e.
    pulmonary e.
    pulmonary e., high-altitude
    pulmonary e., paroxysmal
    pulmonary e., re-expansion
    pulmonary e., solid
    purulent e.
    Quincke's e.
    Reinke's e.
    renal e.
    rheumatismal e.
    salt e.
    solid e.
    terminal e.
    vasogenic e.
    venous e.
    villous e.
    war e.
    cystoid macular e.

edamine

edematigenous

edematization

edematogenic

edematous

EDRF
    endothelium-derived
      relaxing factor

edrophonium
    e. chloride test

EDTA
    ethylenediaminetetraacetic
      acid

EDTA-dependent
  pseudothrombocytopenia

EEE
    eastern equine
      encephalomyelitis
        EEE virus

EF
    ectopic focus
    encephalitogenic factor

effect
    clasp-knife e.
    isomorphic e.
    Mierzejewski e.
    pressure e.
    Somogyi e.
    Staub-Traugott e.

effemination

efflorescence

effluvium
    anagen e.
    telogen e.

affrication

effusion
    chyliform e.
    achylous e.
    hemorrhagic e.
    parapneumonic e.
    pericardial e.
    pleural e.
    pseudochylous e.
    tuberculous e.
    tuberculous pleural e.

EFV
    extracellular fluid volume

egagropilus

EGC
    endocrine granule
      constituent

EGFR
    epidermal growth factor
      receptor

egilops

egobronchophony

egophony

EI
    enzyme inhibitor
    eosinophilic index

Eichhorst corpuscle

Einthoven law

Eisenlohr syndrome

eisanthema

ekiri

elacin

elaioma

elaioplast

E-LAM
    endothelial-leukocyte
      adhesion molecule

elastica-van Giesen stain

elastoidosis
    nodular e.

elastolysis
    generalized e.
    perifollicular e.
    postinflammatory e.

elastolytic

elastoma
    juvenile e.

elastopathy

elastorrhexis

elastosis
    actinic e.
    nodular e. of Favre and
      Racouchot
    e. perforans serpiginosa
    perforating e.
    senile e.
    Isolar e.

elastotic

Elavil

elcosis

electrochromatography

electrofocusing

electrogenic

electron-dense

electron-microscopic

electron-microscopical

electronograph

electropathology

electropherogram

electrophoregram

electrophoresis
    agarose gel e.
    cellulose acetate e.
    disc e.
    gel e.
    moving boundary e.
    paper e.
    polyacrylamide gel e.
    pulsed-field e.
    SDS-polyacrylamide gel e.
    starch gel e.
    two-dimensional gel e.
    ozone e.

electrophoretic

electrophoretogram

electrophotometer

electrosalivogram

electrothanasia

Elek test

eleoma

eleoplast

elephantiasis
    congenital e.
    e. oculi

ELISA
    enzyme-linked
      immunosorbent assay
        ELISA titer assay

elcosis

ellipsin

ellipsoid

elliptocytary

elliptocyte

elliptocytosis
    hereditary e.
    spherocytic e.

elliptocytotic

Ellsworth-Howard test

ELT
    euglobulin lysis time

EM
    ejection murmur
    electron microscope
    erythrocyte mass

Embden-Meyerhof pathway

emboliform

embolism
    air e.
    amniotic fluid e.
    bacillary e.
    bland e.
    bone marrow e.
    capillary e.
    acerebral e.
    coronary e.
    crossed e.
    direct e.
    fat e.
    infective e.
    lymph e.
    lymphogenous e.
    miliary e.
    multiple e.
    oil e.
    pantaloon e.
    paradoxical e.
    pulmonary e.
    retinal e.
    saddle e.
    spinal e.
    trichinous e.
    tumor e.
    venous e.
    cholesterol e.
    cholesterol crystal e.

embolomycotic

embolus
    air e.
    bullet e.
    cancer e.
    fat e.
    foam e.
    obturating e.
    riding e.
    saddle e.
    straddling e.
    tumor e.

embryonization

embryopathy

embryotoxon
    anterior e.
    posterior e.

emeiocytosis

emesia

emetatrophia

emetic

emetogenic

emiocytosis

EMIT
    enzyme-multiplied
        immunoassay technique

emmeniopathy

EMMM
    epirermptropic metastatic
        malignant melanoma

Emmon modification of
    Sabouraud dextrose agar

emphraxis

emphysema
    alveolar duct e.
    atrophic e.
    bullous e.
    centriacinar e.
    centrilobular e.
    chronic hypertrophic e.

emphysema (*continued*)
    compensating e.
    compensatory e.
    cutaneous e.
    acystic e.
    diffuse e.
    distal acinar e.
    ectatic e.
    false e.
    afocal e.
    afocal dust e.
    generalized e.
    glass blower's e.
    hypoplastic e.
    idiopathic unilobar e.
    interlobular e.
    interstitial e.
    intestinal e.
    lobar e.
    lobar e., congenital
    lobar e., infantile
    e. of lungs
    mediastinal e.
    obstructive e.
    obstructive e., localized
    panacinar e.
    panlobular e.
    paracicatricial e.
    paraseptal e.
    pulmonary e.
    pulmonary interstitial e.
    senile e.
    skeletal e.
    small-lunged e.
    subcutaneous e.
    traumatic e.
    unilateral e.
    vesicular e.

emphysematous

Empirin

emprosthotonos

emprosthotonus

empyema
    e. articuli
    e. benignum

empyema (*continued*)
    e. of the chest
    e. of gallbladder
    interlobar e.
    latent e.
    loculated e.
    mastoid e.
    metapneumonic e.
    e. necessitatis
    e. of pericardium
    pneumococcal e.
    pulsating e.
    putrid e.
    streptococcal e.
    synpneumonic e.
    thoracic e.
    tuberculous e.

empyemic

empyesis

empyocele

enameloblast

enameloma

enanthem

enanthema

enanthematous

enarthritis

encanthis

encarditis

encelialgia

enceliitis

encelitis

encephalalgia

encephalatrophy

encephalauxe

encephalitic

encephalitides

encephalitis
    e. A

encephalitis (*continued*)
    acute disseminated e.
    acute necrotizing e.
    Australian X e.
    e. B
    benign myalgic e.
    Binswanger's e.
    e. C
    California e.
    Central European e.
    chronic subcortical e.
    cytomegalovirus e.
    Dawson's e.
    eastern equine e.
    Economo's e.
    epidemic e.
    e. epidemica
    equine e.
    forest-spring e.
    granulomatous amebic e.
    hemorrhagic e.
    herpes e.
    herpes simplex e.
    herpetic e.
    HIV e.
    Ilheus e.
    influenzal e.
    Japanese e.
    Japanese B e.
    La Crosse e.
    lead e.
    Leichtenstern's e.
    lethargic e.
    e. lethargica
    limbic encephalitis
    microglial nodular e.
    Murray Valley e.
    Nipah e.
    e. periaxialis concentrica
    e. periaxialis diffusa
    postinfectious e.
    postvaccinal e.
    Powassan e.
    purulent e.
    pyogenic e.
    Russian autumnal e.
    Russian endemic e.

encephalitis (*continued*)
    Russian forest-spring e.
    Russian spring-summer e.
    Russian tick-borne e.
    Russian vernal e.
    St. Louis e.
    Schilder's e.
    Semliki Forest e.
    Strümpell-Leichtenstern e.
    subacute inclusion
      body e.
    e. subcorticalis chronica
    summer e.
    suppurative e.
    tick-borne e.
    toxoplasmic e.
    van Bogaert's e.
    Venezuelan equine e.
    vernal e.
    vernoestival e.
    Vienna e.
    von Economo's e.
    western equine e.
    West Nile e.
    woodcutter's e.

encephalitogen

encephalitogenic

encephalocele
    basal e.
    frontal e.
    occipital e.

encephaloclastic

encephalocystocele

encephalodialysis

encephalodysplasia

encephaloid

encephalolith

encephaloma

encephalomalacia

encephalomeningitis

encephalomeningocele

encephalomeningopathy

encephalomyelitis
    acute disseminated e.
    acute necrotizing
      hemorrhagic e.
    autoimmune e.
    benign myalgic e.
    eastern equine e.
    equine e.
    postinfectious e.
    postvaccinal e.
    toxoplasmic e.
    Venezuelan equine e.
    viral e.
    virus e.
    western equine e.

encephalomyelocele

encephalomyeloneuropathy

encephalomyelopathy
    postinfection e.
    postvaccinial e.
    subacute necrotizing e.

encephalomyeloradiculitis

encephalomyeloradiculopathy

encephalomyopathy
    mitochondrial e.

encephalonarcosis

encephalopathic

encephalopathy
    AIDS e.
    anoxic e.
    biliary e.
    bilirubin e.
    boxer's e.
    boxer's traumatic e.
    cytomegalovirus e.
    demyelinating e.
    dialysis e.
    hepatic e.
    HIV e.
    HIV-related e.
    hypernatremic e.
    hypertensive e.

encephalopathy (*continued*)
   hypoglycemic e.
   hypoxic e.
   hypoxic-ischemic e.
   lead e.
   metabolic e.
   mitochondrial e.
   multicystic e.
   myoclonic e. of childhood
   portal-systemic e.
   portasystemic e.
   progressive dialysis e.
   progressive subcortical e.
   punch-drunk e.
   saturnine e.
   subacute necrotizing e.
   subacute spongiform e.
   subcortical arteriosclerotic
      e.
   transmissible spongiform e.
   traumatic e.
   uremic e.
   Wernicke's e.

encephalopyosis

encephaloradiculitis

encephalorrhagia
   pericapillary e.

encephalosclerosis

encephalosepsis

encephalosis

encephalothlipsis

enchylema

encopresis

encysted

encystment

endangiitis

endaortitis
   bacterial e.

endarteritis
   Heubner's e.
   e. obliterans
   e. proliferans

endarteropathy
   digital endarteropathy

ending
   annulospiral e.
   club e. of Bartelmez
   encapsulated nerve e.
   epilemmal e.
   flower-spray e.
   free nerve e.
   grape e.
   nerve e.
   nonencapsulated nerve e.
   primary e.
   Ruffini's e.
   secondary e.

end-nucleus

endoangiitis

endoaortitis

endoappendicitis

endoarteritis

endocarditic

endocarditis
   acute bacterial e.
   atypical verrucous e.
   bacterial e.
   Candida e.
   e. benigna
   e. chordalis
   constrictive e.
   fungal e.
   infectious e.
   infective e.
   e. lenta
   Libman-Sacks e.
   Löffler's e.
   Löffler's parietal fibroplastic
      e.
   malignant e.
   marantic e.
   mural e.
   mycotic e.
   native valve e.
   nonbacterial thrombotic e.
   nonbacterial verrucous e.

endocarditis (*continued*)
    parietal e.
    prosthetic valve e.
    rheumatic e.
    rickettsial e.
    right-side e.
    septic e.
    staphylococcal e.
    streptococcal e.
    subacute bacterial e.
    syphilitic e.
    tuberculous e.
    ulcerative e.
    valvular e.
    vegetative e.
    verrucous e.
    viridans e.

endocervicitis

endocolitis

endocraniosis

endocranitis

endocrinopathic

endocrinopathy

endocrinosis

endocyst

endocystitis

endocyte

endocytosis

endoenteritis

endoepidermal

endoesophagitis

endogastritis

endolysis

endomastoiditis

endometrioma

endometriosis
    e. externa
    e. interna

endometriosis (*continued*)
    ovarian e.
    e. ovarii
    stromal e.
    e. vesicae

endometriotic

endometritis
    bacteriotoxic e.
    decidual e.
    exfoliative e.
    glandular e.
    membranous e.
    puerperal e.
    syncytial e.
    tuberculous e.

endometrium
    Swiss-cheese e.

endomitosis

endomitotic

endomyocarditis

endomysial

endomysium

endoneural

endoneurial

endoneuritis

endonuclear

endonucleolus

endopericarditis

endoperimyocarditis

endoperineuritis

endoperitonitis

endophlebitis
    e. hepatica obliterans
    proliferative e.

endophthalmitis
    phacoanaphylactic e.

endoplasmic

endopolyploid

endopolyploidy

endoreduplication

end-organ

endosalpingitis

endosarc

endosepsis

endosome

endosteitis

endostitis

endotendineum

endotenon

endotheliitis

endothelioma
    e. angiomatosum

endotheliosis
    glomerular capillary e.

endothelium
    anterior e. of cornea
    e. anterius corneae
    e. camerae anterioris bulbi
    corneal e.
    e. corneale

endothelium-derived relaxing
    factor

endotoxemia

endotoxin

endotrachelitis

endovasculitis

endovenitis

enervation

enophthalmos

enophthalmus

enostosis

enstrophe

enteraden

enteradenitis

enteralgia

enterectasis

enterepiplocele

enteritis
    choleriform e.
    chronic cicatrizing e.
    e. cystica chronica
    diphtheritic e.
    e. gravis
    mucous e.
    e. necroticans
    e. nodularis
    phlegmonous e.
    e. polyposa
    protozoan e.
    pseudomembranous e.
    radiation e.
    regional e.
    segmental e.
    streptococcus e.
    terminal e.
    tuberculous e.

enteroadherent

enteroaggregative

enterochromaffin

enterocolitis
    antibiotic-associated e.
    hemorrhagic e.
    necrotizing e.
    pseudomembranous e.
    regional e.

enterocutaneous

enterocyst

enterocystocele

enterocystoma

enterocyte

enterodynia

enteroepiplocele

enterogastritis

enterohemorrhagic

enterohepatitis

enterohepatocele

enterohydrocele

enteroinvasive

enterolith

enterolithiasis

enteromegalia

enteromegaly

enteromerocele

enteromycodermitis

enteromycosis
    e. bacteriacea

enteromyiasis

enteroneuritis

enteronitis

enteroparesis

enteropathogen

enteropathogenesis

enteropathogenic

enteropathy
    gluten e.
    protein-losing e.

enteroplegia

enterorrhagia

enterorrhea

enterorrhexis

enterosepsis

enterospasm

enterostasis

enterostaxis

enterostenosis

enterovaginal

enterovenous

enterovesical

enteruria

enthesitis

enthesopathy

enthlasis

entiris

Entner-Doudoroff pathway

entochondrostosis

entochoroidea

entocornea

entocyte

entophthalmia

entopic

entoplasm

entoretina

entosarc

entostosis

entropion
    cicatricial e.
    spastic e.
    e. uveae

entropionize

entropium

enuresis

enuretic

envelope
    egg e.
    nuclear e.

Enzinger tumor classification

enzyme-assisted immunoassay
    technique

enzymopathy
    lysosomal e.

eosin
    e. B
    e. I bluish
    ethyl e.
    water-soluble e.
    e. W or W S
    yellowish e.
    e. Y

eosinopenia

eosinophile

eosinophilia
    Löffler's e.
    pulmonary infiltration e.
    simple pulmonary e.

eosinophilic

eosinophilosis

eosinophilous

eosinophiluria

eparsalgia

EOT
    effective oxygen transport

EP
    ectopic pregnancy
    erythocyte protoporphyrin
        EP test
        EP toxicity

ependopathy

ependymitis

ependymoblast

ependymocyte

ependymopathy

EPF
    exophthalmos-producing
        factor

ephapse

ephaptic

epiblepharon

epicauma

epicondylalgia

epicorneascleritis

epicystitis

epidermatitis

epidermicula

epidermitis

epidermodysplasia

epidermoid

epidermolysis
    e. bullosa
    e. bullosa, acquired
    e. bullosa acquisita
    e. bullosa, junctional
    e. bullosa dystrophica
    e. bullosa dystrophica,
        albopapuloid
    e. bullosa dystrophica,
        dominant
    e. bullosa dystrophica,
        dysplastic
    e. bullosa dystrophica,
        hyperplastic
    e. bullosa dystrophica,
        polydysplastic
    e. bullosa dystrophica,
        recessive
    e. bullosa hereditaria
    e. bullosa letalis
    e. bullosa simplex
    e. bullosa simplex,
        generalized
    e. bullosa simplex,
        localized
    toxic e. epidermolysis

epidermolytic

epidermomycosis

epidermophytid

epidermophytosis

epididymitis
    spermatogenic e.

epididymo-orchitis

epigastralgia

epigastrocele

epiglottiditis

epiglottitis

epilemmal

epiloia

epimenorrhagia

epimenorrhea

epinephrinemia

epineurial

epiorchium

epipharyngitis

epiphora

epiphysiolysis

epiphysiopathy

epiphysis
    slipped e.
    stippled e.

epiphysitis
    e. juvenilis
    vertebral e.

epiplocele

epiploenterocele

epiploitis

epiplomerocele

epiplomphalocele

epiploscheocele

episclera

episcleral

episcleritis
    e. partialis fugax

episclerotitis

epispadia

epispadiac

epispadial

epispadias
    balanic e.
    balanitic e.
    clitoric e.
    complete e.
    glandular e.
    incomplete e.
    penile e.
    penopubic e.
    subsymphyseal e.

episplenitis

epistasis

episthotonos

epitarsus

epitela

epitendineum

epitenon

epithalaxia

epitheliitis

epitheliogenesis
    e. imperfecta

epitheliolysis

epitheliolytic

epithelium
    Barrett's e.
    capsular e.
    e. corneae
    corneal e.
    e. ductus semicircularis
    enamel e.
    false e.
    germinal e.
    gingival e.
    glomerular e.
    junctional e.
    olfactory e.
    respiratory e.
    seminiferous e.
    sense e.
    sensory e.

epithelium (*continued*)
    subcapsular e.
    sulcal e.
    sulcular e.

epitonic

epitrichium

epituberculosis

epityphlitis

EPP
    erythropoietic
        protoporphyria

EPS
    exophthalmos-producing
        substance

epulis
    e. fibromatosa
    fibromatous e.
    e. fissurata

Equanil

equator
    e. of cell

equilibrium
    acid-base e.
    body e.
    fluid e.
    nutritive e.
    water e.

equipotential line

Eranko fluorescence stain

Erb-Charcot disease

ERBF
    effective renal blood flow

Erb-Goldflam disease

ERC
    erythroietin-responsive cell

ergastoplasm

ergoplasm

ergothioneine

erosio
    e. interdigitalis
        blastomycetica

E-rosette test

ERP
    effective refractory period
    equine rhinopneumonitis

ERRT
    extrarenal rhabdoid tumor

eruption
    creeping e.
    drug e.
    fixed e.
    fixed drug e.
    Kaposi's varicelliform e.
    passive e.
    polymorphous light e.
    seabather's e.
    serum e.

erysipelas
    gangrenous e.
    e. grave internum
    malignant e.
    necrotizing e.

erysipelatous

erysipeloid

erysipelotoxin

erythema
    e. annulare
    e. annulare centrifugum
    e. annulare rheumaticum
    e. caloricum
    e. chromicum figuratum
        melanodermicum
    e. circinatum
    e. circinatum rheumaticum
    cold e.
    diaper e.
    e. dyschromicum perstans
    e. elevatum diutinum
    epidemic e.
    figurate e.
    e. figuratum

erythema (*continued*)
    e. figuratum perstans
    e. fugax
    gyrate e.
    e. gyratum
    e. gyratum perstans
    e. gyratum repens
    e. ab igne
    e. induratum
    e. iris
    Jacquet's e.
    e. marginatum
    e. marginatum
      rheumaticum
    e. migrans
    e. multiforme
    e. multiforme majus
    e. multiforme minus
    necrolytic migratory e.
    e. necroticans
    e. nodosum
    e. nodosum leprosum
    e. nodosum migrans
    palmar e.
    e. pernio
    e. streptogenes
    toxic e.
    e. toxicum
    e. toxicum neonatorum
    e. palmare

erythematoedematous

erythematous

erythemogenic

erythralgia

erythrasma

erythremia

erythremomelalgia

erythroblast
    definitive e.
    primitive e.
    primordial e.

erythroblastemia

erythroblastopenia
    transient e. of childhood

erythroblastosis
    e. fetalis
    e. neonatorum

erythroblastotic

erythrocatalysis

erythrochromia

erythroclasis

erythroclast

erythroclastic

erythrocyanosis

erythrocyte
    achromic e.
    basophilic e.
    burr e.
    crenated e.
    hypochromic e.
    Mexican hat e.
    target e.

erythrocythemia

erythrocytolysin

erythrocytolysis

erythrocytopenia

erythrocytorrhexis

erythrocytoschisis

erythrocytosis
    benign e.
    stress e.

erythrocyturia

erythrodegenerative

erythroderma
    congenital ichthyosiform e.,
      bullous
    congenital ichthyosiform e.,
      nonbullous
    e. desquamativum
    e. psoriaticum

erythrodermia

erythrodontia

erythrogen

erythrogenesis
  e. imperfecta

erythrogenic

erythrokatalysis

erythrokeratodermia
  e. variabilis

erythrolein

erythroleukoblastosis

erythroleukothrombocythemia

erythrolitmin

erythrolysin

erythrolysis

erythromelalgia
  e. of the head

erythroneocytosis

erythropenia

erythrophil

erythrophilous

erythrophobic

erythrophore

erythrophose

erythropia

erythroplasia
  Zoon's e.

erythroprosopalgia

erythropsia

erythropyknosis

erythrorrhexis

érythrose
  é. péribuccale pigmentaire
    of Brocq

erythrosin

erythrosis

erythrostasis

erythrothioneine

erythruria

eschar

ESF
  erythropoietic-stimulating
    factor

esocataphoria

esodeviation

esoethmoiditis

esogastritis

esophagalgia

esophagectasia

esophagectasis

esophagism

esophagismus

esophagitis
  Candida e.
  chronic peptic e.
  e. dissecans superficialis
  fungal e.
  pill e.
  reflux e.
  viral e.

esophagocele

esophagodynia

esophagomalacia

esophagomycosis

esophagoptosis

esophagospasm

esophagostenosis

esophagostoma

esophagus
  Barrett's e.
  nutcracker e.

esophoria

esophoric

esosphenoiditis

esotropia

esotropic

ESR
    electron spin resonance
    erythrocyte sedimentation
        rate
            ESR assay

ESS
    endometrial stromal
        sarcoma
    erythrocyte-sensitizing
        substance

esterapenia

esthesioneure

ESTN
    epithelioid soft-tissue
        neoplasm

Estren-Dameshek anemia

état
        é. criblé
        é. lacunaire

é. mammelonné
        é. marbré

ethmoiditis

ethylmalonic-adipicaciduria

etiopathology

eucaryon

eucaryosis

eucaryote

eucaryotic

eugnathia

eugnathic

eukaryon

eukaryosis

eukaryote

eukaryotic

Eulenburg disease

eumorphism

Euproctis

eupyrene

eupyrexia

eupyrous

eustachitis

eusthenuria

eutelolecithal

eventration
        diaphragmatic e.
        umbilical e.

eviration

EWB
    estrogen withdrawal
        bleeding

ExacTech blood glucose meter
    test

exania

exanthem
        Boston e.
        e. subitum

exanthema
        e. subitum

exanthemata

exanthematous

exanthrope

exanthropic

excitation
        reentrant e.

excoriation
        neurotic e.

excrescence
        fungating e.
        fungous e.
        Lambl's e.

excrescent

excretion
    pseudouridine e.

excyclophoria

excyclotropia

exenteritis

exesion

exfetation

exfoliatio
    e. areata linguae

exhumation

exocataphoria

exocolitis

exocytosis

exodeviation

exogastritis

exomphalos

exomysium

exopathic

exopathy

exophoria

exophoric

exophthalmic

exophthalmogenic

exophthalmos
    endocrine e.
    malignant e.
    pulsating e.
    thyrotoxic e.
    thyrotropic e.

exophthalmus

exosepsis

exoserosis

exotropia

exsanguinate

exsanguination

exsanguine

exstrophy
    e. of the bladder
    e. of cloaca
    cloacal e.

extension
    e. per contiguitatem
    e. per continuitatem
    e. per saltam

extracellular

extrachromosomal inheritence

extracorporeal
    e. photophoresis technique

extracystic

extrafusal

extramastoiditis

extranuclear

extraprostatitis

extrasystole
    atrial e.
    atrioventricular (AV) e.
    infranodal e.
    interpolated e.
    junctional e.
    nodal e.
    retrograde e.
    ventricular e.

extravasation
    punctiform e.

extraversion

extrophia

extroversion

exudate
    cotton-wool e.

exudation

exudative

exulcerans

exulceratio
    e. simplex

exumbilication

eyepiece
    comparison e.
    compensating e.

eyepiece (*continued*)
    demonstration e.
    high-eyepoint e.
    huygenian e.
    negative e.
    positive e.
    Ramsden's e.
    widefield e.

F

fabism

facies
    f. abdominalis
    adenoid f.
    f. bovina
    f. dolorosa
    f. hepatica
    f. hippocratica
    Hutchinson f.
    leonine f.
    f. leontina
    Marshall Hall f.
    mitral f.
    mitrotricuspid f.
    moon f.
    myasthenic f.
    myopathic f.
    Parkinson f.
    parkinsonian f.
    Potter f.
    f. scaphoidea

faciocephalalgia

facioplegia

faciostenosis

Facklam classification scheme

FACS
    fluorescence-activated cell
        sorter

FACscan
    fluorescence-activated cell
        sorter scan

factor
    C f.
    chemotactic f.
    C3 nephritic f.
    Simon's septic f.

fagopyrism

fascia
    f. adherens
    fusion f.
    Scarpa's f.

fasciculation
    contraction f.

fasciculus
    maculary f.
    f. of middle cerebellar
        peduncle, deep
    f. of middle cerebellar
        peduncle, inferior
    f. of middle cerebellar
        peduncle, superior

fasciitis
    eosinophilic f.
    necrotizing f.
    perirenal f.

fascitis

faucitis

favid

favism

favus
    f. herpetiformis
    mouse f.
    f. murium

Faxitron x-ray machine

FBE
    fibrinogen breakdown
        product
    full blood examination

F-duction

FECG
    fetal elctrocardiogram

FEL
    familial erythrophagocytic
        lymphomhistiocytosis

febricity

febricula

febris

fecalith

fecaloma

fecaluria

feltwork
Kaes' f.

feminonucleus

femorocele

fenestration
aorticopulmonary f.

FEP, FEPP
free erythrocyte
protoporphyrin

fervescence

festinant

fetopathy

fetus
harlequin f.

fever
adynamic f.
asthenic f.
Brazilian purpuric f.
central f.
cerebrospinal f.
Charcot's f.
childbed f.
continued f.
cotton-mill f.
dehydration f.
desert f.
duck f.
ephemeral f.
eruptive f.
essential f.
exanthematous f.
familial Mediterranean f.
grain f.
hectic f.
humidifier f.
inanition f.
intermittent hepatic f.
land f.
milk f.
mill f.
Murchison-Pel-Ebstein f.
Oroya f.

fever (*continued*)
parrot f.
Pel-Ebstein f.
periodic f.
Pontiac f.
puerperal f.
recurrent f.
remittent f.
salt f.
San Joaquin f.
San Joaquin Valley f.
septic f.
shoddy f.
sthenic f.
thermic f.
threshing f.
uveoparotid f.
valley f.
West Nile f.

fiber
A f.
accelerating f.
accelerator f.
accessory f.
A delta f.
afferent f.
afferent nerve f.
alpha f.
alveolar f.
alveolar crest f.
amygdalofugal f.
apical fibers
arcuate f.
arcuate f., anterior
external
arcuate f., dorsal external
arcuate f., internal
arcuate f., long
arcuate f., posterior
external
arcuate f., short
arcuate f., ventral external
arcuate f. of cerebrum
association f.
association f., long
association f., short
association nerve f.

fiber (*continued*)
   association f. of
     telencephalon
   astral f.
   augmentor f.
   autonomic f.
   autonomic afferent f.
   autonomic efferent f.
   autonomic nerve f.
   auxiliary f.
   axial f.
   B f.
   basilar f.
   Bergmann's f.
   beta f.
   bone f.
   Brücke's f.
   bulbospiral f.
   C f.
   cardiac accelerator f.
   cardiac depressor f.
   cardiac pressor f.
   cemental f.
   cementoalveolar f.
   cerebellovestibular f.
   cerebrospinal f.
   chief f.
   chromatic f.
   chromosomal f.
   cilioequatorial f.
   cilioposterocapsular f.
   circular f.
   circular f. of ciliary muscle
   circular f. of eardrum
   climbing f.
   clinging f.
   commissural f.
   commissural f. of
     telencephalon
   cone f.
   continuous f.
   Corti's f.
   corticobulbar f.
   corticonuclear f.
   corticopontine f.
   corticoreticular f.
   corticorubral f.
   corticospinal f.

fiber (*continued*)
   corticostriate f.
   corticothalamic f.
   dentatorubral f.
   dentatothalamic f.
   dentinal f.
   dentinogenic f.
   depressor f.
   efferent f.
   efferent nerve f.
   endogenous f.
   exogenous f.
   extrafusal f.
   fasciculoventricular f.
   frontopontine f.
   fusimotor f.
   gamma f.
   geniculostriate f.
   Gerdy's f.
   gingival f.
   gingivodental f.
   Gratiolet's radiating f.
   gray f.
   half-spindle f.
   Henle's f.
   Herxheimer's f.
   heterodesmotic f.
   homodesmotic f.
   horizontal f.
   impulse-conducting f.
   interciliary f.
   intercolumnar f.
   internuncial f.
   intersegmental f.
   interzonal f.
   intrasegmental f.
   intrathalamic f.
   James f.
   Korff f.
   f. of lens
   longitudinal f. of ciliary
     muscle
   longitudinal pontine f.
   Luschka's f.
   macular f.
   Mahaim f.
   main f.
   mantle f.

fiber (*continued*)
    Mauthner's f.
    medullated f.
    medullated nerve f.
    meridional f. of ciliary
      muscle
    moss f.
    mossy f.
    motor f.
    Müller's f.
    muscle f.
    muscle f., fast twitch
    muscle f., intermediate
    muscle f., red
    muscle f., slow twitch
    muscle f., type I
    muscle f., type II
    muscle f., white
    myelinated f.
    myelinated nerve f.
    neuroglial f.
    nigrostriate f.
    nodoventricular f.
    nonmedullated f.
    nonmedullated nerve f.
    oblique f.
    oblique f. of ciliary muscle
    oblique f. of stomach
    occipitopontine f.
    odontogenic f.
    orbiculoanterocapsular f.
    orbiculociliary f.
    orbiculoposterocapsular f.
    osteocollagenous f.
    osteogenetic f.
    osteogenic f.
    oxytalan f.
    pallidofugal f.
    parallel f.
    paraventricular f.
    parietopontine f.
    parietotemporopontine f.
    perforating f.
    periventricular f.
    pilomotor f.
    pontocerebellar f.
    postcommissural f.
    postganglionic f.

fiber (*continued*)
    postganglionic nerve f.
    preganglionic f.
    preganglionic nerve f.
    pressor f.
    principal f.
    projection f.
    projection nerve f.
    Prussak's f.
    Purkinje f.
    radial f. of ciliary muscle
    radiating f. of anterior
      chondrosternal ligaments
    radiating f. of eardrum
    radicular f.
    ragged red f.
    Reissner's f.
    retinothalamic projection f.
    Retzius' f.
    Ritter's f.
    rod f.
    Rosenthal f.
    Sappey's f.
    Sharpey's f.
    sinospiral f.
    sinuspiral f.
    somatic f.
    somatic afferent f.
    somatic efferent f.
    somatic nerve fibers
    sphincter f. of ciliary
      muscle
    spindle f.
    Stilling's f.
    f. of stria terminalis
    striatonigral f.
    sudomotor f.
    supraoptic f.
    sustentacular f.
    T f.
    tangential f.
    tangential nerve f.
    temporopontine f.
    tendril f.
    terminal conducting f. of
      Purkinje
    thalamocortical f.
    thalamoparietal f.

fiber (*continued*)
Tomes' f.
traction f.
transseptal f.
transverse pontine f.
trigeminothalamic f.
ultraterminal f.
unmyelinated f.
unmyelinated nerve f.
varicose f.
vasomotor f.
visceral f.
visceral afferent f.
visceral efferent f.
visceral nerve f.
Weissmann's f.
zonular f.

FGT
female genital tract
FGT cytologic smear

FHF
fulminant hepatic failure

FI
fever caused by infection
fibrogen

FIA
fluorescent immunoassay

fibra
f. arcuatae externae
dorsales
f. arcuatae externae
ventrales
f. dentatorubrales
f. parietotemporopontinae
f. pontis profundae
f. pontis superficiales
f. radiales musculi ciliaris
f. supraopticae

fibril
anchoring f.
border f.
dentinal f.
fibroglia f.
muscle f.
muscular f.

fibril (*continued*)
nerve f.
side f. of Golgi
Tomes' f.

fibrillin

fibrilloblast

fibrillolysis

fibrillolytic

fibrinogenemia

fibrinogenopenia

fibrinoplatelet

fibrinopurulent

fibrinorrhea

fibrinoscopy

fibrinuria

fibroadenosis

fibroatrophy

fibroblast

fibrobronchitis

fibrocalcific

fibrocaseous

fibrocellular

fibrochondritis

fibrocystic
f. condition of the breast
f. disease of the pancreas
f. mastitis
f. mastopathy

fibrodysplasia
f. ossificans progressiva

fibroelastoma
papillary f.

fibroelastosis
endocardial f.
primary endocardial f.

fibrofascitis

figure   207

fibrogenesis
    f. imperfecta ossium

fibroglia

fibrohemorrhagic

fibrohistiocytic

fibroma
    f. cavernosum
    f. molle
    f. molluscum
    f. pendulum
    perifollicular f.
    periungual f.
    recurrent digital f. of
        childhood
    soft f.

fibromatosis
    f. colli
    congenital generalized f.
    infantile digital f.
    juvenile hyaline f.
    subcutaneous
        pseudosarcomatous f.

fibropituicyte

fibroplasia
    retrolental f.

fibroplastic

fibropolycystic

fibropolypus

fibropurulent

fibrosis
    African endomyocardial f.
    congenital hepatic f.
    cystic f.
    cystic f. of the pancreas
    diatomite f.
    diffuse interstitial
        pulmonary f.
    endomyocardial f.
    graphite f.
    idiopathic pulmonary f.
    idiopathic retroperitoneal f.
    interstitial f.

fibrosis (*continued*)
    interstitial pulmonary f.
    mediastinal f.
    neoplastic f.
    panmural f. of the bladder
    periureteric f.
    pipestem f.
    pleural f.
    postfibrinous f.
    progressive massive f.
    proliferative f.
    pulmonary f.
    replacement f.
    retroperitoneal f.
    root sleeve f.
    Symmers' f.

fibrositis

fibrothorax

Ficoll-Hypaque technique

FID
    flame ionization detector

field
    Cohnheim f.
    dark- f.
    high-power f.
    low-power f.
    f. of a microscope
    surplus f.
    cribriform f. of vision
    spiral visual f.
    tubular visual f.

FIGLU
    formiminoglutamic
        acid
    formiminoglutamic acid
        test
    FIGLU excretion test

figuratum

figure
    flame f.
    fortification f.
    Minkowski's f.
    mitotic f.

filament
  acrosomal f.
  actin f.
  axial f.
  desmin f.
  glial f.
  intermediate f.
  linin f.
  lymphatic anchoring f.
  meningeal f.
  f. of meninges
  muscle f.
  myosin f.
  pial f. of filum terminale
  root f. of spinal nerve
  spermatic f.
  spinal f.
  terminal f.
  terminal f., dural
  terminal f., external
  terminal f., internal
  terminal f., pial
  terminal f. of spinal dura
    mater
  thick f.
  thin f.

filamin

film
  fixed blood f.

filovaricosis

Filtracheck-UTI
  F.-U. disposible colormetric
    bacteriuria detection
    system
  F.-U. test

filum
  f. anastomotica nervi
    acustici
  f. durae matris spinale
  f. spinale
  f. terminale durale
  f. terminale externum
  f. terminale internum
  f. terminale piale

fimbrin

fimbriocele

fine-needle aspiration biopsy
  (FNAB)

fingeragnosia

Fink-Heimer stain

Finn chamber patch test

fire
  St. Anthony's f.

first-order reaction

Fishberg concentration test

fission
  binary f.
  cellular f.
  multiple f.

fissiparous

fissura
  f. in ano
  f. auris congenita

fissure
  anal f.
  f. in ano
  cutaneous f.
  enamel f.

fistula
  abdominal f.
  anal f.
  f. in ano
  aortocaval f.
  aortoenteric f.
  arteriovenous f.
  f. auris congenita
  biliary f.
  f. bimucosa
  blind f.
  branchial f.
  bronchocavitary f.
  bronchopleural f.
  carotid cavernous f.
  cerebrospinal fluid f.
  cervical f.
  f. colli congenita
  colonic f.

fistula (*continued*)
    complete f.
    f. corneae
    coronary arteriovenous f.
    coronary artery f.
    craniosinus f.
    external f.
    fecal f.
    gastrocolic f.
    genitourinary f.
    hepatic f.
    horseshoe f.
    incomplete f.
    internal f.
    labyrinthine f.
    lacrimal f.
    lymphatic f.
    f. lymphatica
    oroantral f.
    parietal f.
    perianal f.
    perilymph f.
    perilymphatic f.
    perineal f.
    pharyngeal f.
    pilonidal f.
    congenital preauricular f.
    pulmonary f.
    pulmonary arteriovenous f.
    rectovaginal f.
    rectovesical f.
    rectovestibular f.
    salivary f.
    spermatic f.
    stercoral f.
    submental f.
    thoracic f.
    tracheal f.
    tracheocutaneous f.
    umbilical f.
    urethrovaginal f.
    urinary f.
    vesical f.
    vesicouterine f.
    vesicovaginal f.
    vestibular f.

fistulae

fistulous

Fite-Faraco stain

"fitter" cell theory

Fitzgerald factor

Fitz-Hugh and Curtis syndrome

Fitz syndrome

fixation
    Bovin f.
    ossicular f.

fixative
    B5 f.
    Bouin picroformol-acetic f.
    Carnoy f.
    CytoLyt f.
    Gendre f.
    glutaraldehyde f.
    Maximow f.
    Permount slide f.
    picric acid f.
    Zenker f.
    Zenker-formol f.

FJN
    familial juvenile
        nephrophthsis

FJP
    familial juvenile polyp

FK506

flagella

flagellar

flagelliform

flagellum

Flajani disease

Flatau-Schilder disease

flatus
    f. vaginalis

Flaujeac factor

Fleitman test

Flemming
　F. fixative
　F. triple stain

Flexner dysentery

floccillation

flocculation

floccule

flocculent

flocculus

florid oral papillomatosis

Florisil

FLS
　fibrous long-spacing
　(collagen)

FLSA
　follicular lymphosarcoma

flu
　trimellitic anhydride (TMA)
　f.

fluid
　Altmann's f.
　ascitic f.
　Bouin's f.
　decalcifying f.
　Flemming's fixing f.
　formol-Müller f.
　Helly's f.
　Lang's f.
　Müller's f.
　Parker's f.
　Schaudinn's f.
　Thoma's f.
　Zenker's f.
　Carnoy's f.

fluor
　f. albus

fluorane

fluoresceinuria

fluorescence
　secondary f.

fluoronephelometer

fluorosis
　dental f.

flush
　breast f.
　hectic f.
　malar f.

flutter-fibrillation

flux
　celiac f.
　ionic f.

fluxion

FMN
　flavin monomucleotide

FMS
　fat-mobilizing substance

FOAVF
　failure of all vital forces

focus
　Assmann f.
　dysplastic f.
　epileptogenic f.
　epileptogenic f., secondary
　Ghon f.
　mirror f.
　Simon's f.

focusing
　isoelectric f.

fodrin

fogo
　f. selvagem

Folin-Ciocalteu reagent

Folin-Looney test

fold
　opercular f.

follicle
　Montgomery f.
　Naboth's f.
　nabothian f.

folliclis

folliculitis
f. abscedens et suffodiens
agminate f.
f. barbae
f. decalvans
eosinophilic pustular f.
f. gonorrhoeica
gram-negative f.
keloidal f.
f. keloidalis
f. nares perforans
f. ulerythematosa reticulata
f. varioliformis

folliculosis

foot
athlete's f.
broad f.
burning f.
Charcot's f.
cleft f.
club f.
dangle f.
drop f.
end f.
end-f.
flat f.
forced f.
Friedreich's f.
Hong Kong f.
immersion f.
immersion f., tropical
march f.
Morton's f.
mossy f.
pericapillary end f.
perivascular f.
reel f.
rocker-bottom f.
sag f.
spread f.
sucker f.
tabetic f.
taut f.
trench f.
weak f.

foramen
Morgagni f.
morgagnian f.
pleuroperitoneal f.

forceps
Cornet f.

foregilding

formation
coffin f.
Gothic arch f.
palisade f.
rouleau f.
f. of rouleaux

forme
f. fruste
f. tardive

formiminoglutamate

formiminoglutamic acid

formiminotransferase deficiency

formula
Berkow f.
Van Slyke's f.

fossa
implantation f.

fossette

Fowler solution

Fox-Fordyce disease

FPM
filter paper microscopic

FPN reagent

FPP
ferriprotoporphyrin

FR
Fischer-Race (notation)
flocculation reaction
flow rate

fragilitas
f. crinium
f. ossium
f. unguium

fragility
    f. of blood
    capillary f.
    erythrocyte f.
    hereditary f. of bone
    mechanical f.
    osmotic f.

fragilocyte

fragilocytosis

fragment
    Spengler's f.

fragmentation
    f. of myocardium

frame-shift mutagen

Franceschetti-Jadassohn
    syndrome

Frank-Starling disease

Fraser-Lendrum stain for fibrin

freeze-cleaving

freeze-etching

freeze-fracturing

Frei-Hoffmann reaction

fremitus
    bronchial f.
    pericardial f.
    pleural f.
    rhonchal f.

Frenkl anterior ocular traumatic
    syndrome

frenulum
    f. linguae

frenum
    Macdowel f.

Frerichs theory

Fresnal fringe

Friderichsen-Waterhouse
    syndrome

frigorism

frog test

Frohn reagent

Froin syndrome

frolement

front-end processor

frost
    urea f.

fructosazone

fructose-1,6-bisphosphatase
    deficiency

fructosemia

fructosuria
    essential f.

FSF
    fibrin-stabilization factor
    fibrin-stabilizing factor

FSH
    follicle-stimulating
        hormone
            FSH assay

FSP
    fibrinogen split product
    fibrinolytic split product

FSR
    fusiform skin revision

FTI
    free thyroxine index

FU-48 Zenker fixative solution

fuchsin
    acid f.
    basic f.
    new f.

fuchsinophil

fuchsinophilia

fuchsinophilic

fuchsinophilous

fucosidosis

fugue
    epileptic f.

fumaricaciduria

functionalis

fundus
    albinotic f.
    f. albipunctatus
    f. diabeticus
    f. flavimaculatus
    leopard f.
    salt and pepper f.

fungate

fungoid

fungoma

fungosity

fungus
    f. of the brain
    cerebral f.
    f. cerebri
    mosaic f.
    f. testis

funiculitis
    endemic f.
    filarial f.

funiculoepididymitis

funisitis
    necrotizing f.

furfuraceous

Fuhrman system

Fujiwara reaction

functionally patent foramen
  ovale

Fungalase-F stain

FUO
    fever of undetermined
      origin
    fever of unknown origin

furocoumarin

furrow
    Jadelot's f.
    Liebermeister's f.

furuncle

furuncular

furunculoid

furunculosis
    aural f.

furunculus

fusion
    centric f.

fusus
    cortical f.
    fracture f.

FV
    fluid volume

FWR
    Felix-Weil reaction

G

γ (*var. of* gamma)

Gaddum and Schild test

gadolinium

Gailliard syndrome

Gairdner disease

galactacrasia

galactemia

galactocele

galactocrasia

galactoma

galactometastasis

galactophlebitis

galactophlysis

galactophoritis

galactoplania

galactopyra

galactorrhea

galactosazone

galactosemia

galactosialidosis

galactosuria

galacturia

galeropia

galeropsia

Gall body

Gallego differentiating solution

gallein

Gallyas method

GALT
    gut-associated lymphoid
      tissue

galvanism
    dental g.

gamete

gametic

gametocyte

gametoid

gammaglobulinopathy

gammaphoto

gamma-well counter

gammopathy
    monoclonal g.
    benign monoclonal g.

Gamna disease

gampsodactyly

Gamstrop syndrome

gangliocyte

ganglioglioneuroma

ganglion
    Acrel's g.
    Bezold's g.
    compound g.
    diffuse g.
    primary g.
    Remak's g.
    simple g.
    sinoatrial g.
    sinus g.
    synovial g.
    Wrisberg's g.
    wrist g.

ganglionic

ganglionitis
    gasserian g.

gangliosidosis
    generalized g.
    GM1 g.
    GM2 g.

gangliosidosis (*continued*)
- GM2 g., type I
- GM2 g., type II
- GM2 g., type III
- GM2 g., variant 0
- GM2 g., variant AB
- GM2 g., variant B

ganoblast

Ganser syndrome

gap
- anion g.
- chromatid g.
- isochromatid g.
- urinary anion g.

GAPD, GAPDH
- glyceraldehyde phosphate dehydrogenase

gargalanesthesia

gas-liquid chromatography (GLC)

gastradenitis

gastralgia

gastralgokenosis

gastratrophia

gastritis
- antral g.
- antrum g.
- atrophic g.
- atrophic g., diffuse corporal
- atrophic-hyperplastic g.
- autoimmune g.
- catarrhal g.
- chemical g.
- chronic cystic g.
- chronic follicular g.
- corrosive g.
- eosinophilic g.
- erosive g.
- exfoliative g.
- follicular g.
- giant hypertrophic g.
- hemorrhagic g.

gastritis (*continued*)
- hypertrophic g.
- phlegmonous g.
- polypous g.
- pseudomembranous g.
- radiation g.
- superficial g.
- toxic g.
- type A g.
- type B g.
- zonal g.

gastroadenitis

gastroadynamic

gastrocele

gastrocolic

gastrocolitis

gastrocutaneous

gastroduodenitis

gastrodynia

gastroenteralgia

gastroenteritis
- acute infectious g.
- eosinophilic g.
- Norwalk g.

gastroenterocolitis

gastroenteropathy
- allergic g.
- eosinophilic g.

gastroesophagitis

gastrohepatitis

gastroileitis

gastrolith

gastrolithiasis

gastromalacia

gastromegaly

gastromycosis

gastromyxorrhea

gastropancreatitis

gastroparalysis

gastroparesis

gastropathic

gastropathy
    congestive g.

gastroperiodynia

gastroperitonitis

gastrophthisis

gastroplegia

gastroptosis

gastrorrhagia

gastrorrhea

gastrorrhexis

gastrosis

gastrostaxis

gastrostenosis

gastrostomy
    Janeway g.

gastrosuccorrhea
    digestive g.

gastrotoxin

gastrotympanites

GBA
    ganglionic blocking agent

GBIA
    Guthrie bacterial inhibition
        assy

GBM
    glomerular basement
        membrane

GC
    ganglion cell
    gas chromoatography
    granular cast
    guanine cytosine
        GC value

GC-MS
    gas chromatography-mass
        spectrometry

G-CSF
    gramulocyte colony-
        stimulating factor

GCTTS
    giant cell tumor of tendon
        sheath

G/E
    granulocyte-erythroid ratio

gegenhalten

Gieger-Müller counter

gelatin
    g. of Wharton

gelsolin

gemästete

gemination

gemistocyte

gemistocytic

gemmule

gene
    leaky g.
    lethal g.
    mutant g.
    silent g.
    sublethal g.

genoblast

genodermatosis

gentian
    g. violet

gentianophil

gentianophilic

gentianophilous

gentianophobic

gentianophobous

genu
    g. extrorsum
    g. impressum
    g. introrsum
    g. recurvatum
    g. valgum
    g. varum

geroderma
    g. osteodysplastica

gerodermia

geromarasmus

geromorphism
    cutaneous g.

gerontopia

gerontotoxon

gerontoxon

gerüstmark

gestosis

GET
    gastric emptying time

GFAP
    glial fibrillary acidic protein

ghost
    red cell g.

GH-RF
    growth hormone-releasing
        factor

GH-RH
    growth hormone-releasing
        hormone

GH-RIH
    growth hormone-release-
        inhibiting hormone

girdle
    Hitzig g.
    limbus g.
    white limbal g. of Vogt

GITT
    glucose insulin tolerance
        test

gland
    interstitial g.
    Naboth's g.
    nabothian g.
    Philip's g.
    sentinel g.
    splenoid g.

glanderous

glanders

GLC
    gas-liquid chromatography

Glenner-Lillie stain for pituitary

glia
    ameboid g.
    Bergmann's g.
    cytoplasmic g.
    g. of Fañanás
    fibrillary g.

gliacyte

gliadin

glial fibrillary acidic protein
    (GFAP)

glioblast

gliocyte
    retinal g.

gliofibrillary

glioma
    optic g.

gliophagia

gliopil

gliosis
    diffuse g.
    g. endometrii
    hemispheric g.
    hypertrophic nodular g.
    isomorphic g.
    perivascular g.
    unilateral g.
    g. uteri

gliosome

glischrin

glischruria

glissonitis

globular-fibrous transformation

globule
    dentin g.
    Dobie's g.
    Marchi's g.
    Morgagni's g.
    polar g.

globuli

globulinuria

globulus

globus
    g. pharyngeus

glomangiomatous osseous
   malformation syndrome

glomerulose

glomerulus
    g. of kidney
    malpighian g.
    nonencapsulated nerve g.
    olfactory g.
    renal g.
    g. renis
    synaptic g.

glossagra

glossalgia

glossanthrax

glossocele

glossocoma

glossodynia
    g. exfoliativa
    psychogenic g.

glossoncus

glossopathy

glossopexy

glossophytia

glossoptosis

glossopyrosis

glossospasm

glossotrichia

glucocorticoid therapy

glucocorticosteroid

glucogenic amino acid

glucohemia

glucopenia

glucosazone

glucose
    Brun's g.
    g. oxidase paper strip test
    g. tolerance test (GTT)

glucose-6-phosphate
   dehydrogenase deficiency

α-1,4-glucosidase deficiency

glucosuria

Gluge corpuscle

glutomate-pyruvate
   transaminase

γ-glutamylcysteine synthetase
   deficiency

γ-glutamyl transpeptidase
   deficiency

glutaral

glutaraldehyde

glutaric acid

glutaricacidemia

glutaricaciduria

glutathionemia

glutathione (GSH) synthetase
   deficiency

glutathionuria

gluten-sensitive enteropathy
(GSE)

glutitis

glycemia

d-glycericacidemia

l-glycericaciduria

glyceroluria

glycinemia

glycocalyx

glycogenosis
brancher deficiency g.
generalized g.
hepatophosphorylase
deficiency g.
hepatorenal g.
myophosphorylase
deficiency g.

glycogeusia

glycohemia

glycolicaciduria

glycopenia

glycophilia

glycopolyuria

glycoprotein
α1-acid g.

glycoptyalism

glycorrhachia

glycorrhea

glycosemia

glycosialia

glycosialorrhea

glycosphingolipidosis

glycosuria
alimentary g.
benign g.
digestive g.

glycosuria (*continued*)
emotional g.
epinephrine g.
hyperglycemic g.
magnesium g.
nondiabetic g.
nonhyperglycemic g.
normoglycemic g.
orthoglycemic g.
pathologic g.
phlorhizin g.
renal g.
toxic g.

glycuresis

glykemia

GM-CSF
granulocyte-macrophage
colony-stimulating factor

Gmelin test

GMS
Gomori methenamine-
silver stain
GMS stain

gnathalgia

gnathitis

gnathodynia

gnathoschisis

GNID
Gram-negative intracellular
diplococci

GnRH
gonadotropin-releasing
hormone

goitrin

goitrogen

goitrogenic

goitrogenicity

goitrogenous

goitrous

golgiosome

Gomori-Jones periodic acid-methenamine-silver stain

Gomori-Takamatsu stain

gonacratia

gonadoblastoma

gonadopathy

gonadotropin-inhibitory material (GIM)

gonadotropin-producing adenoma

gonagra

gonalgia

gonarthritis

gonarthrocace

gonarthromeningitis

gonarthrosis

gonatocele

gonecystitis

gonecystolith

gonecystopyosis

goneitis

goniodysgenesis

goniosynechia

gonitis
    fungous g.
    g. tuberculosa

gonoblennorrhea

gonocampsis

gonocele

gonococcemia

gonocyte

gonycampsis

gonycrotesis

gonyectyposis

gonyocele

gonyoncus

Gordon
    G. agent
    G. and Sweet stain
    G. test

GPKA
    guinea pig kidney absorption (test)

GRA
    gonadotropin-releasing agent

gradient
    electrochemical g.

Graham-Cole test

Gram-Sure reagent

Gram-Weigert stain

Granger method

granoplasm

granulation
    Bright's g.
    cell g.
    Reilly g.
    Virchow's g.

granule
    acidophil g.
    acrosomal g.
    albuminous g.
    aleuronoid g.
    alpha g.
    amphophil g.
    argentaffin g.
    atrial g.
    Babès-Ernst g.
    basophil g.
    beta g.
    Birbeck g.
    Bollinger's g.
    Bütschli's g.
    chromaffin g.

granule (*continued*)
    chromatic g.
    chromophilic g.
    cone g.
    cortical g.
    cytoplasmic g.
    Ehrlich's g.
    Ehrlich-Heinz g.
    fuchsinophil g.
    Fordyce's g.
    Heinz g.
    iodophil g.
    juxtaglomerular g.
    keratohyalin g.
    Kölliker's interstitial g.
    Kretz' g.
    lamellar g.
    Langerhans g.
    membrane-coating g.
    metachromatic g.
    Much's g.
    Nissl's g.
    oxyphil g.
    Paschen's g.
    perichromatin g.
    proacrosomal g.
    rod g.
    Schrön's g.
    Schrön-Much g.
    Schüffner's g.
    seminal g.
    specific atrial g.
    sphere g.
    sulfur g.
    thread g.
    toxic g.
    trichohyalin g.
    vermiform g.
    volutin g.

granuloadipose

granulocorpuscle

granulocyte-erythroid ratio (G/E)

granulocyte-macrophage
   colony-stimulating factor (GM-CSF)

granulocytopathy

granulocytopenia

granulocytosis

granulofatty

granuloma
    actinic g.
    amebic g.
    g. annulare
    beryllium g.
    Candida g.
    candidal g.
    cholesterol g.
    eosinophilic g.
    g. fissuratum
    foreign-body g.
    g. gangraenescens
    giant cell reparative g.,
      central
    g. gluteale infantum
    laryngeal g.
    lethal midline g.
    lipoid g.
    lipophagic g.
    Majocchi's g.
    malarial g.
    midline g.
    Miescher's g.
    Mignon's eosinophilic g.
    monilial g.
    g. multiforme
    plasma cell g.
    pyogenic g.
    g. pyogenicum
    rheumatic g.
    sarcoid g.
    silicotic g.
    swimming pool g.
    g. telangiectaticum
    trichophytic g.
    g. trichophyticum
    xanthomatous g.
    zirconium g.

granulomatosis
    allergic g.
    bronchocentric g.

granulomatosis (*continued*)
    g. disciformis progressiva et chronica
    eosinophilic g.
    Langerhans cell g.
    lipophagic intestinal g.
    lymphomatoid g.
    necrotizing sarcoid g.
    necrotizing sarcoidal g.
    g. siderotica
    Wegener's g.

granulomatous

granulopenia

granuloplasm

granuloplastic

granulopotent

granulosa

granulosis
    g. rubra nasi

granulovacuolar degeneration

graphitosis

graphospasm

graviditas
    g. examnialis
    g. exochorialis

gravidocardiac

gravimeter

gravimetric

Gravindex pregnany test

gravitometer

Gravlee jet wash

gray
    silver g.
    steel g.

green
    acid g.
    bromcresol g.
    diazin g. S

green (*continued*)
    fast g. FCF
    fast acid g. N
    Hoffman g.
    iodine g.
    Janus g. B
    light g., 2 G or 2 GN
    light g. SF
    light g. SF yellowish
    malachite g.
    methyl g.
    methylene g.
    Victoria g.

GRF
    gonadotropin-releasing factor
    growth hormone-releasing factor

GRH
    growth hormone-releasing hormone

Gridley stain for fungi

grippe
    g. aurique

groove
    Harrison g.
    nail g.

growth
    accretionary g.
    balanced g.
    new g.

Gruber-Widel reaction

grumose

grumous

gryochrome

gryphosis

gryposis
    g. penis

GSC
    gas-solid chromatography
    gravity-settling culture

GSD
    genetically significant dose

GSE
    gluten-sensitive enteropathy

GSR
    galvanic skin response
    generalized Shwartzman
      reaction

GSSR
    generalized Sanarelli-
      Shwartzman reaction

GTH
    gonadotropic hormone

GTT
    glucose tolerance test

guaiac test

guanidinemia

Gulf War syndrome

gumboil

Gumprecht shadow

Gunning-Lieben test

Gutman unit

guttate

gutturotetany

Gutzeit test

GVH
    graft-verus-host
      GVH disease
      GVH reaction

gymnocyte

gymnoplast

gynander

gynandria

gynandrism

gynandroid

gynandromorph

gynandromorphism
    bilateral g.

gynandromorphous

gynandry

gynatresia

gynecopathy

gynesin

gynopathic

gynopathy

gyrospasm

H

H
    Hauch (motile
        microorganism)
    Holzknecht unit
    Hounsfield unit
    hypermetropia
        H agglutination
        H agglutinin
        H antigen
        H chain
        H colony
        cytolipin H
        H and E staining
H-2
    H-2 antigen
    H-2 complex
HA
    hemagglutinating antibody
HA1 virus
HA2 virus
HAA
    hepatitis-associated antigen
Haagensen test
Habermann disease
Haber syndrome
habit
    endothelioid h.
    glaucomatous h.
    leukocytoid h.
Hadfield-Clarke syndrome
haemozoin
Haenszel test
Haffkine vaccine
hafnium
Hahn oxine reagent
HAHTG
    horse antihuman thymus
        globulin

HAI
    hemagglutination inhibition
    hemagglutinin inhibition
Halberstaedter-Prowazek body
Haldane effect
Hale colloidal iron stain
half-life
    drug half-life
half-value layer (HVL)
halisteresis
    h. cerea
halisteretic
hallux
    h. dolorosus
    h. flexus
    h. malleus
    h. rigidus
    h. valgus
    h. varus
halodermia
halogenated hydrocarbon
    assay
halometer
Halon system
haloperidol
    h. assay
halosteresis
halothane
    h. assay
    h. hepatitis
halzoun
HAM-56
    human alveolar
        macrophage-56
        HAM-56 antibody
hamartoma

hamartoma (*continued*)
    cystic adenoid pulmonary h.
    fibrous h. of infancy
    perobiliary gland h.
    pulmonary h.

hamartomatosis
    systemic h.

Hammersten
    H. reagent
    H. test

Hammerschlag method

Ham test

HANE
    hereditary angioneurotic
        edema

Hanger test

hanging-block culture

Hanker-Yates reagent

Hansel stain

Hansemann macrophage

HAP
    heredopathia atactia
        polyneiritiformis

HAPA
    hemagglutinating anti-
        penicillin antibody

haphalgesia

haplomycosis

haplopathy

haplophase

haptenic grouping

harderoporphyria

Hardy-Weinberg law

Harleco synthetic resin

Hartmann solution

HASHD
    hypertensive ateriosclerotic
        heart disease

hashitoxicosis

HATTS
    hemagglutination
        treponemal test for
        syphilis

hawkinsin

hawkinsinuria

HB
    heart block

HCC
    heptacellular carcinoma
    hydroxycholecalciferol

HCP
    hepatocatalase perioxidase
    hereditary coproporphyria

HDCV
    human diploid cell rabies
        vaccine

HDN
    hemolytic disease of
        newborn

HDRA assay

HDW
    reticulocyte hemoglobin
        distribution width

hearing
    double disharmonic h.
    monaural h.

heart
    armored h.
    armour h.
    beer h.
    beriberi h.
    boat-shaped h.
    bony h.
    bovine h.
    chaotic h.
    dynamite h.
    encased h.
    fat h.
    fatty h.
    fibroid h.

heart (*continued*)
   flask-shaped h.
   frosted h.
   hairy h.
   horizontal h.
   hyperthyroid h.
   hypoplastic h.
   icing h.
   myxedema h.
   ox h.
   parchment h.
   sabot h.
   stone h.
   tabby cat h.
   three-chambered h.
   thrush breast h.
   tiger h.
   tiger lily h.
   triatrial h.
   trilocular h.
   vertical h.

HEAT
   human erythrocyte
      agglutination test

hecatomeral

hecatomeric

Heidenhain
   H. azan stain
   H. iron hematoxylin stain

Hektoen enteric agar

helcoid

helcology

helcoma

helcosis

heliosis

Helisal rapid blood test

helium equilibration time (HET)

helminth
   h. identification procedure

heloma
   h. durum
   h. molle

helosis

hemachromatosis

hemadostenosis

hemadsorbent

hemadsorption

hemalum

hemangiectasia

hemangiectasis

hemangioblast

hemangioblastoma

hemangioblastomatosis

hemangioendothelioma
   infantile h.

hemangiofibroma

hemangioma
   capillary h.
   cavernous h.
   h. simplex
   strawberry h.
   venous h.

hemangiomatosis
   disseminated h.

hemangiopericyte

hemapheic

hemaphein

hemapheism

hemarthros

hemarthrosis

hemastrontium

hematapostema

hematemesis
   Goldstein's h.

hematencephalon

Hematest

hematherapy

hematothorax

hematidrosis

hematimeter

hematinemia

hematinuria

hematobilia

hematocele
    parametric h.
    pelvic h.
    retrouterine h.
    scrotal h.
    vaginal h.

hematocelia

hematocephalus

hematochezia

hematochromatosis

hematochyluria

hematocoelia

hematocolpometra

hematocolpos

hematocyst

hematocystis

hematocytolysis

hematocytopenia

hematocyturia

hematohidrosis

hematohyaloid

hematokolpos

hematolysis

hematolytic

hematomediastinum

hematometra

hematomyelia

hematomyelitis

hematomyelopore

hematonephrosis

hematopathology

hematopenia

hematopericardium

hematoperitoneum

hematophilia

hempatopneic index

hematoporphyrinemia

hematoporphyrinism

hematoporphyrinuria

hematorrhachis

hematosalpinx

hematoscheocele

hematosepsis

hematospermatocele

hematospermia

hematospectrocope

hematospectroscopy

hematostatic

hematosteon

hematothorax

hematotoxic

hematotoxicosis

hematotrachelos

hematotympanum

hematoxic

hematoxylin
    alum h.
    Delafield's h.
    iron h.

hematozemia

hematuresis

hematuria

hemeralope

hemeralopia

Hemerocampa

hemiachromatopsia

hemiageusia

hemiageustia

hemialbumin

hemialbumose

hemialbumosuria

hemialgia

hemiamblyopia

hemiamyosthenia

hemianacusia

hemianalgesia

hemianesthesia

hemianopia

hemianopic

hemianopsia

hemianoptic

hemianosmia

hemiapraxia

hemiarthrosis

hemiasomatognosia

hemiasynergia

hemiataxia

hemiataxy

hemiathetosis

hemiatrophy
   facial h.
   progressive lingual h.

hemiballism

hemiballismus

hemicanities

hemicardia

hemichorea

hemichromatopsia

hemichrome

hemicrania
   chronic paroxysmal h.

hemicraniosis

hemidesmosome

hemidiaphoresis

hemidrosis

hemidysergia

hemidysesthesia

hemidystrophy

hemiepilepsy

hemigeusia

hemighost

hemigigantism

hemiglossitis

hemignathia

hemihidrosis

hemihypalgesia

hemihyperesthesia

hemihyperhidrosis

hemihypermetria

hemihyperplasia

hemihypertonia

hemihypertrophy
   facial h.

hemihypesthesia

hemihypoesthesia

hemihypometria

hemihypoplasia

hemihypotonia

hemikaryon

hemimacroglossia

hemineglect

hemiobesity

hemiopalgia

hemiopia

hemiopic

hemiparalysis

hemiparaplegia

hemiparesis

hemiparesthesia

hemiparetic

hemiparkinsonism

hemiplegia
   h. alternans hypoglossica
   alternate h.
   alternating oculomotor h.
   ascending h.
   capsular h.
   cerebral h.
   contralateral h.
   crossed h.
   h. cruciata
   facial h.
   faciobrachial h.
   faciolingual h.
   flaccid h.
   Gubler's h.
   infantile h.
   puerperal h.
   spastic h.
   spinal h.
   Wernicke-Mann h.

hemipyonephrosis

hemirachischisis

hemisacralization

hemiscotosis

hemispasm

hemisphygmia

hemisyndrome

hemitetany

hemithermoanesthesia

hemithorax

hemitonia

hemitremor

hemivagotony

hemivertebra

hemobilia

hemobilinuria

hemocatheresis

Hemoccult

hemocholecyst

hemocholecystitis

hemochromatosis
   acquired h.
   genetic h.
   hereditary h.
   idiopathic h.
   neonatal h.
   perinatal h.
   secondary h.

hemochromatotic

hemoclasis

hemoclastic

hemoconcentration

hemoconiosis

HemaCue glucose meter

hemocytocatheresis

hemocytotripsis

hemodiagnosis

hemodiapedesis

hemodilution

hemodystrophy

hemofuscin

hemoglobin
  h. anti-Lepore
  h. Bart's
  h. C
  h. Chesapeake
  h. Constant Spring
  crossover h.
  h. D
  h. E
  h. G
  h. Gun Hill
  h. H
  h. I
  h. Kansas
  h. Kenya
  h. Köln
  h. Lepore
  h. M
  h. Rainier
  h. S
  h. Seattle
  unstable h.
  h. Yakima

hemoglobinemia

hemoglobinocholia

hemoglobinopathy

hemoglobinuria
  march h.
  paroxysmal cold h.
  paroxysmal nocturnal h.

hemoglobinuric

hemolysate

hemolysin
  bacterial h.
  heterophile h.
  hot-cold h.

hemolysis
  colloid osmotic h.
  contact h.
  venom h.

hemolytic

hemolyzable

hemolyzation

hemolyze

hemomediastinum

hemometra

hemonephrosis

hemopathic

hemopathology

hemopathy

hemopericardium

hemoperitoneum

hemophilia
  h. A
  h. B
  h. B, Leyden
  h. C
  classical h.
  vascular h.

hemophiliac

hemophilic

hemophilioid

hemophthalmia

hemophthalmos

hemophthalmus

hemophthisis

hemopleura

hemopneumopericardium

hemopneumothorax

hemoproctia

hemoptoic

hemoptysic

hemoptysis

hemopyelectasis

HemoQuant fecal blood test

hemorrhachis

hemorrhage
  alveolar h.
  arterial h.
  brain h.
  capillary h.
  capsuloganglionic h.
  cerebral h.
  concealed h.
  Duret's h.
  expulsive h.
  external h.
  extradural h.
  fetomaternal h.
  fibrinolytic h.
  flame-shaped h.
  internal h.
  intracerebral h.
  intracranial h.
  intramedullary h.
  intrapartum h.
  intraventricular h.
  massive h.
  nasal h.
  parenchymatous h.
  h. per rhexin
  petechial h.
  postpartum h.
  pulmonary h.
  punctate h.
  renal h.
  splinter h.
  spontaneous h.
  subarachnoid h.
  subdural h.
  venous h.

hemorrhagenic

hemorrhagic

hemosalpinx

hemosiderinuria test

hemosiderosis
  hepatic h.
  pulmonary h.

hemospermia

hemotherapy

hemothorax

hemotoxic

hemotympanum

hemozoin

HEMPAS

hereditary erythrocytic
  multinuclearity with positive
  acidified serum
    HEMPAS cell

hemuresis

Henderson-Hasselbalch
  equation

HEPA
  high-efficiency particulate
  air (filter)
    HEPA filter

hepar
  h. adiposum
  h. lobatum

heparinemia

hepatalgia

hepatatrophia

hepatatrophy

hepatic phosphorylase
  deficiency

hepatic phosphorylase kinase
  deficiency

hepatism

hepatitides

hepatitis
  h. A
  acute parenchymatous h.
  alcoholic h.
  alcohollike h.
  amebic h.
  anicteric h.
  autoimmune h.

hepatitis (*continued*)
    h. B
    h. C
    cholangiolitic h.
    cholangitic h.
    cholestatic h.
    chronic active h.
    chronic aggressive h.
    chronic interstitial h.
    chronic persisting h.
    h. D
    delta h.
    h. E
    enterically transmitted
      non-A, non-B h.
    epidemic h.
    familial h.
    fatty liver h.
    fulminant h.
    h. G
    giant cell h.
    homologous serum h.
    infectious h.
    inoculation h.
    La Brea h.
    long-incubation h.
    lupoid h.
    MS-1 h.
    MS-2 h.
    neonatal h.
    neonatal giant cell h.
    non-A, non-B h.
    plasma cell h.
    post-transfusion h.
    pseudoalcoholic h.
    serum h.
    short-incubation h.
    subacute h.
    syncytial giant-cell h.
    toxic h.
    transfusion h.
    viral h.

hepatization
    gray h.
    red h.
    yellow h.

hepatocele

hepatocellular

hepatocholangeitis

hepatocholangitis

hepatocirrhosis

hepatocyte
    ground-glass h.

hepatodynia

hepatoid

heptojugular reflux

hepatolienomegaly

hepatolith

hepatolithiasis

hepatolysis

hepatolytic

hepatomalacia

hepatomegalia

hepatomegaly

hepatomelanosis

hepatomphalocele

hepatomphalos

hepatonephritic

hepatonephritis

hepatonephromegaly

hepatopath

hepatopathy

hepatoperitonitis

hepatophlebitis

hepatoptosis

hepatorrhagia

hepatorrhea

hepatorrhexis

hepatosis
   serous h.

hepatosplenitis

hepatosplenomegaly

hepatosplenopathy

hepatotoxic

hepatotoxicity

hepatotoxin

hepatoxic

heptosuria

heredoataxia

heredodegeneration

heredodiathesis

heredoinfection

heredolues

heredoluetic

heredopathia
   h. atactica polyneuritiformis

heredoretinopathia congenita

heredosyphilis

heredosyphilitic

Hermann fixative

hernia
   abdominal h.
   acquired h.
   h. adiposa
   axial hiatal h.
   Barth's h.
   Béclard's h.
   Birkett's h.
   Bochdalek's h.
   cecal h.
   cerebral h.
   h. cerebri
   Cloquet's h.
   complete h.
   concealed h.
   congenital h.

hernia (*continued*)
   Cooper's h.
   crural h.
   diaphragmatic h.
   diaphragmatic h.,
     congenital
   direct h.
   direct inguinal h.
   diverticular h.
   dry h.
   duodenojejunal h.
   encysted h.
   epigastric h.
   external h.
   extrasaccular h.
   fat h.
   femoral h.
   foraminal h.
   gastroesophageal h.
   Grynfeltt h.
   Hesselbach's h.
   Hey's h.
   hiatal h.
   hiatus h.
   Holthouse's h.
   incarcerated h.
   incisional h.
   incomplete h.
   indirect h.
   indirect inguinal h.
   infantile h.
   inguinal h.
   inguinocrural h.
   inguinofemoral h.
   inguinoproperitoneal h.
   inguinosuperficial h.
   intermuscular h.
   internal h.
   interparietal h.
   intersigmoid h.
   interstitial h.
   intra-abdominal h.
   intraperitoneal h.
   h. of the iris
   irreducible h.
   ischiatic h.
   ischiorectal h.
   Krönlein's h.

hernia (*continued*)
    labial h.
    labial h., posterior
    Laugier's h.
    levator h.
    Littre's h.
    lumbar h.
    mesenteric h.
    mesentericoparietal h.
    mesocolic h.
    Morgagni's h.
    oblique h.
    obturator h.
    omental h.
    ovarian h.
    pantaloon h.
    paraduodenal h.
    paraesophageal h.
    paraperitoneal h.
    parasaccular h.
    parietal h.
    pectineal h.
    perineal h.
    Petit's h.
    prevascular h.
    properitoneal h.
    pudendal h.
    pulsion h.
    rectovaginal h.
    reducible h.
    retrocecal h.
    retrograde h.
    retroperitoneal h.
    retrovascular h.
    Richter's h.
    Rieux's h.
    Rokitansky's h.
    rolling h.
    sciatic h.
    scrotal h.
    Serafini's h.
    sliding h.
    sliding hiatal h.
    slip h.
    slipped h.
    spigelian h.
    strangulated h.
    synovial h.

hernia (*continued*)
    tonsillar h.
    Treitz's h.
    umbilical h.
    h. uteri inguinalis
    uterine h.
    vaginal h.
    vaginal h., posterior
    vaginolabial h.
    Velpeau's h.
    ventral h.
    vesical h.
    w h.
    parahiatal h.

hernioid

herpangina

herpes
    h. blattae
    h. corneae
    h. gestationis
    ocular h.
    h. ophthalmicus
    h. zoster auricularis
    h. zoster ophthalmicus
    h. zoster oticus

herpetiform

HET
    helium equilibration time

heterauxesis

heteroalbumose

heteroalbumosuria

heterochromatosis

heterochromia
    heterochromia iridis

heterochromous

heterochylia

heterodesmotic

heterogamete

heterogametic sex

heterogamety

heterogeusia

heteroglobulose

heterokaryon

heterokaryosis

heterokinesis

heterolith

heterologous

heterology

heterolysosome

heteromeral

heteromeric

heteromerous

heterometaplasia

heterometropia

heteropancreatism

heteropathy

heterophagosome

heterophagy

heterophany

heterophil
    h. antibody test
    h. antigen reaction
    h. hemolysin

heterophilic leukocyte

heterophoralgia

heterophoria

heterophoric

heterophthalmia

heterophthalmos

heteroplasia

heteroplasm

heteroplastic

heteroploid

heteroploidy

heteropodal

heteropsia

heteroptics

heterosmia

heterotaxia

heterotaxic

heterotaxis

heterotaxy

heterotonia

heterotonic

heterotopia

heterotopic

heterotopy

heterotrichosis
    h. superciliorum

heterotrophia

heterotrophy

heterotropia

heterotropy

Hexapoda

hexavalent

hexokinase method

hexosazone

hexuronate

hexuronic acid

HF
    Hageman factor
    heart failure
    hemorrhagic fever

HFI
    hereditary fructose
        intolerance

HFR strain

HGF
    hyperglycermic-
        glycogenolytic fever

HHF-35
    muscle-specific actin
        HHF-35 stain

hiatal hernia

Hicks-Pitney thromboplastin
    generation test

hidradenitis
    h. axillaris
    h. suppurativa

hidrosadenitis

hidroschesis

high-molecular-weight
    neutrophil chemotactic factor

high-performance liquid
    chromatography

high-pressure liquid
    chromatography (HPLC)·

high-resolution banding

Higoumenakia sign

hillock
    axon h.

Hill equation

himantosis

Hine-Duley phantom

Hinfl solution

Hinton test

hippurate

hippuria

hippuric acid

hippus

Hirsch-Peiffer stain

hirsuties

hirsutism

Hiss stain

Histalog test

histaminemia

histamine-releasing factor

histanoxia

histidinemia

histidinuria

histiocyte
    cardiac h.
    sea-blue h.

histiocytomatosis

histiocytosis
    Langerhans cell h.
    Langerhans cell h., acute
        disseminated
    Langerhans cell h.,
        multifocal
    Langerhans cell h., unifocal
    sea-blue h.
    sinus h.
    sinus h. with massive
        lymphadenopathy
    h. X

histochemical stain

histochemistry

Histoclad

Histoclear slide processing
    solution

histoculture drug response
    assay (HDRA assay)

histodiagnosis

histodialysis

Histofine staining solution

histogram mode

histohydria

histohypoxia

histology
    pathologic h.

histolysate

histolysis

histolytic

histometaplastic

histoplasmin-latex test

histonuria

histopathology

histoplasmoma

histoplasmosis
    ocular h.

historadiography

historetention

historrhexis

HIT
    hemagglutination-inhibition
        test
    heparin-induced
        thrombocytopenia
    hypertrophic infiltrative
        tendinitis

Hitachi 704 analyzer

HIVAGEN test

HLA-B27

hLT
    human lymphocyte
        transformation

Hm
    manifest hyperopia

HMPS
    hexose monophosphate
        shunt

HOCM
    hypertropic obstructive
        cardiomyopathy

HOECHST 33258

Hofmeister test

Hogben test

holarthritic

holarthritis

Hollander test

Hollenhorst plaque

Hollerith code

hollow cathode lamp

holorachischisis

holoschisis

Holzer method

Holzknecht unit (H)

homeochrome

homeokinesis

homeopathic symbol for
    decimal scale of potencies
    (X)

homeoplasia

homeoplastic

Homer-Wright rosette

homme rouge

homobrachial inversion

homocarnosinosis

homocitrullinuria

homocystinemia

homocystinuria

homodesmotic

homogamete

homogametic sex

homogeneously staining region

homogentisate

homogentisic acid

homogentisic acid oxidase
    deficiency

homogentisuria

homoiopodal

homomorphic

homotopic transplantation

homotransplantation

homotropism

homovanillic acid

homunculus

Hooke law

Hooker-Forbes test

Hopkins-Cole test

Hoppe-Seyler test

hordeolum
    external h.
    internal h.

Horie tumor classification

horizontal transmission

HORM collagen reagent

hormone
    adrenocorticotropic h.
    adrenomedullary h.
    anterior pituitary h. (APH)
    chromatophorotropic h.
    h. demonstration in tissue
    follicule-stimulating h.
      (FSH)
    gonadotropin hormone-
      releasing h.
    interstitial cell-stimulating h.
    melanocyte-inhibiting h.
    prolactin release-inhibiting
      h.
    TSH-releasing h.

hormonoprivia

hormonosis
    exogenous h.

horn
    cicatricial h.

hortobezoar

Hospidex microtiter plate

hospital-acquired penetration
    contact

Hotchkiss-McManus PAS
    technique

Hottentot apron

Howard test

HPF
    heparin-precipitable
      fraction
    high-power field

HPLC
    high-pressure liquid
      chromatography

HRS
    Hamilton Rating Scale

Hüfner equation

Huhner test

humor
    plasmoid h.

Hunter-Schreger line

HUS
    hyaluronidase unit for
      semen

HUTHAS
    human thymus antiserum

HVA
    homovanillic acid
      HVA test

HVSD
    hydrogen-detected
      ventricular septal defect

hyalin
    alcoholic h.
    hematogenous h.

hyalinization
    Crooke's h.

hyalnized stroma

hyalinosis
    h. cutis et mucosae

hyalinuria

hyalitis
    asteroid h.
    h. punctata
    punctate h.
    h. suppurativa
    suppurative h.

hyalogen

hyaloiditis

hyalomitome

hyaloplasm
    nuclear h.

hyaloserositis
    progressive multiple h.

hyalosis
    asteroid h.

hyalosome

hyalotome

Hybond-N-filter

Hybond N+ nylon membrane

hybridization
    somatic cell h.

Hybritech PSA determination
    system

hydatid

hydatidiform

hydatiduria

hydradenitis

hydraeroperitoneum

hydragogue

hydramnion

hydramnios

hydrarthrodial

hydrarthrosis
    intermittent h.

hydrazine-sensitive factor

hydremia

hydrencephalocele

hydrencephalomeningocele

hydrencephalus

hydrencephaly

hydrepigastrium

hydrindicuria

hydroa
    h. estivale
    h. vacciniforme

hydroadipsia

hydroappendix

hydroblepharon

hydrocalycosis

hydrocalyx

hydrocele
    cervical h.
    chylous h.
    h. colli
    communicating h.
    congenital h.
    diffused h.
    Dupuytren's h.
    encysted h.
    h. feminae
    funicular h.
    hernial h.
    Maunoir's h.
    h. of neck
    h. renalis
    scrotal h.
    h. spinalis

hydrocephalic

hydrocephalocele

hydrocephaloid

hydrocephalus
    acquired h.
    communicating h.

hydrocephalus (*continued*)
    congenital h.
    noncommunicating h.
    normal-pressure h.
    normal-pressure occult h.
    obstructive h.
    occult normal-pressure h.
    otitic h.
    posthemorrhagic h.
    primary h.
    secondary h.
    tension h.
    h. ex vacuo

hydrocephaly

hydrocholecystis

hydrocirsocele

hydrocolpos

hydrocyanism

hydrocyst

hydrocytosis

hydrodipsomania

hydrodiuresis

hydroencephalocele

hydrogen-detected ventricular spetal defect (HVSD)

hydrohematonephrosis

hydrohymenitis

hydroma

hydromeningitis

hydromeningocele

hydrometer scale

hydrometra

hydrometrocolpos

hydromphalus

hydromyelia

hydromyelocele

hydromyelomeningocele

hydroparotitis

hydropenia

hydropenic

hydropericarditis

hydropericardium

hydroperinephrosis

hydroperitoneum

hydroperitonia

hydrophilic gel

hydrophthalmia

hydrophthalmos
    h. anterior
    h. posterior
    h. totalis

hydrophthalmus

hydrophysometra

hydropic

hydroplasma

hydropneumatosis

hydropneumopericardium

hydropneumoperitoneum

hydropneumothorax

hydrops
    h. ad matulam
    h. amnii
    h. articuli
    endolymphatic h.
    fetal h.
    h. fetalis
    h. fetalis, immune
    h. fetalis, nonimmune
    h. folliculi
    h. labyrinthi
    labyrinthine h.
    h. spurius
    h. tubae
    h. tubae profluens

hydropyonephrosis

hydrorachis

hydrorrhea
  h. gravidarum

hydrosalpinx
  h. follicularis
  intermittent h.
  h. simplex

hydrosarcocele

hydrosyringomyelia

hydrothionemia

hydrothionuria

hydrothorax
  chylous h.

hydroureter

hydroureteronephrosis

hydroureterosis

hydrouria

hydrovarium

hydroxybutyric acid
  3- h. acid
  4- h. acid
  β- h. acid
  γ-hydroxybutyric acid

4-hydroxybutyricaciduria

γ-hydroxybutyricaciduria

hydroxyformobenzoylic acid

hydroxyglutaric acid

3-hydroxyisovaleric acid

11β-hydroxylase deficiency

17α-hydroxylase deficiency

18-hydroxylase deficiency

21-hydroxylase deficiency

3-hydroxy-3-methylglutaric acid

3-hydroxy-3-
  methylglutaricaciduria

hydroxyprolinemia

3β-hydroxysteroid
  dehydrogenase deficiency

11β-hydroxysteroid
  dehydrogenase deficiency

17β-hydroxysteroid
  dehydrogenase deficiency

hydruria

hydruric

hygroma
  h. colli
  h. praepatellare
  subdural h.

hygromatous

hymenitis

hypacusia

hypacusis

hypalbuminemia

hypalgesia

hypalgesic

hypalgetic

hypalgia

hypamnion

hypamnios

hypanakinesia

hypanakinesis

hypazoturia

hyperabsorption

hyperacanthosis

hyperacidaminuria

hyperacousia

hyperacusia

hyperacusis

hyperacute rejection

hyperadenosis

hyperadrenalism

hyperadrenocorticism

hyperaeration
    focal pulmonary h.

hyperakusis

hyper-β-alaninemia

hyperalbuminemia

hyperalbuminosis

hyperaldosteronemia

hyperaldosteronism

hyperaldosteronuria

hyperalgesia
    auditory h.
    muscular h.

hyperalgesic

hyperalgetic

hyperalgia

hyperalimentosis

hyperallantoinuria

hyperalonemia

hyperalphalipoproteinemia
    familial h.

hyperaminoacidemia

hyperaminoaciduria

hyper-β-aminoisobutyricaciduria

hyperammonemia
    cerebroatrophic h.

hyperammonuria

hyperamylasemia

hyperanacinesia

hyperanakinesia

hyperandrogenism

hyperaphia

hyperaphic

hyperargininemia

hyperazotemia

hyperazoturia

hyperbasophilic

hyperbetalipoproteinemia
    familial h.

hyperbicarbonatemia

hyperbilirubinemia
    h. I
    congenital h.
    conjugated h.
    constitutional h.
    neonatal h.
    unconjugated h.

hyperbradykininemia

hyperbradykininism

hypercalcemia
    familial hypocalciuric h.
    idiopathic h.

hypercalcinemia

hypercalcinuria

hypercalcipexy

hypercalcitoninemia

hypercalciuria
    absorptive h.

hypercapnia

hypercapnic

hypercarbia

hypercarotenemia

hypercatabolism

hypercatharsis

hypercathartic

hypercellularity

hyperchloremia

hyperchloremic

hyperchlorhydria

hyperchloruration

hyperchloruria

hypercholesteremia

hypercholesterolemia
   familial h.
   polygenic h.

hypercholesterolemic

hypercholesterolia

hypercholia

hyperchondroplasia

hyperchromaffinism

hyperchromasia

hyperchromatic

hyperchromatin

hyperchromatism

hyperchromatosis

hyperchromia

hyperchromic

hyperchylia

hyperchylomicronemia
   familial h.
   familial h. with
     hyperprebetalipo-
     proteinemia

hypercinesia

hypercoagulability

hypercoagulable

hypercoria

hypercorticalism

hypercorticism

hypercortisolism

hypercreatinemia

hypercryalgesia

hypercryesthesia

hypercupremia

hypercupriuria

hypercyanotic

hypercythemia

hypercytochromia

hypercytosis

hyperdiploid

hyperdipsia

hyperdiuresis

hyperdynamia
   h. uteri

hypereccrisia

hypereccrisis

hypereccritic

hyperelectrolytemia

hyperemia
   collateral h.
   passive h.
   reactive h.
   venous h.

hypereosinophilia

hyperepinephrinemia

hyperequilibrium

hypererythrocythemia

hyperesophoria

hyperesthesia
   acoustic h.
   auditory h.
   cerebral h.
   gustatory h.
   muscular h.
   olfactory h.

hyperesthesia (*continued*)
  oneiric h.
  optic h.
  tactile h.

hyperesthetic

hyperestrogenemia

hyperestrogenism

hyperestrogenosis

hyperevolutism

hyperexcretory

hyperexophoria

hyperexplexia

hyperferremia

hyperferremic

hyperferricemia

hyperfibrinogenemia

hyperflexion

hypergalactia

hypergalactosis

hypergalactous

hypergammaglobulinemia
  monoclonal h.
  polyclonal h.

hypergastrinemia

hypergenesis

hypergenetic

hypergenitalism

hypergeusesthesia

hypergeusia

hyperglandular

hyperglobulinemia

hyperglucagonemia

hyperglycemia
  rebound h.

hyperglycemic

hyperglycemic-glycogenolytic
  factor

hyperglyceridemia

hyperglyceridemic

hyperglycerolemia

hyperglycinemia
  ketotic h.
  nonketotic h.

hyperglycinuria

hyperglycistia

hyperglycogenolysis

hyperglycorrhachia

hyperglycosemia

hyperglycosuria

hyperglycystia

hypergonadism

hypergonadotropic

hyperguanidinemia

hyperhemoglobinemia

hyperheparinemia

hyperhepatia

hyperhidrosis
  axillary h.
  emotional h.
  h. unilateralis
  volar h.
  palmar h.

hyperhidrotic

hyperhydration

hyperhydrochloria

hyperhydrochloridia

hyperhydroxyprolinemia

hyperidrosis

hyperimidodipeptiduria

hyperimmunoglobulinemia
   h. E

hyperinsulinar

hyperinsulinemia

hyperinsulinism

hyperinvolution

hyperiodemia

hyperirritability

hyperkalemia

hyperkaliemia

hyperkeratinization

hyperkeratosis

hyperketonemia

hyperketonuria

hyperketosis

hyperkinemia

hyperkinesia

hyperkinesis

hyperkinetic

hyperkoria

hyperlactacidemia

hyperlactation

hyperlecithinemia

hyperleptinemia

hyperleukocytosis

hyperleydigism

hyperlipemia
   carbohydrate-induced h.
   combined fat- and
     carbohydrate-induced h.
   endogenous h.
   essential familial h.
   exogenous h.
   familial fat-induced h.
   mixed h.

hyperlipidemia
   combined h.
   familial combined h.
   mixed h.
   multiple lipoprotein-type h.
   remnant h.

hyperlipidemic

hyperlipoproteinemia
   acquired h.
   familial h.

hyperliposis

hyperlithemia

hyperlithic

hyperlithuria

hyperlordosis

hyperluteinization

hyperlysinemia

hypermagnesemia

hypermastia

hypermelanosis

hypermelanotic

hypermenorrhea

hypermetamorphosis

hypermetaplasia

hypermethioninemia

hypermetria

hypermetrope

hypermetropia

hypermineralization

hypermobility

hypermorph

hypermotility

hypermyotonia

hypermyotrophy

hypernatremia
   hypodipsic h.

hypernatremic

hypernatronemia

hyperneocytosis

hypernitremia

hyperonychia

hyperope

hyperopia

hyperopic

hyperorchidism

hyperorexia

hyperornithinemia

hyperorthocytosis

hyperosmia

hyperosmolality

hyperosmolarity

hyperosphresia

hyperosteogeny

hyperostosis
   h. corticalis deformans
      juvenilis
   h. corticalis generalisata
   h. cranii
   flowing h.
   h. frontalis interna
   infantile cortical h.
   senile ankylosing h. of
      spine

hyperostotic

hyperovarianism

hyperovarism

hyperoxaluria
   enteric h.
   primary h.

hyperoxemia

hyperoxia

hyperoxic

hyperpallesthesia

hyperpancreorrhea

hyperparathyroidism
   primary h.
   secondary h.
   tertiary h.

hyperpathia

hyperpepsia

hyperpepsinemia

hyperpepsinia

hyperpepsinuria

hyperperistalsis

hyperpermeability

hyperpexia

hyperpexy

hyperphagic

hyperphenylalaninemia
   malignant h.
   maternal h.
   persistent h.
   transient h.

hyperphoria

hyperphosphatasemia
   chronic congenital
      idiopathic h.
   h. tarda

hyperphosphatasia

hyperphosphatemia

hyperphosphaturia

hyperphosphoremia

hyperpigmentation

hyperpinealism

hyperpipecolatemia

hyperpituitarism

hyperplasia
    adenomatous h.
    adrenal h., congenital
    adrenal h., lipoid
    adrenal h., nodular
    adrenal cortical h.
    adrenocortical h.
    adrenocortical h., nodular
    chronic perforating pulp h.
    endometrial h.
    h. endometrii
    fibrous inflammatory h.
    follicular h.
    focal nodular h.
    giant follicular h.
    giant lymph node h.
    inflammatory h.
    intimal h.
    juxtaglomerular cell h.
    lipoid h.
    lymphoid h.
    neoplastic h.
    nodular lymphoid h.
    nodular h. of the prostate
    nodular regenerative h.
    ovarian stromal h.
    benign prostatic h.
    pseudoepitheliomatous h.
    Swiss-cheese h.

hyperplasmia

hyperploid

hyperploidy

hyperpnea

hyperpneic

hyperpolypeptidemia

hyperponesis

hyperponetic

hyperposia

hyperpotassemia

hyperpraxia

hyperprebetalipoproteinemia
    familial h.

hyperpresbyopia

hyperproinsulinemia

hyperprolactinemia

hyperprolactinemic

hyperprolinemia

hyperproteinemia

hyperproteosis

hyperpselaphesia

hyperptyalism

hyperpyremia

hyperpyretic

hyperpyrexia

hyperpyrexial

hyperreactio luteinalis

hyperreflexia
    autonomic h.
    detrusor h.

hyperreninemia

hyperreninemic

hyperresponsive

hypersalemia

hypersalivation

hypersarcosinemia

hypersecretion

hypersegmentation
    hereditary h. of neutrophils

hyperserotonemia

hypersomatotropism

hypersomia

hypersomnia

hypersomnolence

hypersphyxia

hypersplenia

hypersplenism

hyperspongiosis

hypersteatosis

hypersthenuria

hypersuprarenalism

hypersusceptibility

hypersympathicotonus

hypertarachia

hypertelorism
   ocular h.
   orbital h.

hyperthecosis

hyperthermal

hyperthermalgesia

hyperthermesthesia

hyperthermia
   h. of anesthesia
   malignant h.

hyperthermoesthesia

hyperthrombinemia

hyperthymism

hyperthyrea

hyperthyroidism
   iodine-induced h.
   masked h.

hyperthyroidosis

hyperthyroxinemia
   familial dysalbuminemic h.

hypertonia
   h. polycythaemica

hypertrichosis
   h. lanuginosa
   h. pinnae auris
   h. universalis

hypertriglyceridemia
   familial h.
   sporadic h.

hypertrophy
   adaptive h.
   asymmetrical septal h.
   Billroth h.
   compensatory h.
   concentric h.
   eccentric h.
   false h.
   hemifacial h.
   Marie's h.
   numeric h.
   benign prostatic h.
   pseudomuscular h.
   simple h.
   true h.
   unilateral h.
   ventricular h.
   vicarious h.

hypertropia

hypertyrosinemia

hyperuresis

hyperuricacidemia

hyperuricaciduria

hyperuricemia

hyperuricemic

hyperuricosuria

hyperuricuria

hypervalinemia

hypervariable region

hypervascular

hyperviscosity

hypervolemia

hypervolemic

hypervolia

hypesthesia

hyphema

hyphemia

hyphidrosis

hypnalgia

hypnocyst

hypoacusis

hypoadrenocorticism

hypoalbuminemia

hypoalbuminosis

hypoaldosteronemia

hypoaldosteronism
    hyporeninemic h.
    isolated h.

hypoaldosteronuria

hypoalgesia

hypoalimentation

hypoalonemia

hypoalphalipoproteinemia

hypoaminoacidemia

hypoandrogenism

hypoazoturia

hypobarism

hypobaropathy

hypobetalipoproteinemia
    familial h.

hypobilirubinemia

hypobromite

hypobromous acid

hypocalcemia

hypocalcemic

hypocalcia

hypocalcipectic

hypocalcipexy

hypocalciuria

hypocapnia

hypocapnic

hypocarbia

hypocarbonemia

hypocatalasia

hypocellular

hypocellularity

hypochloremia

hypochloremic

hypochlorhydria

hypochloridation

hypochloridemia

hypochloruria

hypocholesteremia

hypocholesteremic

hypocholesterolemia

hypocholesterolemic

hypocholuria

hypochondroplasia

hypochromasia

hypochromatic

hypochromatism

hypochromatosis

hypochromia

hypochromic

hypochromotrichia

hypochylia

hypocinesia

hypocitraturia

hypocitremia

hypocitruria

hypocoagulability

hypocoagulable

hypocomplementemia

hypocomplementemic

hypocorticalism

hypocorticism

hypocupremia

hypocyclosis

hypocythemia

hypocytosis

hypoderm

hypodermis

hypodermolithiasis

hypodermosis

hypodiploid

hypodiploidy

hypodipsia

hypodipsic

hypodontia

hypodynamia
   h. cordis

hypodynamic

hypoeccrisia

hypoeccrisis

hypoeccritic

hypoelectrolytemia

hypoeosinophilia

hypoepinephrinemia

hypoequilibrium

hypoergic

hypoesophoria

hypoesthesia
   acoustic h.
   auditory h.
   gustatory h.
   olfactory h.
   tactile h.

hypoesthetic

hypoestrogenemia

hypoevolutism

hypoexophoria

hypoferremia

hypoferrism

hypofertility

hypofibrinogenemia

hypofunction

hypogalactia

hypogalactous

hypogammaglobulinemia
   acquired h.
   common variable h.
   X-linked h.
   X-linked infantile h.

hypoganglionosis

hypogenitalism

hypogeusesthesia

hypogeusia

hypoglandular

hypoglucagonemia

hypoglycemia
   alimentary h.
   autoimmune h.
   factitial h.
   factitious h.
   fasting h.
   insulin-induced h.
   ketotic h.
   leucine-induced h.
   mixed h.

hypoglycemia (*continued*)
    neonatal h.
    postprandial h.
    reactive h.

hypoglycemic

hypoglycemosis

hypoglycogenolysis

hypoglycorrhachia

hypogonadism
    eugonadotropic h.
    hypergonadotropic h.
    hypogonadotropic h.
    primary h.
    secondary h.

hypogonadotropic

hypogranulocytosis

hypohepatia

hypohidrosis

hypohidrotic ectodermal
  dysplasia

hypohydrochloria

hypoidrosis

hypoinsulinemia

hypoinsulinism

hypoiodidism

hypokalemia

hypokalemic

hypokaliemia

hypokinemia

hypokinesia

hypokinesis

hypokinetic

hypolactasia

hypolemmal

hypoleydigism

hypolipemia

hypolipoproteinemia

hypoliposis

hypolymphemia

hypomagnesemia

hypomastia

hypomelanosis
    idiopathic guttate h.
    h. of Ito

hypomenorrhea

hypometabolic

hypometabolism

hypomethioninemia

hypometria

hypomineralization

hypomorph

hypomotility

hypomyxia

hyponatremia
    depletional h.
    dilutional h.

hyponatruria

hyponeocytosis

hyponitremia

hyponychon

hypo-orchidism

hypo-orthocytosis

hypo-osmolality

hypo-ovarianism

hypopallesthesia

hypopancreatism

hypopancreorrhea

hypoparathyroid

hypoparathyroidism

hypopepsia

hypopepsinia

hypoperfusion

hypoperistalsis

hypopexia

hypopexy

hypophagia

hypophoria

hypophysis staining method

hypophosphatasia

hypophosphatemia
    familial h.
    X-linked h.

hypophosphatemic

hypophosphaturia

hypophosphoremia

hypophyseoprivic

hypophysioprivic

hypophysitis
    lymphocytic h.

hypopiesia

hypopiesis

hypopietic

hypopigmentation

hypopinealism

hypopituitarism

hypoplastic

hypoplasty

hypoploid

hypopnea

hypopneic

hypoponesis

hypoporosis

hypoposia

hypopotassemia

hypopotassemic

hypopotentia

hypopraxia

hypoproteinemia
    prehepatic h.

hypoproteinia

hypoproteinic

hypoproteinosis

hypoprothrombinemia

hypopselaphesia

hypoptyalism

hypopyon

hyporeactive

hyporeflexia

hyporeninemia

hyporeninemic

hyposalemia

hyposalivation

hyposarca

hyposialosis

hyposmia

hyposmolarity

hyposomatotropism

hyposomia

hypospadia

hypospadiac

hypospadias

hyposplenism

hypostasis

hypostatic

hyposteatolysis

hyposthenia

hypostheniant

hyposthenic

hyposthenuria
  tubular h.

hypostosis

hyposuprarenalism

hyposympathicotonus

hyposynergia

hypotelorism
  ocular h.
  orbital h.

hypotension
  chronic orthostatic h.
  chronic idiopathic
    orthostatic h.
  idiopathic orthostatic h.
  orthostatic h.
  postural h.
  vascular h.

hypothermia
  accidental h.
  endogenous h.
  mild h.
  moderate h.
  severe h.

hypothermic

hypothermy

hypothesis
  response-to-injury h.

hypothrepsia

hypothrombinemia

hypothymism

hypothyrea

hypothyroid

hypothyroidism

hypothyrosis

hypotonia
  benign congenital h.
  h. oculi

hypotrichiasis

hypotrichosis

hypotrophy

hypotropia

hypotryptophanic

hypouremia

hypouresis

hypouricemia

hypouricuria

hypourocrinia

hypovarianism

hypovenosity

hypovitaminosis

hypovolemia

hypovolemic

hypovolia

hypoxemia

hypoxia
  anemic h.
  fetal h.
  hypoxic h.
  stagnant h.

hypoxia-ischemia

hypoxic

hypoxidosis

hypsicephaly

hypsokinesis

hysteralgia

hysteratresia

hysteresis
    protoplasmic h.

hysterobubonocele

hysterocele

hysterodynia

hysterolith

hysteropathy

hysteroptosia

hysteroptosis

hysterorrhexis

hysterospasm

hysterovagino-enterocele

IASD
  interatrial septal defect
IAT
  invasive activity test
  iodine-azide test
IB
  inclusion body
IBF
  immunoglobulin-binding
    factor
ICF
  intracellular fluid
ichthyosiform
ichthyosis
  i. congenita
  congenital i.
  harlequin i.
  i. hystrix
  lamellar i.
  i. linearis circumflexa
  i. palmaris et plantaris
  i. simplex
  i. uteri
  i. vulgaris
  X-linked i.
ichthyotic
ICSH
  interstitial cell-stimulating
    hormone
ICT
  inflammation of connective
    tissue
  insulin coma therapy
icteric
icteritious
icteroanemia
icterogenic
icterogenicity
icterohematuria

icterohematuric
icterohemoglobinuria
icterohepatitis
icteroid
icterus
  chronic familial i.
  congenital familial i.
  congenital hemolytic i.
  i. gravis neonatorum
  i. neonatorum
  nuclear i.
  i. prae cox
ictus
  i. epilepticus
  i. paralyticus
  i. sanguinis
  i. solis
IDA
  image display and analysis
IDDM
  insulin-dependent diabetes
    mellitus
Ide test
idioglossia
idioglottic
idiolalia
idiosome
idiospasm
IDR
  intradermal reaction
IDS
  immunity deficiency state
iduronidase
ileitis
  distal i.
  regional i.
  terminal i.

ileocolitis
    tuberculous i.
    i. ulcerosa chronica

ileus
    adynamic i.
    dynamic i.
    hyperdynamic i.
    mechanical i.
    meconium i.
    occlusive i.
    paralytic i.
    i. paralyticus
    spastic i.
    i. subparta

IFC
    intrinsic factor concentrate

IFRA
    indirect fluorescent rabies
      antibody (test)

IGGNU
    intratubular germ cell
      neplasia of the
      unclassified type

IGV
    intrathoracic gas volume

IgM

ILA
    insulin-like activity

illacrimation

illness
    compressed-air i.

Ilosvay reagent

illumination
    axial i.
    central i.
    critical i.
    darkfield i.
    dark-ground i.
    direct i.
    focal i.
    Köhler i.
    lateral i.
    oblique i.
    through i.

illuminator
    Abbe's i.

IMC
    immunohistochemical

imbibition

Imerslund-Grasbeck syndrome

IMH
    idiopathic myocardial
      hypertrophy

imidazolepyruvic acid

imidodipeptiduria

iminoglycinuria

immersion
    homogeneous i.
    oil i.
    water i.

imminent abortion

IMMU-MARK immunostaining kit

immunochemical assay

immunocompromised

immunoconcentration assay

immunodeficiency
    antibody i.
    cellular i.
    combined i.
    common variable i.
    common variable
      unclassifiable i.
    i. with elevated IgM
    i. with hyper-IgM
    severe combined i.
    i. with short-limbed
      dwarfism
    i. with thymoma

immunodeficient

immunoelectro-osmophoresis
  (IEOP)

immunoglobulinopathy
    monoclonal i.

index (*continued*)
Colour i.
degenerative i.
mitotic i.
nucleoplasmic i.
uricolytic i.

indicanemia

indicanmeter

indicanorachia

indicanuria

indicarmine

indicator
anaerobic i.
redox i.

indicophose

indigitation

indigo-carmine test

indigopurpurine

indigotin

indigotindisulfonate sodium

indirubin

indirubinuria

indisposition

indolaceturia

indole test

indollactic acid

indoluria

indophenol

indoxylemia

indoxyluria

indulin

indulinophil

indulinophilic

INE
infantile necrotizing
encephalomyelopathy

inert electrode

infarct
anemic i.
bilirubin i.
bland i.
bone i.
Brewer's i.
calcareous i.
cystic i.
embolic i.
hemorrhagic i.
lacunar i.
pale i.
red i.
septic i.
thrombotic i.
uric acid i.
white i.
i. of Zahn

infarction
acute myocardial i.
anterior myocardial i.
anteroinferior myocardial i.
anterolateral myocardial i.
anteroseptal myocardial i.
apical myocardial i.
atrial i.
cardiac i.
cerebral i.
cortical i.
diaphragmatic myocardial i.
extensive anterior
myocardial i.
forebrain i.
high lateral myocardial i.
inferior myocardial i.
inferolateral myocardial i.
intestinal i.
lacunar i.
lateral myocardial i.
maternal floor i.
mesenteric i.
migrainous i.
myocardial i.
non-Q wave i.
nonocclusive mesenteric i.
nontransmural myocardial
i.

infarction (*continued*)
    posterior myocardial i.
    pulmonary i.
    Q wave i.
    right ventricular i.
    septal myocardial i.
    silent myocardial i.
    subendocardial myocardial
      i.
    transmural myocardial i.
    watershed i.

infection
    ascending i.
    chronic Epstein-Barr virus i.
    germinal i.
    hematogenous i.
    perinatal i.
    TORCH i.
    transcervical i.
    transplacental i.

infection-immunity

infectiosity

infiltrate
    Assmann's tuberculous i.

infiltration
    adipose i.
    calcareous i.
    calcium i.
    cellular i.
    epituberculous i.
    fatty i.
    gelatinous i.
    glycogen i.
    gray i.
    inflammatory i.
    pulmonary i. with
      eosinophilia
    sanguineous i.
    serous i.
    tuberculous i.
    urinous i.

infinitely miscible

infinitesimal

inflamed ulcer

inflammagen

inflammation
    acute i.
    adhesive i.
    atrophic i.
    catarrhal i.
    chronic i.
    cirrhotic i.
    diffuse i.
    disseminated i.
    exudative i.
    fibrinous i.
    fibrosing i.
    focal i.
    granulomatous i.
    hyperplastic i.
    hypertrophic i.
    interstitial i.
    metastatic i.
    necrotic i.
    obliterative i.
    parenchymatous i.
    plastic i.
    productive i.
    proliferous i.
    pseudomembranous i.
    purulent i.
    sclerosing i.
    seroplastic i.
    serous i.
    simple i.
    specific i.
    subacute i.
    suppurative i.
    toxic i.
    traumatic i.
    ulcerative i.

infraction
    Freiberg's i.

infravergence

ingravescent

inguinodynia

inhalation pneumonia

inhibin

iniasis

initiating agent

initis

inoblast

inochondritis

inoglia

inolith

inomyositis

inophragma

inosclerosis

inosculate

inosculation

inosemia

inositis

inositoluria

inosituria

inosuria

inotagma

INR
    International Normalized
      Ratio

INS
    idiopathic nephrotic
      syndrome

insidious

insolation
    asphyxial i.
    hyperpyrexial i.

instant thin-layer
    chromatography

instructive theory

insudate

insufficiency
    active i.
    adrenal i.

insufficiency (*continued*)
    adrenal i., primary
    adrenal i., secondary
    adrenocortical i.
    adrenocortical i., acute
    adrenocortical i., chronic
    adrenocortical i., primary
    adrenocortical i., secondary
    aortic i.
    basilar i.
    cardiac i.
    coronary i.
    i. of the externi
    i. of the eyelids
    gastric i.
    gastromotor i.
    hepatic i.
    ileocecal i.
    i. of the interni
    mitral i.
    muscular i.
    myocardial i.
    parathyroid i.
    placental i.
    pulmonary i.
    renal i.
    respiratory i.
    thyroid i.
    tricuspid i.
    uterine i.
    i. of the valves
    valvular i.
    velopharyngeal i.
    venous i.
    vertebrobasilar i.

insular sclerosis

insulated gate field effect
    transistor

insulinemia

insulinlipodystrophy

insulinopathy

insulinopenic

insulitis

intergranular

integrating microscope

interactive processing

inter alpha trypsin inhibitor

interatrial septal defect (IASD)

interchromosomal aberration

intercoronary anastomosis
    i. anastomosis

intercristal space

intercurrent disease

interelectrode distance

interference
    anion i.
    bacterial i.
    cation i.
    centromere i.
    i. filter
    hemplysis i.
    icterus i.
    ionization i.
    i. microscope
    spectral i.

interkinesis

interlobitis

intermediary metabolism

intermeningeal

intermitotic

internode
    i. of Ranvier

internuncial

interocclusal clearance

interpapillary ridge

interparoxysmal

interphyletic

interpial

interpleural

interpolation

interspecific graft

intertriginous

intertrigo
    i. labialis

interval
    coupling i.
    escape i.
    lucid i.
    reference i.

intervening sequence

interventricular septal defect
(IVSD)

intestinalization

intestine
    iced i.

intimitis

intolerance
    disaccharide i.
    fructose i., hereditary
    lactose i.
    lactose i., congenital
    lysine i., congenital
    lysinuric protein i.
    sucrose i., congenital

intracellular
    i. accumulation(s)
    i. fluid volume (ICF)
    i. parasite
    i. toxin
    i. water (ICW)

intracutaneous reaction

intracytoplasmic

intradermal
    i. nevus
    i. reaction (IDR)
    i. test (IT)

intraductal
    i. carcinoma (IDC)
    i. hyperplasia
    i. papillary carcinoma (IPC)
    i. papilloma
    i. papillomatosis

intraepidermal

intraepidermic bulla

intraesophageal pH test

intrafistular

intrafusal

intraictal

intralesional

intramembranous space

intraneural

intraoperative cell salvage

intraovular

intrapulmonary spindle cell
    thymoma

intraprotoplasmic

intrapyretic

intravasation

intravascular
    i. agglutination
    i. coagulation screen
    i. consumption
        coagulopathy (IVCC)
    i. hemolysis
    i. papillary endothelial
        hyperplasia

intravital stain

introsusception

intumesce

intumescence

intumescent

intussusception
    agonic i.
    postmortem i.
    retrograde i.
    appendiceal i.

intussusceptum

intussuscipiens

inulin clearance

inundation fever

invagination

invermination

inverse-square law

inversion
    paracentric i.
    pericentric i.
    i. of uterus
    visceral i.

inverting enzyme

invert sugar

inveterate

involucre

involucrum

involute

iodate reaction of epinephrine

iod-Basedow

iodine
    Lugol's i.

iodine-131 uptake test

iodine-azide test (IAT)

iodine-131-6 beta iodomethyl-
    19-norcholesterol

iodinophil

iodinophilous

iododerma

iodomethane

iodophil

idotyrosine deiodinase defect

ioduria

ionizing radiation

ionophose

ion-selective electrode (ISE)

IPS
   initial prognostic score

IRBBB
   incomplete right bundle-
      branch block

IRG
   immunoreactive glucagon

iridalgia

iridauxesis

iridectropium

iridemia

iridentropium

irideremia

iridization

iridoavulsion

iridocapsulitis

iridocele

iridochoroiditis

iridocoloboma

iridocyclitis
   heterochromic i.

iridocyclochoroiditis

iridodialysis

iridodiastasis

iridodonesis

iridokeratitis

iridoleptynsis

iridomalacia

iridoncus

iridoparalysis

iridopathy

iridoperiphakitis

iridoplegia
   accommodation i.

iridoplegia (*continued*)
   complete i.
   reflex i.
   sympathetic i.

iridoptosis

iridorhexis

iridoschisis

iridosteresis

iris
   i. bombé
   detached i.
   tremulous i.
   umbrella i.

irisopsia

iritic

IRMA
   immunoradiometric assay

iron
   i. citrate

iron-positive pigment
   demonstration

iron-sulfide protein

irreducible hernia

irritability
   i. of the bladder
   i. of the stomach
   tactile i.

IRS
   infrared spectrophotometry

Isamine blue

ISC
   irreversibly sickled cell

ischesis

ischialgia

ischiocele

ischiodynia

ischionitis

ischogyria

ischuria
    i. paradoxa
    i. spastica

ISH
    icteric serum hepatitis
    in situ hybridization

ISI
    International Sensitivity
        Index

island
    blood i.
    i. of Calleja
    cartilage i.
    i. of Langerhans
    olfactory i.
    i. of pancreas
    Pander's i.

islet
    blood i.
    Calleja i.
    i. of Langerhans
    pancreatic i.
    Walthard i.

isochromatic

isochromatophil

isochromosome

isochroous

isocytosis

isoeugenol

isohydric

isoiodeikon test

isoleucyl-RNA synthetase

isomorphic response

isonicotinic acid hydrazine
    (INH)

isoprostane

isopyknic

isorubin

isoserum treatment

isosulfan blue

isothermognosis

isovaleric acid

isovalericacidemia

isovalerylglycine

isovolumic contraction (IC)

IST
    insulin sensitivity test
    insulin shock therapy

isthmitis

isthmoparalysis

isthmoplegia

IT
    implantation test
    intradermal test
    intratumoral test
    isomeric transition

ithycyphos

ithylordosis

ithyokyphosis

ITLC
    instant thin-layer
        chromatography

Ito-Reenstierna test

ITP
    idiopathic thromocytopenic
        purpura

ITT
    insulin tolerance test

IUD
    intrauterine death

IUGR
    intratuerine growth rate

IVAP
    in vivo adhesive platelet

Ivemark syndrome

IVGTT
    intravenous glucose
        tolerance test

ivory exostosis

IVTTT
    intravenous tolbutamide
        tolerance test

Ivy
    I. bleeding time

Ivy (*continued*)
    I. method
    I. method of bleeding time
    I. template bleeding time

ixodiasis

ixodic

ixodid

Ixodidae

Ixodoidea

J

jaagsiekte

Jacobsson method

Jacod syndrome

Jacquemin test

jactatio

jactation

jactitation

Jaffe
    J. assay
    J. reaction

Jamestown Canyon virus

Janeway lesion

janiceps

Jansky human blood group
  classification

Janus green b.

jar
    anaerobic j.
    Coplin j.

jargonaphasia

Jass staging system

jaundice
    acholuric j.
    acholuric familial j.
    acute febrile j.
    anhepatic j.
    anhepatogenous j.
    black j.
    breast milk j.
    catarrhal j.
    cholestatic j.
    chronic acholuric j.
    congenital hemolytic j.
    Crigler-Najjar j.
    epidemic j.
    familial acholuric j.
    familial nonhemolytic j.
    hematogenous j.
    hemolytic j.
    hepatocellular j.
    hepatogenic j.
    hepatogenous j.
    homologous serum j.
    human serum j.
    infectious j.
    infective j.
    latent j.
    mechanical j.
    neonatal j.
    j. of the newborn
    nonhemolytic j.
    nonhemolytic j., congenital
    nonhemolytic j., congenital
      familial
    nonhemolytic j., familial
    nuclear j.
    obstructive j.
    physiologic j.
    regurgitation j.
    retention j.
    Schmorl's j.
    spherocytic j.
    toxemic j.

JC virus

Jeanselme nodule

jejunitis

jejunoileitis

jelly
    Wharton's j.

Jenner stain

Jerne plaque assay

jet lesion

Jk antigen

Jobbins antigen

jodbasedow

Johne
    J. bacillus
    J. disease

joint
    bleeder's j.
    j. calculus
    Charcot's j.
    Clutton's j.
    false j.
    flail j.
    fringe j.
    hemophilic j.
    irritable j.
    von Gies j.

Jolles test

Js antigen

Junin virus

Juniperus

juvenile-onset diabetes

juxta-articular nodule

juxtacortical
    j. chondroma
    j. osteogenic sarcoma

juxtaglomerular
    j. cell tumor
    j. granulation index

juxtanuclear

juxtapulmonary-capillary
    j-c. receptor

K

ketoacidosis

kabure

Kahn test

Kaiserling fixative

kakosmia

kakotrophy

Kala azar

kalemia

kaliemia

kalimeter

kaliopenia

kaliopenic

kaliuresis

kaliuretic

kallak

kallikrein system

kaluresis

kaluretic

Kanagawa phenomenon

kanyemba

kaodzera

Kaolin clotting time

kaolinosis

kaolin partial thromboplastin
    time

Kaplan-Meier staining method

Kaposi
    K. sarcoma
    K. varicelliform eruption

karyapsis

karyenchyma

karyochrome

karyochylema

karyoclasis

karyoclastic

karyocyte

karyogamic

karyogamy

karyogenesis

karyogenic

karyokinesis
    asymmetrical k.
    hyperchromatic k.
    hypochromatic k.

karyokinetic

karyoklasis

karyoklastic

karyolymph

karyolysis

karyolytic

karyomegaly

karyomere

karyometry

karyomitosis

karyomitotic

karyomorphism

karyon

karyophage

karyoplasm

karyoplasmic

karyoplasmolysis

karyoplast

karyoplastin

karyopyknosis

karyopyknotic

karyoreticulum

karyorrhectic

karyorrhexis

karyostasis

karyotheca

karyotin

karyotype
    k. aberration
    numerical k.
    X k.
    XO k.
    XX k.
    XXX k.
    XXY k.
    XY k.
    XYY k.

karyotyping

karyozoic

Katayama test

Kato thick smear technique

katophoria

katotropia

KB
    ketone body

K capture

Kelev stain rabies virus

Kenyon stain

kerasin-type histiocytosis

keratalgia

keratectasia

keratin
    α-k.
    alpha k.
    hard k.
    k. pearl
    soft k.

keratin (*continued*)
    k. stain
    k. staining

keratinization

keratinocyte

keratinosome

keratinous

keratitis
    Acanthamoeba k.
    acne rosacea k.
    actinic k.
    aerosol k.
    alphabet k.
    annular k.
    k. arborescens
    artificial silk k.
    aspergillus k.
    band k.
    band-shaped k.
    k. bandelette
    k. bullosa
    catarrhal ulcerative k.
    deep k.
    deep pustular k.
    dendriform k.
    dendritic k.
    desiccation k.
    Dimmer's k.
    disciform k.
    k. disciformis
    epithelial diffuse k.
    epithelial punctate k.
    exfoliative k.
    exposure k.
    fascicular k.
    k. filamentosa
    furrow k.
    herpetic k.
    hypopyon k.
    interstitial k.
    interstitial k., nonsyphilitic
    lagophthalmic k.
    lattice k.
    marginal k.
    metaherpetic k.

keratitis (*continued*)
    microbial k.
    mycotic k.
    neuroparalytic k.
    neurotrophic k.
    k. nummularis
    parenchymatous k.
    peripheral ulcerative k.
    k. petrificans
    phlyctenular k.
    k. profunda
    k. punctata
    k. punctata leprosa
    k. punctata profunda
    k. punctata subepithelialis
    punctate k.
    punctate k., deep
    punctate k., superficial
    purulent k.
    k. pustuliformis profunda
    reaper's k.
    reticular k.
    ribbonlike k.
    rosacea k.
    sclerosing k.
    scrofulous k.
    secondary k.
    serpiginous k.
    k. sicca
    striate k.
    suppurative k.
    trachomatous k.
    trophic k.
    ulcerative k.
    vascular k.
    vesicular k.
    xerotic k.
    zonular k.

keratocele

keratoconjunctivitis
    epidemic k.
    flash k.
    herpetic k.
    phlyctenular k.
    shipyard k.
    k. sicca
    superior limbic k.
    viral k.

keratoconus

keratocyst

keratocyte

keratoderma
    k. acquisitum
    k. blennorrhagicum
    k. climactericum
    k. palmare et plantare
    mutilating k.
    palmoplantar k.
    palmoplantar k., diffuse
    punctate k.
    senile k.

keratodermatocele

keratodermia

keratoectasia

keratoglobus

keratohelcosis

keratohemia

keratohyalin

keratoiditis

keratoiridocyclitis

keratoiritis
    hypopyon k.

keratoleukoma

keratolysis
    pitted k.
    k. plantare sulcatum

keratoma
    k. hereditarium mutilans
    k. plantare sulcatum

keratomalacia

keratomata

keratomycosis
    k. nigricans

keratonosus

keratopathy
    band k.

keratopathy (*continued*)
    band-shaped k.
    bullous k.
    climatic k.
    filamentary k.
    Labrador k.
    lipid k.
    striate k.
    vesicular k.

keratorhexis (keratorrhexis)

keratoscleritis

keratosis (pl. keratoses)
    actinic k.
    arsenic k.
    k. blennorrhagica
    k. follicularis
    k. follicularis contagiosa
    inverted follicular k.
    lichenoid k.
    k. linguae
    k. nigricans
    k. obturans
    k. palmaris et plantaris
    k. pharyngea
    k. pilaris
    k. punctata
    seborrheic k.
    k. seborrheica
    senile k.
    solar k.
    stucco k.
    tar k.
    k. vegetans

keratotic
    k. papilloma
    k. precipitate

keratotorus

kerectasis

kerion

kernicterus

keroid

ketoacidosis (KA)

α-keto acid dehydrogenase
    deficiency

α-ketoadipicacidemia

α-ketoadipicaciduria

ketoaminoacidemia

β-ketobutyric acid

ketoconazole

Keto-Diastix

ketogenesis

ketogenetic

ketogenic

17-ketogenic
    17-K steroid assay test
    17-K steroids

ketohexose

ketone
    k. body
    k. body stabilization
    dimethyl k.
    methyl butyl k.

ketonemia

ketonuria

ketoplasia

ketoplastic

ketosis

ketosuria

β-ketothiolase deficiency

ketotic hyperglycemia

kg-cal
    kilogram-calorie

kidney
    abdominal k.
    amyloid k.
    Armanni-Ebstein k.
    arteriosclerotic k.
    atrophic k.
    cake k.

kidney (*continued*)
    cicatricial k.
    clump k.
    congested k.
    contracted k.
    crush k.
    cyanotic k.
    cystic k.
    disk k.
    doughnut k.
    fatty k.
    flea-bitten k.
    floating k.
    Formad's k.
    fused k.
    Goldblatt k.
    horseshoe k.
    hypermobile k.
    lardaceous k.
    large red k.
    lumbar k.
    lump k.
    medullary sponge k.
    movable k.
    mural k.
    myelin k.
    myeloma k.
    Page k.
    pelvic k.
    polycystic k.
    Rose-Bradford k.
    sacciform k.
    sigmoid k.
    sponge k.
    supernumerary k.
    thoracic k.
    wandering k.
    waxy k.
    surgical k.

Ki-FDC1p antibody

kilocalorie (kc)

kilohertz (kHz)

kilojoule (kJ)

KIMIP antibody

Ki-M4p antibody

kinanesthesia

kinase
    aspartate k.
    creatine k.
    pyruvate k.

kinesalgia

kinesia

kinesialgia

kinesin

kinesioneurosis

kinetocyte

kinetoplasm

kinetosis

kinin system

kinocentrum

kinocilium

kinosphere

Kinyoun carbol fuchsin stain

Kitasato broth

Kjeldahl method

kleeblattschädel

Kleihauer
    K. acid elution test
    K. stain

Klenow fragment

knob
    olfactory k.
    surfers' k.
    synaptic k.

knot
    enamel k.
    Hensen's k.
    primitive k.
    protochordal k.
    surfers' k.
    syncytial k.

Kober test

Kohn one-step staining
   technique

koilocyte

koilocytosis

koilocytotic

koilonychia

koilorrhachic

koilosternia

kolypeptic

kopiopia

Kossa stain

kraurosis
   k. vulvae

kresofuchsin

krypton

krypton-85

kubisagari

kubisgari

Kupffer
   K. cell
   K. cell hypertrophy

kuru

kwashiorkor
   marasmic k.

kwaski

kyllosis

kymatism

kynurenic acid

kyphos

kyphoscoliosis

kyrtorrhachic

L

L26 antibody

LA
    latex agglutination

labiochorea

labiomycosis

labyrinthitis
    bacterial l.
    hematogenic l.
    meningogenic l.
    l. ossificans
    acute suppurative l.
    tympanogenic l.

Lacis

lacrimal calculus

lactaciduria

lactase deficiency

lactational mastitis

lactenin

lacticacidemia

lacticemia

lactoacidemia

lactobacillary milk

lactocele

lactoferrin

lactogen
    human placental l.

lactophenol cotton blue

lactorrhea

lactose-litmus broth

lactosuria

lactotrope

lactotroph

lacuna
    Blessig's l.
    chondrocyte l.
    Howship's l.
    intervillous l.
    trophoblastic l.

lacune

lag
    anaphase l.
    nitrogen l.

lagophthalmos

lagophthalmus

laiose

LAIT
    latex agglutination-
      inhibition t.

lambda
    l. chain

lame foliacée

lamella (pl. lamellae)
    annulate l.
    concentric l.
    cornoid l.
    elastic l.
    enamel l.
    ground l.
    haversian l.
    intermediate l.
    interstitial l.
    posterior border l. of Fuchs

lamellipodia

lamellipodium

lameness

lamin

laminated thrombus

Lan antigen

lancet fluke

Langerhans
    L. cell
    islets of L.

langerhansian hormone

Lansing virus

lanthanic

lanugo hair

laparocele

laparomyitis

larva (pl. larvae)
    l. currens
    fly l.
    l. migrans

larval

larvate

larvicide

larviphagic

laryngalgia

laryngitis

laryngomalacia

laryngoparalysis

laryngopathy

laryngopharyngitis

laryngoplegia

laryngoptosis

laryngopyocele

laryngorrhagia

laryngorrhea

laryngoscleroma

laryngotracheitis

laryngotracheobronchitis

Laségue disease

Lash casein hydrolysate-serum
    medium

latah

late-phase response

laterotorsion

latex
    l. agglutination test
    l. fixation test
    l flocculation t.

lathyrism

lathyrus protein

lauric acid

lauryl sulfate broth

law
    Allen's paradoxic l.
    Ambards l.
    Ángstrom l.
    Bastian's l.
    Bastian-Bruns l.
    Beer l.
    Bohring's l.
    Coulomb's l.
    Courvoisier's l.
    Dalton's l.
    Einthoven's l.
    Faraday l. of electrolysis
    Farr's l.
    Fick's l.
    Gay-Lussac l.
    Gerhardt-Semon l.
    Godélier's l.
    Graham's l.
    Gudden's l.
    Gull-Toynbee l.
    Jackson's l.
    Halsted's l.
    Hardy-Weinberg l.
    inverse-square l.
    Joule's l.
    Kirchoff's l.
    Koch's l.
    Küstner's l.
    Lambert's l.
    Louis' l.
    Marfan's l.
    Newton's l. of cooling

law (*continued*)
- Nysten's l.
- Ollier's l.
- Planck's radiation l.
- Prévost's l.
- Profeta's l.
- l. of referred pain
- Snell's l.
- Sterling's l.
- Stokes' l.
- Teevan's l.
- Toynbee's l.
- Virchow's l.

layer
- ameloblastic l.
- bacillary l.
- basal l. of endometrium
- basal l. of epidermis
- Bechterew's l.
- Bekhterev's l.
- Bernard's glandular l.
- blastodermic l.
- Bowman's l.
- cambium l.
- capillary l. of choroid
- cerebral l. of retina
- l. of cerebral cortex
- Chievitz l.
- choriocapillary l.
- circular l. of muscular coat of colon
- circular l. of muscular coat of rectum
- circular l. of muscular coat of small intestine
- circular l. of muscular coat of stomach
- circular l. of tympanic membrane
- clear l. of epidermis
- columnar l.
- compact l. of endometrium
- cutaneous l. of tympanic membrane
- depletion l.
- Dobie's l.
- enamel l., inner

layer (*continued*)
- enamel l., outer
- ependymal l.
- epitrichial l.
- fibrous l. of articular capsule
- fibrous l. of tympanic membrane
- Floegel's l.
- functional l. of endometrium
- fusiform l. of cerebral cortex
- ganglion cell l.
- ganglionic l. of cerebellum
- ganglionic l. of cerebral cortex
- ganglionic l. of optic nerve
- ganglionic l. of retina
- germ l.
- germinative l.
- germinative l. of epidermis
- germinative l. of nail
- glomerular l.
- granular l. of cerebellum
- granular l. of cerebral cortex, external
- granular l. of cerebral cortex, internal
- granular l. of epidermis
- granular l. of follicle of ovary
- granular l. of olfactory bulb, external
- granular l. of olfactory bulb, internal
- granular l. of Tomes
- granule l. of cerebellum
- gray and white l. of rostral colliculus
- gray l. of superior colliculus, deep
- gray l. of superior colliculus, intermediate
- gray l. of superior colliculus, superficial
- gray and white l. of superior colliculus

layer (*continued*)
    Henle's l.
    Henle's fiber l.
    horny l. of epidermis
    horny l. of nail
    Huxley's l.
    inner l. of glomerular
      capsule
    Kaes-Bekhterev l.
    Langhans' l.
    limiting l., internal
    longitudinal l. of muscular
      coat of colon
    longitudinal l. of muscular
      coat of rectum
    longitudinal l. of muscular
      coat of small intestine
    longitudinal l. of muscular
      coat of stomach
    malpighian l.
    mantle l.
    marginal l.
    medullary l. of thalamus,
      external
    medullary l. of thalamus,
      internal
    membranous l. of
      subcutaneous tissue
    Meynert's l.
    mitral cell l.
    molecular l., external
    molecular l., inner
    molecular l., internal
    molecular l., outer
    molecular l. of cerebellum
    molecular l. of cerebral
      cortex
    molecular l. of olfactory
      bulb
    mucous l.
    mucous l. of tympanic
      membrane
    multiform l. of cerebral
      cortex
    nerve fiber l.
    nervous l. of retina
    neuroepithelial l. of retina
    Nitabuch's l.

layer (*continued*)
    nuclear l., external
    nuclear l., inner
    nuclear l., internal
    nuclear l., outer
    nuclear l. of cerebellum
    odontoblastic l.
    olfactory nerve fiber l.
    Ollier's l.
    optic l. of superior
      colliculus
    oriens l. of hippocampus
    osteogenetic l.
    outer l. of glomerular
      capsule
    Pander's l.
    papillary l. of corium
    papillary l. of dermis
    parietal l. of tunica vaginalis
      of testis
    peripheral l. of cerebral
      cortex
    pigmented l. of ciliary
      body
    pigmented l. of eyeball
    pigmented l. of iris
    pigmented l. of retina
    piriform neuronal l.
    plasma l.
    plexiform l., external
    plexiform l., inner
    plexiform l., internal
    plexiform l., outer
    plexiform l. of cerebellum
    plexiform l. of cerebral
      cortex
    polymorphic l. of cerebral
      cortex
    prickle cell l.
    Purkinje l.
    Purkinje cell l.
    pyramidal l. of cerebral
      cortex, external
    pyramidal l. of cerebral
      cortex, internal
    pyramidal l. of
      hippocampus
    radiate l. of hippocampus

layer (*continued*)
　　radiate l. of tympanic
　　　membrane
　　reticular l. of corium
　　reticular l. of dermis
　　l. of rods and cones
　　Rohr's l.
　　sclerotogenous l.
　　skeletogenous l.
　　somatic l.
　　spinous l. of epidermis
　　splanchnic l.
　　spongy l. of endometrium
　　subendocardial l.
　　subendothelial l.
　　subepicardial l.
　　submantle l.
　　submucous l. of bladder
　　submucous l. of bronchi
　　submucous l. of colon
　　submucous l. of esophagus
　　submucous l. of pharynx
　　submucous l. of small
　　　intestine
　　submucous l. of stomach
　　submucous l. of urinary
　　　bladder
　　submucous l. of uterine
　　　tube
　　subserous l. of bladder
　　subserous l. of gallbladder
　　subserous l. of liver
　　subserous l. of peritoneum
　　subserous l. of small
　　　intestine
　　subserous l. of stomach
　　subserous l. of urinary
　　　bladder
　　subserous l. of uterine tube
　　subserous l. of uterus
　　l. of superior colliculus
　　suprachoroid l.
　　synovial l. of articular
　　　capsule
　　Tomes' granular l.
　　visceral l. of glomerular
　　　capsule

layer (*continued*)
　　visceral l. of tunica vaginalis
　　　of testis
　　Weil's l. layer
　　white l. of superior
　　　colliculus, deep
　　white l. of superior
　　　colliculus, intermediate
　　Zeissel's l.
　　zonal l. of superior
　　　colliculus
　　zonal l. of thalamus
　　parietal l. of glomerular
　　　capsule

LCAD deficiency

LCAT deficiency

LDL-C
　　low density lipoprotein-
　　　cholesterol

L-dopa
　　levodopa

lean body mass

lechopyra

lecithinemia

lecithoblast

Lederer anemia

Legionella urinary antigen
　(LUA) ELISA test kit

left-to-right ratio

legionellosis

Legionnaire's disease

leiasthenia

leiodermia

leiodystonia

leiomyoma

leiomyosarcoma

leishmoniasis
　　anergic l.

leishmoniasis (*continued*)
    cutaneous l.
    lupoid l.
    mucocutaneous l.
    visceral l.

Leitz image analysis system

lemic

lemma

lemmoblast

lemmocyte

lens
    achromatic l.
    aplanatic l.
    apochromatic l.
    electron l.
    oil immersion l.

lens-induced uveitis

lenticonus

lenticula

lentiginosis

lentiginous

lentiglobus

lentigo (pl. lentigenes)
    nevoid l.
    senile l.
    malignant l.
    l. senilis
    l. simplex
    solar l.

leontiasis
    l. ossea
    l. ossium

lepidic

Lepidoptera

lepocyte

lepori pox virus

lepra cell

leprid

lepride

leproma

lepromatous

leprosarium

leprosery

leprosy
    dimorphous l.
    histoid l.
    lepromatous l.
    Malabar l.
    tuberculoid l.

leptochromatic

leptocyte

leptocytosis

leptodactylous

leptodactyly

leptomeningeal

leptomeningitis

leptomeningopathy

leptonema

leptoscope

leptospirosis

leptotene

leptotrichosis
    l. conjunctivae

lesion
    angiocentric proliferative l.
    Armanni-Ebstein l.
    Baehr-Löhlein l.
    Bankart l.
    benign lymphoepithelial l.
    birds' nest l.
    Blumenthal l.
    Bracht-Wächter l.
    central l.
    coin l.
    cold l.
    Councilman's l.

lesion (*continued*)
Ebstein's l.
extracapillary l.
fibrohistiocytic l.
Ghon's primary l.
gross l.
Hill-Sachs l.
histologic l.
hystocytoid hemangioma-like l.
impaction l.
indiscriminate l.
initial syphilitic l.
irritative l.
Janeway l.
jet l.
Kimmelstiel-Wilson l.
Lennert l.
local l.
Löhlein-Baehr l.
Mallory-Weiss l.
molecular l.
nonexophytic l.
onionskin l.
organic l.
papulonodular l.
partial l.
peripheral l.
precancerous l.
precursor l.
primary l.
ring-wall l.
spontaneous l.
squamous intraepithelial l.
structural l.
systemic l.
target l.
total l.
trophic l.
verrucopapillary external genital l.
wire-loop l.

Leu
L. antibody (#s 2, 3, 4, 7, 8, 12, 14, 22)
L. antigen
M. M1 antibody

leucinosis

leucinuria

leucitis

leukemia
acute granulocytic l.
acute lymphoblastic l.
acute megaloblastic l.
acute monoblastic l.
acute monocytic l.
acute myelocytic l.
acute myelogenous l.
acute nonlymphocytic l.
acute undifferentiated l.
adult T-cell l.
aleukemic granulocytic l.
aleukemic lymphocytic l.
aleukemic monocytic l.
basophilic l.
basophilocytic l.
blast cell l.
chronic cell l.
chronic granulocytic l.
chronic lymphatic l.
chronic lymphocytic l.
chronic lymphosarcoma l.
chronic monoblastic l.
chronic monocytic l.
chronic myelocytic l.
chronic myelogenous l.
chronic myelomonocytic l.
l. cutis
embryonal l.
eosinophilic l.
erythromyeloblastic l.
hairy cell l.
histiocytic l.
leukopenic l.
lymphatic l.
lymphoid l.
lymphosarcoma cell l.
lymphoid l.
mast cell l.
mature cell l.
megakaryocytic l.
meningeal l.

leukemia (*continued*)
    micromyeloblastic l.
    mixed cell l.
    monoblastic l.
    monocytic l.
    murine l.
    myeloblastic l.
    myelocytic l.
    myelogenic l.
    myelogenous l.
    myeloid l.
    myelomonocytic l.
    Naegeli type of monocytic l.
    neutrophilic l.
    plasma cell l.
    polymorphocytic l.
    Rieder cell l.
    Schilling type of monocytic l.
    smoldering l.
    stem cell l.
    subleukemic
    thrombocytic l.
    thymic l.

leukemid

leukemoid

leukencephalitis

leukin

leukoblast

leukocoria

leukocyte
    acidophilic l.
    l. acid phosphatase stain
    l. adherence assay test
    agranular l.
    l. alloantibodies
    l. antigen
    basophilic l.
    l. common antigen
    cystinotic l.
    endothelial l.
    eosinophilic l.
    l. esterase

leukocyte (*continued*)
    globular l.
    granular l.
    heterophilic l.
    hyaline l.
    l. inclusion
    l. inhibitory factor
    l. interferon
    lymphoid l.
    mast l.
    nonfilament polymorphonuclear l.
    oxyphilic l.
    polymorphonuclear l.
    polynuclear l.
    segmented l.
    transitional l.
    Türk's irritation l.

leukocytolysin

leukocytolysis

leukocytolytic

leukocytoma

leukocytopenia

leukocytosis
    absolute l.
    agonal l.
    basophilic l.
    eosinophilic l.
    lymphocytic l.
    monocytic l.
    mononuclear l.
    neutrophilic l.
    pathologic l.
    physiologic l.
    pure l.
    relative l.
    terminal l.
    toxic l.

leukocyturia

leukoderma
    l. colli
    occupational l.
    postinflammatory l.
    syphilitic l.

leukodermatous

leukodermia

leukodermic

leukodystrophy
    Alexander l.
    globoid cell l.
    hereditary adult-onset l.
    hereditary cerebral l.
    Krabbe's l.
    metachromatic l.
    spongiform l.
    sudanophilic l.

leukoedema

leukoencephalitis
    acute hemorrhagic l.
    acute hemorrhagic l. of
      Weston Hurst
    l. periaxialis concentrica
    subacute sclerosing l.
    van Bogaert's
      sclerosing l.

leukoencephalopathy
    metachromatic l.
    multifocal progressive l.
    necrotizing l.
    progressive multifocal l.
    subacute sclerosing l.

leukoencephaly

leukoerythroblastic

leukoerythroblastosis

leukokeratosis

leukokinetic

leukokinin

leukokoria

leukokraurosis

leukolymphosarcoma

leukolysis

leukolytic

leukoma
    adherent l.

leukomalacia
    periventricular l.

leukoma

leukomatous

leukomyelitis

leukomyelopathy

leukonecrosis

leukonychia

leukopathia
    acquired l.
    l. punctata reticularis
      symmetrica
    l. unguium

leukopathy

leukopenia
    autoimmune l.
    basophil l.
    basophilic l.
    congenital l.
    malignant l.
    pernicious l.

leukopenic
    l. factor

leukoplakia
    atrophic l.
    l. buccalis
    hairy l.
    l. lingualis
    oral l.
    oral hairy l.
    l. vulvae

leukorrhagia

leukorrhea

leukosarcoma

leukosis

leukostasis

leukotrichia

levocardia
    isolated l.
    mixed l.

levoclination

levodopa

levothyroxine

levulose tolerance test

lichen
    l. amyloidosus
    l. annularis
    atrophic l. planus
    bullous l. planus
    l. corneus hypertrophicus
    l. fibromucinoidosus
    hypertrophic l. planus
    l. myxedematosus
    l. nitidus
    l. obtusus corneus
    l. pilaris
    l. planopilaris
    l. planus
    l. planus, bullous
    l. planus, vesiculobullous
    l. planus actinicus
    l. planus annularis
    l. planus atrophicus
    l. planus erythematosus
    l. planus follicularis
    l. planus hypertrophicus
    l. planus subtropicum
    l. planus tropicum
    l. planus verrucosus
    l. ruber moniliformis
    l. ruber planus
    l. sclerosus
    l. sclerosus et atrophicus
    l. scrofulosorum
    l. scrofulosus
    l. simplex chronicus
    l. spinulosus
    l. striatus
    l. syphiliticus
    l. tropicus
    l. urticatus

lichenoid
    l. dermatitis
    l. eczema

lien
    l. mobilis

lienitis

lienocele

lienomalacia

lienomyelomalacia

lienopathy

lienotoxin

lienteric

lientery

ligandin

light
    l. microscopy
    polarized l.
    strobe l.

light-scattering immunoassay

Lignac
    L. syndrome
    Lignac-Fanconi syndrome

lignoid

Lillie
    L. allochrome connective
      tissue staub
    L. azure-eosin stain
    L. sulfuric acid bile blue
      stain

limit
    assimilation l.
    l. dextrin
    Hayflick's l.
    l. of flocculation
    quantum l.
    saturation l.

limophthisis

limosis

line
  accretion l.
  Aldrich-Mees lines
  l. of Amici
  anocutaneous l.
  anorectal l.
  Beau's l.
  Blaschko's l.
  Brücke's l.
  calcification l.
  cell l.
  cement l.
  contour l.
  Czermak's l.
  l. of demarcation
  dentate l.
  De Salle's l.
  Dobie's l.
  Eberth's l.
  l. of Ebner
  ectental l.
  embryonic l.
  equipotential l.
  established cell l.
  Frommann's l.
  Futcher's l.
  genal l.
  Gubler l.
  Hensen's l.
  imbrication l. of cementum
  imbrication l. of Pickerill
  incremental l.
  incremental l. of cementum
  incremental l. of Ebner
  intraperiod l.
  Jadelot's l.
  l. of Kaes
  Krause's line
  labial line
  major dense lines
  major period lines
  Mees' l.
  Morgan's l.
  mucogingival l.
  nasal l.
  neonatal l.
  oculozygomatic l.
  l. of Owen

line (*continued*)
  pectinate l.
  period l.
  Pickerill's imbrication l.
  primitive l.
  Raji l.
  Reid base l.
  resonance l.
  Retzius' l.
  Salter's l.
  Sampaolesis's wavy line
  simian l.
  Sydney l.
  Trümmerfeld l.
  Ullmann's l.
  Z l.
  l. of Zahn

linea (pl. lineae)
  l. albicantes
  l. atrophicae

lingua (pl. linguae)
  l. frenata
  l. geographica
  l. nigra
  l. plicata
  l. villosa nigra

linguopapillitis

linin

linitis

linnean system of nomenclature

lipacidemia

lipaciduria

liparocele

liparodyspnea

lipase
  l. assay
  lipoprotein l.
  pancreatic l.

lipedema

lipemia
  absorptive l.

lipemia (*continued*)
    diabetic l.
    postprandial l.
    l. retinalis

lipemic

lipidemia

lipidosis (pl. lipidoses)
    cerebroside l.
    galactosylceramide l.
    glucosylceramide l.
    glycolipid l.
    sphingomyelin l.
    sulfatide l.

lipiduria

lipoamide dehydrogenase
  deficiency

lipoarthritis

lipoatrophy
    insulin l.

lipocardiac

lipocele

lipoceratous

lipocere

lipochromemia

lipocyanine

lipodystrophia
    l. intestinalis
    l. progressiva

lipodystrophy
    congenital generalized l.
    congenital progressive l.
    generalized l.
    intestinal l.
    partial l.
    progressive l.
    progressive congenital l.
    progressive partial l.
    total l.

lipoedema

lipofibroma

lipofuscin

lipofuscinosis
    ceroid-l.
    neuronal ceroid-l.

lipogenic

lipogranuloma

lipogranulomatosis
    disseminated l.
    Farber's l.

lipohemia

lipohemarthrosis

lipohyalin

lipohypertrophy
    insulin l.

lipoic acid

lipoid
    l. degeneration
    l. dystrophy
    l. nephrosis
    l. proteinosis

lipoidemia

lipolipoidosis

lipoma
    l. annulare colli
    diffuse l.
    l. dolorosa
    epidural l.

lipomatoid

lipomatosis (pl. lipomatoses)
    l. atrophicans
    congenital l. of pancreas
    diffuse l.
    l. dolorosa
    encephalocraniocutaneous
     l.
    m. gigantea
    macrodystrophia l.
    mediastinal l.
    l. neurotica

lipomatosis (*continued*)
    nodular circumscribed l.
    renal l.
    l. renis
    symmetrical l.

lipomelanin

lipomeningocele

lipomyelomeningocele

liponephrosis

lipopathy

lipopeliosis

lipopenia

lipopenic

lipophagia
    l. granulomatosis

lipophagy

lipophanerosis

lipophilic

lipophilin

lipoprotein
    floating beta l.

lipoproteinemia

lipoprotein-X (Lp-X)

lipoproteinosis

liposis

lipotrophic

lipoxeny

lippa

lippitude

lipuria

lipuric

liquifacient

liquifactive

liquid
    l. chromotography
    l. scintillation counter
    l. scintillator

Lison-Dunn stain

lissencephalia

lissencephalic

lissencephaly
    Walker's l.

listeriosis, listerosis

lithiasis
    appendicular l.
    l. conjunctivae
    pancreatic l.
    uric acid l.
    urinary l.

lithic

lithium
    l. assay
    l. carbonate
    l. tungstate

lithocholate

lithogenesis

lithogenic

lithogenous

lithonephritis

lithuresis

littoral cell

littritis

livedo
    postmortem l.
    l. racemosa
    livedo reticularis
    l. reticularis, idiopathic
    l. reticularis, symptomatic
    l. telangiectatica

livedoid

liver
    albuminoid l.
    amyloid l.
    biliary cirrhotic l.
    brimstone l.
    bronze l.
    l. cell adenoma
    cirrhotic l.
    degraded l.
    fatty l.
    floating l.
    l. flocculation test
    foamy l.
    frosted l.
    l. function test
    hobnail l.
    icing l.
    infantile l.
    iron l.
    nutmeg l.
    pigmented l.
    polycystic l.
    sago l.
    sugar-icing l.
    wandering l.
    waxy l.

liver phosphorylase deficiency

liver phosphorylase kinase
  deficiency

lividity
    postmortem l.

livor
    l. mortis

lixiviation

lobe
    polyalveolar l.

lobulation
    fetal l.
    portal l.

lobule

lochiocolpos

lochiometra

lochiometritis

lochiorrhagia

lochiorrhea

lochioschesis

lochiostasis

lochometritis

locoregional

loculated

loculus (pl. loculi)

locus (pl. loci)
    l. minoris resistentiae

logagraphia

logarithm

logic
    CMOS l.
    emitter-coupled l.
    tristate l.

logit transformation

lophotrichous

Losch nodule

loupe

louse (pl. lice)

louse-borne typhus

low-density
    l-d. lipoprotin
    l-d. lipoprotein-cholesterol

Lowenthal reaction

loxarthron

loxarthrosis

loxia

L-phase variant

Lu antigen

lues

luetic
   l. aneurysm
   m. aortitis

Lugol solution

lumbago
   ischemic l.

lumbarization

lumbodynia

lumbrical

lumbricidal

lumbricoid

lumbricosis

Lumi-Phos solution

Luna-Ishak stain

lunatomalacia

lung
   accessory l.
   acinic cell tumor of l.
   air conditioner l.
   arc welder's l.
   bauxite l.
   bilobed l.
   bird breeder's l.
   bird fancier's l.
   bird handler's l.
   black l.
   brown l.
   cadmium l.
   cardiac l.
   cheese handler's l.
   cheese washer's l.
   coal miner's l.
   cobalt l.
   corundum smelter's l.
   cystic disease of l.
   eosinophilic l.
   epoxy resin l.
   farmer's l.
   fibroid l.
   grain handler's l.
   harvester's l.
   honeycomb l.

lung (continued)
   humidifier l.
   hyperlucent l.
   Labrador l.
   malt worker's l.
   mason's l.
   meat wrapper's l.
   miller's l.
   miner's l.
   mushroom worker's l.
   pigeon breeder's l.
   pseudovascular adenoid
      squamous cell carcinoma
      of the l. (PASSCL)
   rudimentary l.
   shock l.
   silo filler's l.
   silver finisher's l.
   silver polisher's l.
   thresher's l.
   uremic l.
   vanishing l.
   vineyard sprayer's l.
   welder's l.
   wet l.
   white l.

lupiform

lupinine

lupoid

lupous

lupus
   l. band test
   chilblain l.
   chronic discoid l.
      erythematosus
   cutaneous l. erythematosus
   disseminated l.
      erythematosus
   drug-induced l.
   l. erythematosus
   l. erythematosus, chilblain
   l. erythematosus inhibitor
   l. erythematosus, discoid
   l. erythematosus,
      hypertrophic

lupus (*continued*)
  l. erythematosus, systemic
  l. erythematosus, systemic,
    ANA-negative
  l. erythematosus, systemic,
    transient neonatal
  l. erythematosus profundus
  l. erythematosus tumidus
  l. hypertrophicus
  l. miliaris disseminatus
    faciei
  neonatal l.
  l. nephritis
  l. pernio
  l. profundus
  l. tumidus
  l. verrucosus
  l. vulgaris
  m. vulgaris erythematoides

Luse body

lutein body

luteinization

leuteinizing follicular cyst

luteotropic hormone

lutetium

luteum
  cystis corpus l.

luxatio
  l. coxae congenita
  l. erecta
  l. imperfecta
  l. perinealis

luxation
  Malgaigne's l.

Luxol fast blue stain

luxuriant

17,20-lyase deficiency

lycopenemia

lycoperdonosis

lycopodium

Lyme
  L. borreliosis
  L. disease serology

lymph
  aplastic l.
  corpuscular l.
  croupous l.
  euplastic l.
  fibrinous l.
  glycerinated l.
  inflammatory l.
  intercellular l.
  intravascular l.
  l. node biopsy
  l. varix

lymphadenitis
  Kikachi l.
  paratuberculous l.
  regional granulomatous l.
  tuberculous l.

lymphadenocele

lymphadenocyst

lymphadenopathy
  angioimmunoblastic l.
  angioimmunoblastic l. with
    dysproteinemia
  dermatopathic l.
  immunoblastic l.
  silicone l.

lymphadenopathy-associated
virus

lymphadenosis

lymphadenovarix

lymphangeitis

lymphangiectasia
  intestinal l.

lymphangiectasis
  cavernous l.
  cystic l.
  intestinal l.
  simple l.

lymphangiectatic

lymphangiitis

lymphangioendothelial sarcoma

lymphangiomatosis

lymphangiomycomatosis

lymphangiomyomatosis

lymphangiophlebitis

lymphangiosarcoma

lymphangitic

lymphangitis

lymphapheresis

lymphatism

lymphatitis

lymphatolysis

lymphatolitic

lymphectasia

lymphedema
    congenital l.
    hereditary l.
    l. praecox
    primary l.

lymphemia

lymphenteritis

lymphnoditis

lymphoblast

lymphoblastic
    l. leukemia
    l. lymphoma
    l. lymphosarcoma

lymphocele

lymphocyst

lymphocytapheresis

lymphocyte
    atypical l.
    cytologic T. l.
    Downey-type l.

lymphocyte (*continued*)
    l. function associated
        antigen
    mantle-zone l.
    l. mitogenic factor
    nodular poorly
        differentiated l.
    l. predominance Hodgkin
        disease (LPHD)
    l. subset enumeration
    l. transfer test
    tumor-infiltrating l. (TIL,
        TILS)

lymphocyte-activating factor

lymphocyte-stimulating
    hormone

lymphocythemia

lymphocytic
    l. adenohypophysitis
    l. choriomeningitis
    l. hypophysitis
    l. infiltration of skin
    l. interstitial pneumonitis
    l. leukemoid reaction
    l. leukocytosis
    l. leukopenia
    l. thymoma
    l. transformation

lymphocytoblast

lymphocytolysis

lymphocytopenia

lymphocytopoiesis

lymphocytorrhexis

lymphocytosis
    acute infectious l.
    neutrophilic l.

lymphocytotoxicity

lymphocytotoxin

lymphoderma

lymphogenous

lymphogranuloma
    benign l.
    inguinal l.
    malignant l.
    Schaumann l.
    venereal l.

lymphogranulomatosis

lymphohematopoiesis

lymphohistiocytosis
    erythrophagocytic l.
    hemophagocytic l.

lymphoma
    adult T-cell l.
    adult T-cell leukemia/l.
    anaplastic l.
    B-cell l.
    benign l.
    biphenotypic l.
    Burkitt l.
    centrocytic l.
    cutaneous l.
    diffuse histiocytic l.
    discordant l.
    extranodal l.
    giant follicular l.
    histiocytic l.
    Hodgkin l.
    immunoblastic l.
    l. immunophenotyping
    large cell l.
    Lennert l.
    lymphoblastic l.
    lymphocytic l.
    lymphoplasmacytoid l.
    microfollicular l.
    malignant l.
    mantle cell l.
    marginal zone l.
    Mediterranean l.
    monocytoid B-cell l.
    nodular histiocytic l.
    non-Hodgkin l.
    non-MALT l.
    parafollicular B-cell l.
    poorly-differentiated
      lymphocytic l.

lymphoma (*continued*)
    prethymic lymphoblastic l.
    pyothorax-associated l.
    respiratory angiocentric l.
    small cell lymphocytic l.
    stem cell l.
    T cell rich, B-cell l.
    undifferentiated l.
    Waldeyer ring l.
    well-differentiated
      lymphocytic l.

lymphomatosis
    avian l.
    visceral l.

lymphomatous

lymphomyeloma

lymphomyxoma

lymphopathia

lymphopathy
    ataxic l.

lymphopenia

lymphopenic thymic dysplasia

lymphophagocytosis

lymphoplasmapheresis

lymphopoietic

lymphoproliferative

lymphoreticular

lymphoreticulosis

lymphorrhage

lymphorrhagia

lymphorrhea

lymphostasis

lymphotism

lymphotrophy

lysate

lysergic acid

lysidin
    l. bitartrate

lysin

lysine-ketoglutarate reductase
    deficiency

l-lysine: NAD oxidoreductase
    deficiency

lysinuria

lysosomal

lysosomal α-glucosidase
    deficiency

lysosome
    primary l.
    secondary l.

lysozymuria

M

μ

mA
milliampere

Mac387 antibody

Macchiavello stain

macerate

maceration

Mache unit

macrencephalia

macrencephaly

macroamylase

macroamylasemia

macroamylasemic

macroaggregate

macroaggregated albumin
(MAA)

macroamylase

macrobiote

macroblast

macroblepharia

macrobrachia

macrocephaly

macrocheilia, macrochilia

macrocheiria

macrochilia

macrochiria

macroclitoris

macrocolon

macroconidium (pl.
macroconidia)

macrocornea

macrocrania

macrocryoglobulin

macrocyst

macrocyte

macrocythemia

macrocytic

macrocytosis

macrodactylia

macrodactyly

macrodont

macrodontia

macrodontic

macrodontism

macrodystrophia
m. lipomatosa progressiva

macroencephaly

macroerythroblast

macroesthesia

macrofollicular

macrogamete

macrogametocyte

macrogenitosomia
m. praecox

macroglia

macroglobulin

macroglobulinemia
Waldenström's m.

macroglossia

macrognathia

macrographia

macrography

macrogyria

macrolides

macrolymphocyte

macromastia

macromazia

macromerozoite

macromonocyte

macromyeloblast

macronodular

macronormoblast

macronucleus

macronucleoli

macronychia

macroorchidism

macro-ovalocyte

macroparasite

macropathology

macrophage
    m. activation factor
    m. agglutination factor
    alveolar m.
    m. chemotactic factor
    m. colony-stimulating factor
    m. growth factor
    Hansemann m.
    inflammatory m.
    m. inflammatory protein
    m. migration inhibition
      factor
    m. migration inhibition test
    m. pulmonary alveolar m.
    tingible body m.

macrophage-56

macrophage-activating factor

macrophage-derived growth
  factor

macrophage-inhibiting factor

macrophagocyte

macrophallus

macrophthalmia

macroplasia

macroplastia

macropodia

macropolycyte

macropromyelocyte

macroreticulocyte

macropsia

macroscopic agglutination

macroshock

macrosigmoid

macrosis

macrosomatia
    m. adiposa congenita

macrosomia
    fetal m.
    neonatal m.

macrospore

macrosteatosis

macrostereognosia

macrothrombocyte

macrotia

macrotome

macula (pl. maculae)
    m. albida, m. albidae
    m. atrophica
    cerebral m.
    m. ceruleae
    m. densa
    m. gonorrhoeica
    m. lactea
    mongolian m.
    Saenger's m.
    m. tendineae

macule
    ash-leaf m.
    coal m.
    lance-ovate m.

maculopapular

maculopathy
   bull's eye m.

maculovesicular

madarosis

maduromycosis

magenta
   m. 0
   m. I
   m. II
   m. III
   acid m.
   basic m.

MAggF
   macrophage agglutination
      factor

magnesemia

magnesium
   m. ammonium phosphate
   m. assay

main
   m. d'accoucheur
   m. en crochet
   m. en griffe
   m. en lorgnette
   m. en singe
   m. en squelette
   m. succulente

MAK6 immunohistochemical
   reagent

malabsorption
   congenital lactose m.
   glucose-galactose m.
   sucrose-isomaltose m.,
      congenital
   m. syndrome

malacia
   metaplastic m.
   myeloplastic m.
   porotic m.
   m. traumatica

malacic

malacoma

malacoplakia
   renal m.
   m. vesicae

malacosis

malacosteon

malacotic

maladie
   m. des jambes
   m. de Roger
   m. des tics

malakoplakia

malaria
   algid m.
   benign tertian m.
   bovine m.
   falciparum m.
   hemolytic m.
   hemorrhagic m.
   malariae m.
   ovale m.
   pernicious m.
   quartan m.
   quotidian m.
   remittent m.
   vivax m.

malariacidal

malarious

Malassez disease

malate dehydrogenase

malathion

maldigestion

malformation
   Arnold-Chiari m.
   arteriovenous m. (AVM)
   cardiac valvular m.
   cerebral arteriovenous m.
   Chiari's m.
   cutaneous m.

malformation (*continued*)
    cystic adenomatoid m.
    Dandy-Walker m.
    Ebstein m.
    Mondini's m.

malleation

mallein test

Mallory
    M. aniline blue stain
    M. collagen stain
    M. iodine stain
    M. phloxine stain
    M. phosphotungstic acid
      hematoxylin stain
    M. stain for actinomyces
    M. stain for hemofuchsin
    M. trichrome stain
    M. triple stain

malpighii
    stratum m.

malt
    m. agar
    n. extract broth

MALT
    mucosa-associated
      lymphoid tissue

maltosuria

malum
    m. articulorum senilis
    m. coxae senile
    m. vertebrale suboccipitale

mammary
    m. duct ectasia
    m. dysplasia
    m. Paget disease
    m. tumor virus

mamma
    m. areolata

mammalgia

mammatroph

mammillitis

mammitis

mammosomatotropic

mammotroph

manchette

maneuver
    Gowers' m.
    Valsalva m.

manganism

manganous

mange
    sarcoptic m.

manifesting heterozygote

mannans

mannosazone

mannosidosis

mantle cell

mantle zone lymphocyte

Mantoux skin test

manus
    m. cava
    m. extensa
    m. flexa
    m. plana
    m. superextensa
    m. valga
    m. vara

manuum

map
    chromosome m.
    cytogenic m.
    linkage m.

mapping
    g. mapping

maprotiline

marantic
    m. atrophy
    m. endocarditis
    n. thrombosis

marasmatic

marasmic

marasmoid

marasmus
    nutritional m.

marbleization

Marburg
    M. virus

marcescens
    m. marcescens

marche
    m. à petits pas

Marchesani syndrome

Marchi
    M. fixative
    M. reaction
    M. stain

Marcy agent

Marfan
    M. disease
    M. syndrome

margaritoma

margin
    costal m.
    dentate m.

marginated chromatin

Margolis syndrome

maritonucleus

Marituba virus

mark
    pock m.
    Pohl's m.
    Pohl-Pinkus m.
    port-wine m.
    strawberry m.
    Unna m.

marker
    allotypic m.

marker (*continued*)
    B-cell m.
    cell surface m.
    DNA marker
    endocrine m.
    enzyme m.
    genetic m.
    HMB-45 m.
    immunohistochemical m.
    myogen m.
    polymorphic genetic m.
    rhabdomyosarcoma m.
    S-100 m.
    utrophin m.

Marme reagent

marmoratus
    status m.

marmoreal

marmoset virus

Marquis reagent

marrow
    aplastic bone m.
    basophilic m.
    depressed m.
    erythrocytic m.
    leukocytic m.
    lymphocytic m.
    gelatinous m.
    monocytic m.
    neutrophilic m.
    reticulocytic m.

Marseilles fever

marsh fever

Martin-Lester agar

MASCT/MAS cytology test

mass
    m. action law
    achromatic m.
    appendiceal m.
    appendix m.
    m. attenuation coefficient
    carbon gelatin m.

mass (*continued*)
    critical m.
    erythrocyte m.
    fibrillar m. of Flemming
    filar m.
    m. fragmentography
    red blood cell m.
    m. spectrograph
    tigroid m.

Masson
    M. argentaffin stain
    M. trichrome method
    M. trichrome stain

Masson-Fontana ammoniacal
    silver stain

mast cell

mastadenitis

mastadenoma

mastalgia

mastatrophia

mastatrophy

mastauxe

masthelcosis

mastitis
    acute m.
    bovine m.
    cystic m.
    fibrocystic m.
    gargantuan m.
    glandular m.
    granulomatous m.
    interstitial m.
    lactational m.
    m. neonatorum
    parenchymatous m.
    periductal m.
    plasma cell m.
    puerperal m.
    retromammary m.
    submammary m.
    stagnation m.
    suppurative m.

mastocytogenesis

mastocytoma

mastocytosis
    diffuse m.
    systemic m.

mastoiditis

mastoidea

mastodynia

mastoidalgia

mastoiditis
    Bezold's m.
    sclerosing m.
    silent m.

mastomenia

mastopathia
    m. cystica

mastopathy
    cystic m.

mastoptosis

mastorrhagia

mastoscirrhus

material
    biuret reactive m.
    calibration m.
    Cotasil silicone slide
        coating m.
    cross-reacting m.
    extra-cellular m.
    fluorescent m.
    gonadotropin-inhibitory m.
    Matrix Reference m.
    neurosecretory m.
    particulate crystalline m.
    Simulated Matrix Reference
        m.

matrix
    bone m.
    m. calculus
    cytoplasmic m.
    hair m.

matrix (*continued*)
    mitochondrial m.
    myxoid m.
    sarcoplasmic m.

maturate

maxillitis

Maximow stain for bone
  marrow

mayweed

mazamurra

mazodynia

mazoplasia

MCAD deficiency

MCI/MI

McGadey syndrome

MCH
    mean corpuscular
      hemoglobin

MCHC
    mean corpuscular
      hemoglobin concentration

mCi
    millicurie

McLeod phenotype

McPhail test

MCV
    mean corpuscular volume

M-DES stain

Mecke reagent

meconiorrhea

media (pl. of medium)

mediastinitis
    acute m.
    chronic m.
    fibrosing m.
    fibrous m.
    granulomatous m.
    indurative m.

mediastinopericarditis
    adhesive m.

medionecrosis
    m. of aorta

medium (pl. media)
    aerotitis m.
    aqueous mounting m.
    Bactalert FAN culture m.
    Balamuth culture m.
    Cyto-Gel embedding m.
    culture m.
    dermatophyte test m.
    Epon tissue embedding m.
    Farrant m.
    glycerol gelatin m.
    Lash casein-hydrolysate-
      serum m.
    Loffler blood culture m.
    Loffler coagulated serum
      m.
    mounting m.
    nonpermissive culture m.
    oxidation-fermentation m.
    Petragnani m,
    PVA lacto-phenol m.
    radiopaque m.
    Rees culture m.
    serous otitis m.
    tellurite m.
    thioglycolate m.
    tissue culture m.

medorrhea

medullization

medulloblast

medulloepithelioma

Medusa head

megabladder

megacalycosis

megacecum

megacephalic

megacholedochus

megacolon
  aganglionic m.
  chronic idiopathic m.
  congenital m.
  idiopathic m.
  toxic m.

megacystis

megacystic syndrome

megaesophagus

megakaryocyte
  basophilic m.

megalencephalon

megalencephaly

megalgia

megaloblast

megaloblastoid

megaloblastosis

megalocephalia

megalocephalic

megalocephaly

megalocheiria

megaloclitoris

megalocornea

megalocystis

megalocyte

megalocythemia

megalocytosis

megalodactylia

megalodactylism

megalodactylous

megalodactyly

megalodontia

megaloesophagus

megalogastria

megaloglossia

megalographia

megalohepatia

megalonychia

megalopenis

megalophthalmos

megalopia

megalopodia

megalopsia

Megalopyge

megalosplenia

megalothymus

megaloureter

megalourethra

megamitochondria

meganucleus

megarectum

megasigmoid

megasoma

megaspore

megathrombocyte

megaureter

megaurethra

megavolt

megophthalmos

mehlnährschaden

meibomian
  m. cyst
  m. stye

meibomianitis

meibomitis

meiogenic

meiosis

meiotic

Meissel stain

meissnerian differentiation

melagra

melalgia

melanemesis

melanemia

melanicterus

melaniferous

melanin
    artificial m.
    m. bleaching method
    m. pigmentation
    m. staining method

melanoblastosis

melanocyte
    dendritic m.

melanocyte-inhibiting hormone

melanocyte-stimulating
  hormone

melanocytic

melanocytosis
    oculodermal m.

melanoderma
    parasitic m.
    senile m.

melanodermatitis
    m. toxica lichenoides

melanogen

melanoglossia

melanoleukoderma
    m. colli

melanoma
    acral lentiginous m.
    benign juvenile m.
    cutaneous malignant m.
    desmoplastic m.

melanoma (*continued*)
    epitheloid m.
    lentigo maligna m.
    malignant m.
    nodular m.
    subungual m.
    superficial spreading m.

melanomastosis

melanonychia

melanophore-stimulating
  hormone

melanoplakia

melanoptysis

melanosis
    m. bulbi
    m. circumscripta
    m. coli
    m. iridis
    m. of the iris
    m. oculi
    oculocutaneous m.
    oculodermal m.
    Riehl's m.
    m. sclerae
    tar m.
    transient neonatal pustular
      m.
    vagabond's m.

melanosome

melanotrichia
    m. linguae

melanotroph

melanuria

melanuresis

melanuria

melanuric

melasma

Melasyn (water-soluble
  synthetic melanin)

melena
    m. neonatorum
    m. spuria
    m. vera

melenic

melicera

meliceris

melitis

melituria

melorheostosis

melosalgia

meloschisis

membrane
    accidental m.
    acute inflammatory m.
    acute pyogenic m.
    adamantine m.
    alveolar-capillary m.
    alveolocapillary m.
    antral m.
    asphyxial m.
    basal m. of semicircular
      duct
    basement m.
    Bichat's m.
    Bowman's m.
    Bruch m.
    m. capacitance
    capsular m.
    capsulopupillary m.
    cell m.
    chromatic m.
    croupous m.
    cyclitic m.
    cytoplasmic m.
    decidual m.
    dentinoenamel m.
    Descemet's m.
    diphtheritic m.
    egg m.
    elastic m.
    elastic m., external
    elastic m., internal

membrane (*continued*)
    enamel m.
    endoneural m.
    epithelial basement m.
    erythrocyte m.
    excitable m.
    exocoelomic m.
    false m.
    fenestrated m.
    m. filter technique
    glassy m.
    glomerular m.
    glomerular capillary m.
    ground m.
    Haller's m.
    Hannover's intermediate m.
    Henle's m.
    Henle's elastic m.
    Henle's fenestrated m.
    Heuser's m.
    Huxley's m.
    hyaline m.
    hyaloid m.
    Hybond N+ nylon m.
    inflammatory m.
    Jackson's m.
    Jacob's m.
    Kölliker's m.
    Krause's m.
    limiting m., external
    limiting m., inner
    limiting m., internal
    limiting m., outer
    Mauthner's m.
    medullary m.
    Nasmyth's m.
    nuclear m.
    otolithic m.
    periorbital m.
    photoreceptor m.
    plasma m.
    postsynaptic m.
    m. potential
    premature rupture of fetal
      m's.
    presynaptic m.
    proper m. of semicircular
      duct

membrane (*continued*)
   prophylactic m.
   m. protein
   pupillary m.
   pyloric m.
   pyogenic m.
   pyophylactic m.
   reticular m.
   Ruysch's m.
   ruyschian m.
   Schwann's m.
   semipermeable m.
   m. of Slavianski
   slit m.
   striated m.
   synaptic m.
   undulating m.
   unit m.
   vernix m.
   vitelline m.
   vitreous m.
   Volkmann's m.
   Wachendorf's m.
   Zinn's m.

membranolysis

membranoproliferative
  glomerulonephritis

membranous-proliferative
  glomerulonephritis

memory
   cache m.
   core m.
   magnetic core m.

menadione

menalgia

menaquinone

mendelevium

mendelian genetics

Mendel law

menhidrosis

menidrosis

meningeal

meningioma
   cutaneous m.
   fibroblastic m.
   meningothelial m.
   mucinous m.
   psammomatous m.

meningematoma

meninghematoma

meningismus

meningitic

meningitis (pl. meningitides)
   acute aseptic m.
   amebic m.
   aseptic m.
   bacterial m.
   basilar m.
   benign lymphocytic m.
   cerebral m.
   cerebrospinal m.
   chronic m.
   cryptococcal m.
   eosinophilic m.
   epidemic cerebrospinal m.
   external m.
   gummatous m.
   Haemophilus influenzae m.
   internal m.
   lymphocytic m.
   meningococcal m.
   Mollaret's m.
   mumps m.
   occlusive m.
   m. ossificans
   otitic m.
   pneumococcal m.
   purulent m.
   pyogenic m.
   m. serosa circumscripta
   serous m.
   spinal m.
   sterile m.
   subacute m.
   m. sympathica
   syphilitic m.

meningitis (*continued*)
tubercular m.
tuberculous m.
viral m.

meningoarteritis

meningocele
anterior m.
cranial m.
sacral m.
spinal m.
spurious m.
traumatic m.

meningocephalitis

meningocerebral
cicatrix

meningocerebritis

meningococcemia
acute fulminating m.

meningocyte

meningoencephalitis
acute primary hemorrhagic
m.
amebic m.
eosinophilic m.
herpetic m.
mumps m.
primary amebic m.
toxoplasmic m.
syphilitic m.

meningoencephalocele

meningoencephalomyelitis

meningoencephalomyelopathy

meningoencephalopathy

meningomalacia

meningomyelitis
syphilitic m.

meningomyelocele

meningomyeloencephalitis

meningomyeloradiculitis

meningo-osteophlebitis

meningopathy

meningopolyneuritis

meningoradiculitis

meningorrhagia

meningorrhea

menischesis

meniscitis

meniscocyte

meniscocytosis

meniscus (pl. menisci)
degenerated m.
discoid m.
discoid lateral m.
m. tactus

menolipsis

menometrorrhagia

menoplania

menorrhagia

menorrhalgia

menoschesis

menostaxis

menouria

mephitic

mephitis

meralgia
m. paresthetica

2-mercaptoethanol

merisis

meristic variation

Merkel
M. cell
M. corpuscle

merocoxalgia

merogony
    diploid m.
    parthenogenetic m.

meromelia

meromyosin

meropia

merorachischisis

merosmia

merotomy

mesangial

mesangiocapillary

mesangiolysis

mesangium
    extraglomerular m.

mesarteritis
    Mönckeberg's m.

mesaxon

mesectoderm

mesencephalitis

mesenchymal
    m. differentiation
    m. hemartoma
    n. hyloma

mesenchyme

mesenchymoma

mesenteritis
    retractile m.

mesiodens

mesiodentes

mesoaortitis
    m. syphilitica

mesoappendicitis

mesobilin

mesoblastema

mesocardia

mesochondrium

mesochoroidea

mesocornea

mesophlebitis

mesophragma

mesorachischisis

mesostroma

metabisulfate test

metabolic
    m. antagonism
    m. clearance rate
    m. detoxification
    m. equivalent
    m. pathway

metabolism
    divalent m.
    glucose m.
    propionate m.

metachromatic-type
    leukodystrophy

metachromasia

metachromatic

metachromatin

metachromatism

metachromatophil

metachromia

metachromic

metachromophil

metachromophile

metacresol
    m. purple
    m. sulfonphthalein

metacyesis

metafemale

metagenesis

metagglutinin

metaicteric

metakinesis

metallophilic

metamorphopsia

metamorphotic

metaneutrophil

metanucleus

metaphase

metaphosphoric acid

metaphysitis

metaplasia
    agnogenic myeloid m.
    apocrine m.
    autoparenchymatous m.
    cartilaginous m.
    chondroid m.
    decidual m.
    endothelial m.
    epidermoid m.
    glandular m.
    Hurthle cell m.
    myeloid m.
    myeloid m., primary
    myeloid m., secondary
    osseous m.
    pseudopyloric m.
    squamous m.
    tuboendometrioid m.

metaplastic
    m. columnar epithelium
    m. keratinization
    m. ossification

metapneumonic

metastasize

metastasis (pl. metastases)
    biochemical m.
    hematogenous m.
    lymphogenous m.

metasynapsis

metasyncrisis

metasyndesis

metatarsalgia
    Morton's m.

metatypical carcinoma

metaxeny (var. of metoxeny)

Metazoa

Metchnikoff theory

meter
    AccuData Easy glucose m.
    d'Arsonval m.
    HemoCue glucose m.
    Miles Encore QA glucose
      m.

meteorism

methacrylate
    butyl m.
    glycol m.

methamphetamine

methemalbumin

methemalbuminemia

methemoglobinemia
    acquired m.
    m. assay
    congenital m.
    hereditary m.
    toxic m.

methemoglobinemic

methemoglobinuria

methenamine
    m. hippurate
    m. mandelate
    m. silver

method
    acid anhydride m.
    acid fast staining m.
    agar diffusion m.
    Ashley differential
      agglutination m.
    autoclave m.
    axon staining m.

method (*continued*)

bacterial agar m.
bacterial antigen detection m.
Baker sudan black m.
Barger's m.
Baumgartner m.
Beaver direct smear m.
Bengston m.
benzo sky blue m.
Berg chelate removal m.
biotin streptavidin detection m.
Bodian m.
calcium m. for
cellophane tape m.
cell separation m.
Chang aniline-acid fuchsin m.
chloranilate m.
cholesterol staining m.
chromolytic m.
Clark-Collip m.
clean-catch collection m.
cobaltinitrite m.
Coblenz test m.
collagen staining m.
cooled knife m.
copper sulfate m.
Couette m.
creatine, m. for
creatinine, m. for
cysteic acid m.
Denis and Leche's m.
diazo staining m.
diffusion m.
digitonin m.
Ellinger's m.
enzyme digestion m.
esterase staining m.
Fishberg's m.
Fiske's m.
Fiske and Subbarow's m.
fixed base, m. for
fixed sediment m.
flat substrate m.
Folin's m.
Folin and Wu's m.

method (*continued*)

formaldehyde-induced fluorescence m.
formalin-ether sedimentation m.
frozen section m.
Givens' m.
glucose oxidase m.
glycerin m.
Gram's m.
Hammerschlag m.
Heublein m.
hexokinase m.
HSU m.
immunofluorescence m.
immunoperoxidase staining m.
indican, m. for
indole, m. for
indophenol m.
iodine, m. for
Jendrassik-Grof m.
Jenner m.
Jones m.
Kjeldahl's m.
Klüver-Barrera m.
Lee-White clotting time m.
Lillie allochrome m.
macro-Kjeldahl m.
Millipore m.
Monte Carlo m.
melanin bleaching m.
melanin staining m.
Nichols m.
Nuclepore m.
panoptic m.
Papanicolaou m.
Penfield m.
peptic activity, m. for
periodic acid-Schiff m.
peroxidase staining m.
plasma thrombin clot m.
protein separation m.
PVA fixative m.
reference m.
Romanovsky's (Romanowsky's) m.
Sahli m.

method (*continued*)
    Salzman m.
    Schick m.
    Shaffer-Hartmann m.
    Somogyi m.
    special reference m.
    streptavidin-biotin
        peroxidase m.
    suction m.
    sugar, m. for
    sulfosalicylic acid m.
    sulfur, total, m. for
    Sumner's m.
    Sweet m.
    thermodilution m.
    two-slide m.
    ultropaque m.
    urea, m. for
    urease, m. for
    uric acid, m. for
    Van Slyke's m.
    Westergren sedimentation
        rate m.
    Whipple m.
    Wintrobe sedimentation
        rate m.
    zeta sedimentation ratio m.
    Ziehl-Neelsen m.
    ZSR m.

methodology

methyl
    m. acetate
    m. aldehyde
    m. blue
    m. bromide
    m. butyl ketone
    m. green
    m. hydroxy-furfural
    m. isobutyl ketone
    m. iodide
    m. mercury
    m. orange
    m. parathion
    m. red test
    m. violet
    m. yellow

α-methylacetoaceticaciduria

methylchloroisothiazolinone

3-methylcrotonic acid

3-methylcrotonyl CoA
    carboxylase deficiency

3-methylcrotonylglycine

β-methylcrotonylglycinuria

methylene
    m. azure
    m. blue
    m. dichloride
    m. violet
    m. white

methylenetetrahydrofolate
    (THF) reductase deficiency

methylenophil

methylenophilous

3-methylglutaconic acid

3-methylglutaconicaciduria

3-methylglutaric acid

methylglyoxalidin

3-methylhistidine

methylisothiazolinone

methylmalonic acid

methylmalonicacidemia

methylmalonicaciduria

methylrosaniline chloride

methylthionine chloride

Metopirone test

metopism

metoxenous

metratonia

metratrophia

metrectopia

X MG/Lambert-Eaton panel

metria

metritis
    m. dissecans
    dissecting m.
    puerperal m.

metrocele

metrocolpocele

metrocystosis

metrocyte

metroendometritis

metroleukorrhea

metrolymphangitis

metromalacia

metromenorrhagia

metroparalysis

metropathy

metroperitonitis

metrophlebitis

metroptosis

metrorrhagia
    m. myopathica

metrorrhea

metrorrhexis

metrosalpingitis

metrostaxis

metrostenosis

mevalonicaciduria

X micatosis

microabscess
    Munro m.

microalbuminuria

microanalysis

microaneurysm

microangiopathic

microangiopathy
    diabetic m.
    thrombotic m.

microbioassay

microblast

microblepharia

microblepharism

microblephary

microcalcification

microcardia

microcentrum

microcheilia

microcinematography

microcolon

microcoria

microcornea

microcurie-hour

microcyst

microcyte
    hypochromic m.

microcythemia

microcytic

microcytosis

microdactylia

microdactyly

microdont

microdontia

microdontic

microdontism

microdrepanocytic

microdrepanocytosis

microdysgenesia

microelectrode

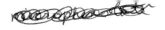

microelectrophoresis

microelectrophoretic

microembolus

microerythrocyte

microfilament

microfluorometry

microfracture

microgastria

microgenia

microgenitalism

microglia

microgliacyte

microglial

microgliocyte

microglobulin

microglossia

micrognathia

micrograph
   electron m.

micrographia

micrography

microgyrus

microhematocrit

microhematuria

microhepatia

microincineration

microinfarct

microliter

microlith

microlithiasis
   m. alveolaris pulmonum
   pulmonary alveolar m.

micrology

micromandible

micromanometer

micromanometric

micromastia

micromaxilla

micromazia

micromegalopsia

micromere

micrometer
   eyepiece m.
   filar m.
   ocular m.
   stage m.

micrometry

micromyeloblast

micronodular

micronormoblast

micronucleus

micronychia

micro-orchidia

micro-orchidism

micropannus

micropathology

micropenis

microphakia

microphallus

microphthalmia

microphthalmos

micropinocytosis

micropituicyte

microplasia

Micro-Plate EIA (enzyme
   immunoassay) kit

micropolariscope

microprecipitation

micropsia

microptic

microrchidia

microrhinia

microscelous

microscope
  acoustic m.
  beta ray m.
  BHTU m.
  binocular m.
  centrifuge m.
  color-contrast m.
  comparison m.
  compound m.
  dark-field m.
  electron m.
  fluorescence m.
  infrared m.
  integrating m.
  interference m.
  ion m.
  JEOL 100 S transmission
    electron m.
  JEOL 1200 S transmission
    electron m.
  laser m.
  light m.
  Nomarski m.
  Olympus BH2 m.
  opaque m.
  phase m.
  phase-contrast m.
  Philips 301 electron m.
  polarizing m.
  polarizing m., rectified
  projection x-ray m.
  reflecting m.
  Rheinberg m.
  scanning m.
  scanning electron m.
  schlieren m.
  simple m.
  stereoscopic m.
  stroboscopic m.

microscope (*continued*)
  transmission electron m.
  trinocular m.
  ultra-m.
  ultrasonic m.
  ultraviolet m.
  x-ray m.
  Zeiss Axiophot fluorescent
    m.
  Zeiss Axioplan m.
  Zeiss LSM-10 laser m.
  Zeiss transmission electron
    m.

microscopist

microscopy
  clinical m.
  electron m.
  fluorescence m.
  immunofluorescence m.
  television m.
  epifluorescence m.

microsoma

microsomal

microsome

microsomia

microspectrophotometer

microsphere

microspherocyte

microspherocytosis

microspherolith

microsplenia

microsplenic

microsporosis
  m. nigra

microsteatosis

Microstix-3

Microtainer lancets

microthelia

microthrombus

microtonometer

microtransfusion

microtropia

microtubule

microvascular

microvasculature

microvasculopathy
    retinal m.

microvoltometer

microxycyte

microxyphil

micrurgic

micrurgy

Middlebrook agar

Middlebrook-Dubos
    hemagglutinin test

migrans
    larva m.

migration
    external m.
    internal m.
    retrograde m.
    transperitoneal m.

Mikulicz cell

milia (pl. of milium)

miliaria
    m. alba
    apocrine m.
    m. crystallina
    m. profunda
    m. rubra

miliary

milium (pl. milia)
    colloid m.

milliampere (mA)

millibar (mbar)

millicoulomb

millicurie

milliequivalent (mEq)

millifarad (mF)

millihenry (mH)

millilambert (mL)

milphosis

mimesis

mimetic

mimosis

miopragia

miosis
    irritative m.
    paralytic m.
    spastic m.
    spinal m.

miotic

miryachit

mitapsis

mitochondria

mitochondrial

mitochondrion

mitogenesia

mitogenesis

mitogenetic

mitogenic

mitokinetic

mitome

mitoplasm

mitoschisis

mitoses

mitosis (pl. mitoses)
    heterotypic m.

mitosis (*continued*)
    homeotypic m.
    multicentric m.
    pathologic m.
    pluripolar m.

mitosome

mitotic
    m. cycle
    m. index

Mitsuda antigen

mittelschmerz

Mittendorf dots

mixture
    dextrose solution m.
    Gunning's m.
    Mayer's glycerin-albumin
      m.
    racemic s.
    toxoid-antitoxin m.

mobility
    electrophoretic m.

mole
    blood m.
    Breus' m.
    cystic m.
    false m.
    fleshy m.
    hydatid m.
    hydatidiform m.
    stone m.
    true m.
    tubal m.
    vesicular m.

molecule
    accessory m.
    adhesion m.
    cell adhesion m.
    intercellular
      adhesion m.
    middle m.
    neural cell adhesion m.

molimen

molimina

Molisch test

mollities
    m. ossium

molluscum (pl. mollusca)
    m. contagiosum
    m. fibrosum
    m. sebaceum virus
    m. verrucum

molybdate

monad

monarthritis
    m. deformans

monaster

monathetosis

monavitaminosis

monerula

monilated

monilethrix

moniliform

moniliid

monoblepsia

monochorea

monochromacy

monochromasy

monochromat

monochromatic

monochromatism
    cone m.
    rod m.

monochromatophil

monochromophilic

monochromatopsia

monocorditis

monocytopenia

monoclonal IgM cápita

monocytosis

Mono-Diff test

monodiplopia

monogenesis

monogenetic

monogenic character

monokine

monoleptic fever

monolocular

monomer

monomorphous

monomorphism

monomyoplegia

monomyositis

mononeuritis
    m. multiplex

mononeuropathy
    cranial m.
    multifocal m.
    multiple m.
    m. multiplex

mononuclear

mononucleate

mononucleosis
    chronic m.

mono-osteitic

monoparesis

monoparesthesia

monopathy

monopenia

monoplegia

monoplegic

monorchia

monorchid

monorchidic

monorchidism

monorchis

monorchism

monosomic

monosomy

monosymptomatic

morbific

morbigenous

morbilliform

morbus
    m. coxae senilis
    m. moniliformis

mordant
    m. solution

morgue

moribund

morphea
    m. acroterica
    m. alba
    generalized m.
    guttate m.
    linear m.
    m. linearis
    m. pigmentosa

morpholysis

morphoplasm

mors
    m. thymica

morsus
    m. humanus

morula

mosaicism
    erythrocyte m.
    confined placental m.
    gonadal m.

moth
  brown-tail m.
  flannel m.
  io m.

motoneuron
  alpha m.
  beta m.
  gamma m.
  heteronymous m.
  homonymous motoneurons
  lower motoneurons
  peripheral motoneuron
  upper motoneurons

moulage

mount
  India ink m.
  wet m.

mountant

mounting medium

mouse-specific lymphocyte
  antigen

mouth
  Ceylon sore m.
  denture sore m.
  dry m.
  glass-blowers' m.
  purse-string m.
  tapir m.
  trench m.
  white m.

6-MP
  6-mercaptopurine

MRSA
  methicillin-resistant
    Staphylococcus aureus

MSB trichome stain

mucicarmine stain

mucicarminophilic

mucigen granules

mucihematein
  Mayer's m.

mucinosis
  cutaneous focal m.
  follicular m.
  localized m.
  metabolic m.
  papular m.
  reticular emphysematous
    m.

mucinuria

mucitis

mucocele
  suppurating m.

mucocolitis

mucocolpos

mucoenteritis

Mucolexx

mucolipidosis
  m. I, m. II, m. III, m. IV

mucopolysaccharidosis
  m. I
  m. IH
  m. IH/S
  m. IS
  m. II
  m. III
  m. IV
  m. V
  m. VI
  m. VII

mucopolysacchariduria

mucoprotein assay

mucopurulent
  m. exudate

mucopus

mucormycosis
  cutaneous m.
  pulmonary m.

mucosanguineous

mucositis

mucosulfatidosis

mucous
   m. cast
   m. cyst
   m. plaque
   m. threads

mucoviscidosis

Mucuna

mucus
   m. extravasation
   m. retention

Müller fixative

multichannel analyzer

multicystic

multiform

multiforme
   glioblastoma m.

multilocular

multinodular

multinucleate

multituberculate

mummification

mumps
   m. antibody titer
   m. serology
   m. skin test antigen
   m. virus vaccine

mumu

muramic acid

muramidase

murexide

murrina

musca
   m. volitantes

muscarine

muscegenetic

muscle phosphofructokinase
   deficiency

muscle phosphorylase
   deficiency

muscle-specific actin (HHF-35)

musculamine

musicogenic

mussitation

Musto stain

mutagen

mutagenicity test

mutant
   m. gene

mutarotation

mutation
   auxotrophic m.
   clear plaque m.
   cold-sensitive m.
   conditional lethal m.
   frame shift m.
   host-range m.
   K-*ras* m.
   phage-resistant m.
   pleiotropic m.
   rapid-lysis m.
   somatic m.
   suppressor m.
   ultra-violet light-induced m.

MVE virus

MY-10 clone stain

myalgia
   m. abdominis
   m. capitis
   m. cervicalis
   m. myalgia

myasthenia
   m. gastrica
   m. gravis
   m. gravis pseudoparalytica
   m. gravis, familial infantile

mycophenolate

myasthenia (*continued*)
    m. laryngis
    neonatal m.

myasthenic

myatonia

myatony

myatrophy

mycelial
    m. fungus
    m. pathogen

mycelial (pl. mycelium)
    aerial m
    nonseptate m.
    septate m.

mycete

mycid

mycoagglutinin

mycobacterial adjuvant

mycobacterium (pl.
    mycobacteria)

mycodermatitis

mycomyringitis

mycopathology

X mycopus

mycosis (pl. mycoses)
    m. cutis chronica
    m. fungoides
    Gilchrist m.
    m. intestinalis
    m. leptothrica
    splenic m.

mycteroxerosis

mydriasis
    alternating m.
    bounding m.
    paralytic m.
    spasmodic m.
    spastic m.
    spinal m.
    springing m.

myectopia

myectopy

myelalgia

myelapoplexy

myelatelia

myelatrophy

myelauxe

myelemia

myelencephalitis

myelin

myelinated

myelinic

myelinoclasis
        acute perivascular m.
        postinfection perivenous m.

myelinolysis
    central pontine m.

myelinopathy

myelinosis

myelinotoxic

myelinotoxicity

myelitic

myelitis
    acute m.
    ascending m.
    bulbar m.
    cavitary m.
    central m.
    chronic m.
    compression m.
    concussion m.
    cornual m.
    diffuse m.
    disseminated m.
    hemorrhagic m.
    neuro-optic m.
    periependymal m.
    postinfectious m.

myelitis (*continued*)
    postvaccinal m.
    subacute m.
    subacute necrotic m.
    syphilitic m.
    transverse m.
    m. vaccinia
    viral m.

myeloablation

myeloablative

myeloblastemia

myeloblastosis

myelocele

myeloclast

myelocyst

myelocystic

myelocystocele

myelocystomeningocele

myelocythemia

myelocytoma

myelocytosis

myelodysplasia

myelodysplastic

myeloencephalitis
    eosinophilic m.

myeloencephalopathy

myelofibrosis
    osteosclerosis m.
    m. with myeloid metaplasia

myeloidin

myeloidosis

myelolysis

myelolytic

myeloma
    indolent m.
    localized m.

myeloma (*continued*)
    multiple m.
    plasma cell m.
    solitary m.

myelomalacia

myelomatoid

myelomatosis

myelomenia

myelomeningitis

myelomeningocele

myelomonocytic

myeloneuritis

myelo-opticoneuropathy
    subacute m.

myelopathic

myelopathy
    anterior m.
    ascending m.
    carcinomatous m.
    cervical m.
    cervical spondylotic m.
    chronic progressive m.
    compression m.
    concussion m.
    cystic m.
    descending m.
    focal m.
    funicular m.
    hemorrhagic m.
    HTLV-1-associated m.
    necrotizing m.
    paracarcinomatous m.
    paraneoplastic m.
    radiation m.
    spondylotic cervical m.
    systemic m.
    transverse m.
    traumatic m.
    vacuolar m.

myeloperoxidase (MPO)
    deficiency

myelophthisic

myelophthisis

myeloplegia

myelopoiesis
    ectopic m.
    extramedullary m.

myeloproliferative

myeloradiculitis

myeloradiculodysplasia

myeloradiculopathy

myelorrhagia

myelosarcoma

myelosarcomatosis

myeloschisis

myelosclerosis

myelosis
    aleukemic m.
    chronic nonleukemic m.
    nonleukemic m.

myelosuppression

myelosuppressive

myelosyphilis

myelotome

myelotoxic

myelotoxicity

myiasis
    creeping m.
    cutaneous m.
    dermal m.
    intestinal m.
    m. linearis
    nasal m.

myiocephalon

myiocephalum

myiodesopsia

myitis

myoadenylate deaminase
   deficiency

myoatrophy

myoblast

myoblastic

myobradia

myocardiopathy

myocarditic

myocardium
    hibernating m.
    stunned m.

myocele

myocelialgia

myocelitis

myocellulitis

myochosis

myoclonia
    m. epileptica
    m. fibrillaris multiplex
    fibrillary m.
    pseudoglottic m.

myoclonic

myoclonus
    action m.
    Baltic m.
    cortical m.
    cortical reflex m.
    epileptic m.
    essential m.
    intention m.
    m. multiplex
    palatal m.
    reflex m.

myocolpitis

myocyte
    Anichkov m.
    Anitschkow's m.

myocytolysis
    coagulative m.
    focal m. of heart

myodegeneration

myodesopsia

myodiastasis

myodynia

myodystonia

myodystony

myodystrophia
    m. fetalis

myodystrophy

myoedema

myoendocarditis

myofascitis

myofiber

myofibril

myofibrilla

myofibrillar

myofibroma
    infantile m.

myofibromatosis
    juvenile m.

myofibrosis
    m. cordis

myofibrositis

myofilament

myogelosis

myogenous

myoglia

myoglobinuria
    familial m.
    idiopathic m.
    spontaneous m.

myoglobulinuria

myohypertrophia
    m. kymoparalytica

myoid
    visual cell m.

myoidem

myoidema

myoischemia

myokymia

myolemma

myolysis
    m. cardiotoxica

myomalacia

myomelanosis

myometritis

myon

myonecrosis
    clostridial m.

myoneural

myonosus

myopachynsis

myopalmus

myoparalysis

myoparesis

myopathia
    m. infraspinata

myopathic

myopathy

myope

myopericarditis

myophage

myophagism

myophosphorylase deficiency

myoplasm

myopsis

myorrhexis

myosalgia

myosalpingitis

myosclerosis

myosinuria

myositic

myositis
    acute disseminated m.
    acute progressive m.
    m. a frigore
    m. clostridial
    m. fibrosa
    inclusion body m.
    infectious m.
    interstitial m.
    multiple m.
    orbital m.
    m. ossificans
    m. ossificans circumscripta
    m. ossificans progressiva
    m. ossificans traumatica
    parenchymatous m.
    primary multiple m.
    progressive ossifying m.
    m. purulenta
    rheumatoid m.
    m. serosa

myospasm

myospasmia

myospherulosis

myostroma

myosuria

myosynizesis

myotenositis

myotonia

myotonoid

myotonus

myotube

myotubular

myotubule

myriachit

myringitis
    m. bullosa
    bullous m.

myringodermatitis

myringomycosis

myxadenitis
    m. labialis

myxangitis

myxasthenia

myxedema
    circumscribed m.
    congenital m.
    infantile m.
    nodular m.
    operative m.
    papular m.
    pituitary m.
    pretibial m.
    primary m.
    secondary m.

myxedematoid

myxedematous

myxiosis

myxocystitis

myxoglobulosis

myxolipoma

myxoma, (pl. myxomas,
   myxomata)
    atrial m.
    cardiac m.
    cystic m.
    m. fibrosum
    lanceolate m.
    odontogenic m.
    vascular m.

myxospore

myxovirus

Myxozoa

N

N
    newton
    normal

N High Sensitivity C-reactive
    protein (CRP) assay

NA
    neutralizing antibody

nabothian
    n. cyst
    o. follicle

NAD
    nicotinamide adenine
        dinucleotide

Nadi reaction

Naeglaria

NAF
    neutrophil activating factor

Nakanishi stain

naked virus

nanism
    mulibrey n.
    pituitary n.
    senile n.

Nannizzia

nanocurie (Nci)

nanofarad (nF)

nanogram (ng)

nanoid

nanoliter (nl)

nanometer (nm)

nanomole (nmol)

nanophthalmia

nanophthalmos

Nanophyetus salmincola

nanosoma

nanosomia

nanous

nanukayami

nanus

NAP
    neutrophil activating
        protein

Napier formed-gel test

naperian logarithm

napthol

narcolepsy

narcose

narcosis
    nitrogen n.

narcous

native albumin

natremia

natriuresis

natriuretic

natruresis

natruretic

natural
    n. antibody
    n. focus of infection
    n. killer cell-stimulating
        factor

Nauta stain

navel
    blue n.

NBS
    normal blood serum

NBT
    nitroblue tetrazolium

NCAM
    neural cell adhesion
        molecule

NCI
 National Cancer Institute

nCi
 nanocurie

NCL-ARm monoclonal antibody

NCL-ARp polyclonal antibody

NCL-ER-LH2 monoclonal antibody

NCL-PCR monoclonal antibody

nebenkern

nebulous urine

Necator americans

neck
 bull neck
 Madelung's neck
 neck of spermatozoon
 webbed neck
 wry neck

necklace
 Casal's necklace

necrencephalus

necrobiosis
 n. lipoidica
 n. lipoidica diabeticorum

necrobiotic

necrocytosis

necrocytotoxin

necrogenic

necrogenous

necrolysis
 toxic epidermal n.

necropsy

necroscopy

necrose

necrosis (pl. necroses)
 acidophilic n.
 acute tubular n. (ATN)

necrosis (pl. necroses)
 (*continued*)
 arteriolar n.
 aseptic n.
 avascular n.
 avascular n. of bone
 Balser's fatty n.
 bridging n.
 caseation n.
 caseous n.
 central hemorrhagic n.
 cheesy n.
 coagulative n.
 colliquative n.
 contraction band n.
 cystic medial n.
 enzymatic fat n.
 epiphyseal ischemic n.
 Erdheim's cystic medial n.
 exanthematous n.
 fibrinoid n.
 gangrenous n.
 hyaline n.
 ischemic n.
 liquefaction n.
 massive hepatic n.
 mummification n.
 Paget's quiet n.
 piecemeal n.
 postpartum pituitary n.
 pressure n.
 n. progrediens
 progressive emphysematous n.
 n. of renal papillae
 renal cortical necrosis
 subacute hepatic n.
 subcutaneous fat n.
 submassive hepatic n.
 syphilitic n.
 Zenker's n.

necrospermia

necrospermic

necrotic

necrotizing
 n. fasciitis

necrotizing (*continued*)
    n. sialometaplasia
    n. vasculitis

necrotomy

necrozoospermia

needle
    n. aspiration cytology

Neethling virus

nefluorophotometer

Negeshi virus

Neisser
    diplococcus of N.
    N. stain

nematoblast

nematocidal

nematospermia

neocytosis

neomembrane

neomort

neoplasia
    multiple endocrine n.
    multiple endocrine n., type
        I
    multiple endocrine n., type
        II
    multiple endocrine n., type
        IIA
    multiple endocrine n., type
        IIB
    multiple endocrine n., type
        III

neopterin

nephelometer

nephelometry

nephralgia

nephralgic

nephrapostasis

nephrauxe

nephrectasia

nephrectasis

nephrectasy

nephredema

nephrelcosis

nephremia

nephritides

nephritis
    arteriosclerotic n.
    azotemic n.
    Balkan n.
    capsular n.
    n. caseosa
    caseous n.
    cheesy n.
    chloro-azotemic n.
    n. dolorosa
    dropsical n.
    exudative n.
    fibrolipomatous n.
    glomerular n.
    glomerulocapsular n.
    n. gravidarum
    hemorrhagic n.
    Heymann's n.
    indurative n.
    interstitial n.
    Lancereaux's n.
    lupus n.
    parenchymatous n.
    chronic parenchymatous n.
    pneumococcus n.
    n. repens
    salt-losing n.
    scarlatinal n.
    suppurative n.
    syphilitic n.
    tubular n.
    tuberculous n.
    tubulointerstitial n.
    anti-GBM n.
    anti-GBM antibody n.

nephritis (*continued*)
    anti-glomerular basement membrane n.
    Henoch-Schönlein purpura n.

nephritogenic

nephroangiosclerosis

nephrocalcinosis

nephrocele

nephrocolic

nephrocoloptosis

nephrocystitis

nephrocystosis

nephroerysipelas

nephrohemia

nephrohydrosis

nephrohypertrophy

nephrolith

nephrolithiasis

nephromalacia

nephromegaly

nephron

nephronophthisis
    familial juvenile n.

nephropathia

nephropathic

nephropathy
    AIDS n.
    analgesic n.
    Balkan n.
    contrast n.
    diabetic n.
    gouty n.
    HIV-associated n.
    hypazoturic n.
    IgA n.
    IgM n.

nephropathy (*continued*)
    ischemic n.
    light chain n.
    potassium-losing n.
    reflux n.
    sickle cell n.
    thin basement membrane n.
    urate n.
    uric acid n.
    vasomotor n.

nephrophagiasis

nephrophthisis

nephroptosia

nephroptosis

nephropyelitis

nephrorrhagia

nephrosclerosis
    arteriolar n.
    benign arteriolar n.
    hyaline arteriolar n.
    hyperplastic arteriolar n.
    intercapillary n.
    malignant n.

nephrosis (pl. nephroses)
    amyloid n.
    cholemic n.
    Epstein's n.
    glycogen n.
    hydropic n.
    hypokalemic n.
    larval n.
    lipid n.
    lipoid n.
    lower nephron n.
    necrotizing n.
    osmotic n.
    vacuolar n.

nephrosonephritis

nephrospasis

nephrotic

nephrotoxic

nephrotoxicity
    contrast agent n.
    contrast medium n.

nephrotoxin

nephrotuberculosis

nesidioblast

nesidioblastosis

nesslerization

nest
    birds' n.
    Brunn's epithelial n
    Walthard cell n.

net
    achromatic n.
    chromidial n.

neuragmia

neuralgia
    cervicobrachial n.
    cervico-occipital n.
    cranial n.
    n. facialis vera
    geniculate n.
    glossopharyngeal n.
    Hunt's n.
    idiopathic n.
    intercostal n.
    mammary n.
    migrainous n.
    Morton's n.
    nasociliary n.
    occipital n.
    otic n.
    postherpetic n.
    red n.
    Sluder's n.
    sphenopalatine n.
    supraorbital n.
    trifacial n.
    trifocal n.
    trigeminal n.
    Vail's n.
    vidian n.

neuralgic

neuralgiform

neurapraxia

neurarthropathy

neure

neurectopia

neurectopy

neurepithelial

neurepithelium

neurilemma

neurilemmal

neurilemmitis

neurilemoma
    acoustic n.

neurinoma
    acoustic n.
    acoustic n., bilateral

neuritic

neuritis
    alcoholic n.
    brachial n.
    dietetic n.
    fallopian n.
    Gombault's n.
    hypertrophic n., interstitial
    intraocular n.
    lead n.
    leprous n.
    n. migrans
    migrating n.
    multiple n.
    n. multiplex endemica
    optic n.
    periaxial n.
    n. puerperalis traumatica
    radiation n.
    radicular n.
    retrobulbar n.
    n. saturnina
    sciatic n.
    syphilitic n.
    toxic n.
    vestibular n.

neuroacanthocytosis

neuroallergy

neuroamebiasis

neuroarthropathy

neuroblast
   sympathetic n.

neuroborreliosis

neuroceptor

neurochorioretinitis

neurochoroiditis

neurocysticercosis

neurocytology

neurocytoma

neurodealgia

neurodeatrophia

neurodegenerative

neurodendrite

neurodendron

neurodermatitis
   circumscribed n.
   disseminated n.
   exudative n.
   localized n.
   nummular n.

neurodynia

neuroencephalomyelopathy

neuroepithelial

neuroepithelioma

neuroepithelium

neurofiber
   afferent n.
   autonomic n.
   hypertensive n.

neurofibra
   n. associationis
   n. commissuralis

neurofibra (*continued*)
   n. postganglionares
   n. preganglionares
   n. projectionis
   n. viscerales

neurofibril

neurofibrilla

neurofibrillar

neurofibromatosis
   n. 1
   n. 2
   bilateral acoustic n.
   central n.
   peripheral n.

neurofibromin

neurofilament

neurogangliitis

neuroglia
   interfascicular n.
   peripheral n.

neuroglial

neurogliocyte

neuroglycopenia

neurohistology

neuroid

neuroinflammation

neurokeratin

neurolabyrinthitis

neurolemma

neurolipomatosis
   n. dolorosa

neurolues

neurolymphomatosis

neuroma
   acoustic n.
   traumatic n.

neuromalacia

neuromalakia

neuromatous

neuromyasthenia
    epidemic n.

neuromyelitis
    n. optica

neuromyopathic

neuromyopathy
    carcinomatous n.

neuromyositis

neuromyotonia

neuron
    afferent n.
    bipolar n.
    central n.
    connector n.
    efferent n.
    fusimotor n.
    Golgi type I n.
    Golgi type II n.
    intercalary n.
    intercalated n.
    internuncial n.
    local circuit n.
    motor n.
    multiform n.
    multipolar n.
    peripheral sensory n.
    piriform n.
    polymorphic n.
    postganglionic n.
    preganglionic n.
    premotor n.
    primary sensory n.
    projection n.
    pseudounipolar n.
    Purkinje n.
    pyramidal n.
    secondary sensory n.
    sensory n.
    spiny n.
    unipolar n.

neuronal

neurone

neuronitis
    vestibular n.

neuronopathy

neuronophage

neuronophagia

neuropapillitis

neuropathic

neuropathogenesis

neuropathogenicity

neuropathology

neuropathy
    acrodystrophic n.
    alcoholic n.
    amyloid n.
    angiopathic n.
    arsenic n.
    autonomic n.
    axonal n.
    brachial plexus n.
    compression n.
    Dejerine-Sottas n.
    Denny-Brown's sensory n.
    Denny-Brown's sensory
        radicular n.
    descending n.
    diabetic n.
    entrapment n.
    femoral n.
    giant axonal n.
    hepatic n.
    hereditary hypertrophic n.
    progressive hypertrophic n.
    hypertrophic interstitial n.
    ischemic n.
    isoniazid n.
    Leber's optic n.
    lumbosacral plexus n.
    motor n.
    hereditary motor and
        sensory n.
    nitrofurantoin neuropathy
    hereditary optic n.

neuropathy (*continued*)
    paraneoplastic n.
    periaxial n.
    porphyric n.
    sacral plexus n.
    sarcoid n.
    segmental (demyelination) n.
    sensorimotor n.
    sensory n.
    sensory and autonomic n.
    sensory and motor n.
    sensory radicular n.
    serum n.
    serum sickness n.
    suprascapular n.
    tomaculous n.
    toxic n.
    vasculitic n.

neuropil

neuropile

neuroplasm

neuroplasmic

neuropodion

neuropodium

neuroretinitis

neuroretinopathy

neurosome

neurosyphilis
    asymptomatic n.
    commisural n.
    meningovascular n.
    parenchymatous n.
    paretic n.
    tabetic n.

neurotendinous

neuroterminal

neurothele

neurotmesis

neurotrauma

neurotrosis

neurotubule

neurovaricosis

neurovirulence

neurovirulent

Neusser granule

neutralization test

neutralizing antibody

neutral protein Hegadorn (NPH)
    NPH insulin

neutral red

neutropenia
    autoimmune n.
    chronic hypoplastic n.
    congenital n.
    cyclic n.
    drug-induced n.
    familial benign chronic n.
    hypersplenic n.
    idiopathic n.
    Kostmann's n.
    malignant n.
    neonatal n., alloimmune
    neonatal n., isoimmune
    periodic n.
    peripheral n.
    primary splenic n.
    severe congenital n.

neutrophil
    giant n.
    n. activating factor (NAF)

neutrophilia

neutrophilic

nevoblast

nevocellular

nevocyte

nevocytic

nevolipoma

nevus (pl. nevi)
    achromic n.
    acquired n.
    n. anemicus
    n. angiomatodes
    n. araneus
    Becker's n.
    blue rubber bleb n.
    capillary n.
    cellular blue n.
    choroidal n.
    chromatophore n. of
        Naegeli
    n. comedonicus
    connective tissue n.
    n. depigmentosus
    n. elasticus
    n. elasticus of
        Lewandowsky
    epidermal n.
    epithelial n.
    n. flammeus
    n. fuscoceruleus
        acromiodeltoideus
    n. fuscoceruleus
        ophthalmomaxillaris
    hepatic n.
    n. of Ito
    n. lipomatosus
    n. lipomatosus cutaneus
        superficialis
    melanocytic n.
    nuchal n.
    Ota's n.
    pigmented hairy epidermal
        n.
    port-wine n.
    spider n.
    n. spilus
    n. spilus tardus
    n. spongiosus albus
        mucosae
    stellar n.
    strawberry n.
    n. unius lateris
    Unna's n.
    uveal n.
    vascular n.

nevus (*continued*)
    n. vascularis
    n. vasculosus
    white sponge n.

Newcastle-Manchester bacillus

Newcomer fixative

newton
    N. law of cooling

NIA
    nephelometric inhibition
        assay

niacin test

Nickerson-Kveim
    N-K. test

Nicol prism

nidal

nidus (pl. nidi)

nigrities
    n. linguae

nigrosin

Nile blue
    N. b stain

ninhydrin-Schiff
    n-S. reaction
    n-S. stain for proteins

Nissl
    N. bodies
    N. stain

nitrate
    n. agar
    n. broth
    n. reduction test
    n. utilization test

nitrifying bacterium

nitremia

nitrituria

nitroanilene poisoning

Nitrobacteraceae

nitroblue
    n. tetrazolim
    n. tetrazolim dye
    n. tetrazolim stain

nitro dye

nitrogen
    alkali-soluble n.
    amino acid n.
    blood urea n. (BUN)
    n. balance
    n. equivalent
    n. narcosis
    serum urea n. (SUN)

nitrophenol

nitropropiol test

nitroprusside

nitroso dye

nitrosurea agent

NMR LipoProfile

N-Multistix

Noble stain

nocardiosis
    pulmonary n.

nociassociation

noci-influence

noctalbuminuria

node
    Aschoff-Tawara n.
    atrioventricular n.
    Babès' n.
    Bouchard's n.
    Delphian n.
    Dürck's n.
    gouty n.
    Haygarth's n.
    Heberden's n.
    Hensen's n.
    hilar n.
    jugulodigastric n.
    mesenteric n.

node (*continued*)
    Meynet's n.
    Osler's n.
    Parrot's n.
    primitive n.
    n. of Ranvier
    Rotter's n.
    Roüviere's n.
    SA (sinoatrial) n.
    Schmorl's n.
    sentinel n.
    singer's n.
    sinoatrial n.
    syphilitic n.
    teacher's n.
    Troisier's n.
    Virchow's n.

nodosa
    arteriitis n.
    arthritis n.
    periarteritis n.
    salpingitis isthmica n.

nodose
    n. ganglion
    n. rheumatism

nodositas

nodosity

nodular
    n. amyloidosis
    n. body
    n. glomerulosclerosis
    n. nonsuppurative
      panniculitis
    n. sclerosing Hodgkin's
      disease (NSHD)
    n. tuberculid
    n. vasculitis

nodulate

nodulated

nodulation

nodule
    apple jelly n.
    Aschoff's n.

nodule (*continued*)
    Babès' n.
    Busacca n.
    Caplan n.
    cirrhotic n.
    cold n.
    cortical n.
    Dalen-Fuchs n.
    dysplastic n.
    fibrosiderotic n.
    Fraenkel's n.
    Gandy-Gamna n.
    Gamna n.
    Hoboken n.
    Jeanselme's n.
    juxta-articular n.
    Kimmelstiel-Wilson n.
    Koeppe n.
    Losch n.
    Lutz-Jeanselme n
    macroregenerative n.
    microglial n.
    Morgagni's n.
    parenchymal n.
    regenerative n.
    regenerative n.,
        monoacinar
    regenerative n., multiacinar
    rheumatic n.
    rheumatoid n.
    Schmorl n.
    siderotic n.
    surfers' n.
    n. tabac
    teacher's n.
    thyroid n.
    typhoid n.
    Wohlbach's n.

nodulous

noma
    n. vulvae

Nomarski microscope

nomenclature
    binary n.
    binomial n.
    chromosome n.

nonagglutinating vibrio

nonbacterial

non-B hepatitis

nonconjugative plasmid

nondisjunction

nonelectrolyte

nonestrified fatty acid

noninvolution

nonmedullated

nonmotile

nonmyelinated

non-neuronal

non-nucleated

nonoliguric

nonpermissive culture media

nonsecretor

nonseptate

nonstructural gene

normoblastosis

normocalcemia

normocholesterolemia

normocholesterolemic

normochromasia

normokalemia

normokalemic

normolipidemic

normoskeocytosis

normouricemia

normouricemic

normouricuria

normouricuric

NOS
    not otherwise specified

nosazontology

nosetiology

nosography

nosologic

nosology

nosonomy

nosotaxy

nosotoxin

notalgia

notation
    scientific n.

notch
    Kernohan's n.

notencephalocele

NOVA Celltrak 12 hematology
    analyzer

Now Legionella urinary antigen
    test

Now Streptococcus
    pneumoniae urinary antigen
    test

noxa

NP
    normal plasma
    nucleoplasmic index

NPH
    neutral protamine
        Hegadorn (insulin)

NPT
    nonprecipitin test

NRBC
    nucleated red blood cell

NRS
    normal reference serum

NS
    nonspecific
    not significant
    not sufficient

NSE
    neuron-specific enolase

NSM
    neurosecretory material

NTAB
    nephrotoxic antibody

NTG
    nontoxic goiter

nubecula

nuclear-cytoplasmic ratio

nucleated
    n. red blood cell

nucleation
    heterogenous n.

nucleic acid

nucleiform

nucleocapsid

nucleochylema

nucleochyme

nucleocytoplasmic

nucleofugal

nucleohyaloplasm

nucleoid

nucleolar

nucleoli

nucleoliform

nucleolin

nucleolinus

nucleoloid

nucleololus

nucleolonema

nucleoloneme

nucleolonucleus

nucleolus
    secondary n.

nucleolymph

nucleopetal

nucleophile

nucleoplasm

nucleoprotein

nucleoreticulum

nucleosome

nucleosis

nucleospindle

nucleotide
    cyclic n.
    pyridine n.

nucleotoxin

nucleus (pl. nuclei)
    cellular n.
    compact n.
    conjugation n.
    daughter n.
    diploid n.
    droplet n.
    fertilization n.
    free n.
    germinal n.
    gonad n.
    haploid n.
    hyperchromatic n.
    polymorphic n.
    reproductive n.
    sanded n.
    Schwann's n.
    segmentation n.
    shadow n.
    stripped n.
    vesicular n.
    wrinkled n.
    zygote n.

NucliSens HIV-1 QT assay

nullisomic

number
    atomic n.
    Avogardo n.

number (*continued*)
    color index n.
    CT n.
    dibucaine n.
    diploid n.
    fluoride n.
    haploid n.
    Polenske n.
    random n.
    Reichert-Meissl n.
    Reynold n.

numerical
    n. karyotype
    n. taxonomy

nummiform

nummular
    n. dermatitis
    n. sputum

nummulation

N-Uristix

nutation

nutatory

nutrient
    n. agar
    n. broth
    n. medium

nyctalgia

nyctalope

nyctalopia

nycturia

nymphitis

nymphoncus

nystagmic

nystagmiform

nystagmoid

nystagmus
    amaurotic n.
    amblyopic n.
    ataxic n.

nystagmus (*continued*)
    aural n.
    central n.
    Cheyne's n.
    Cheyne-Stokes n.
    convergence n.
    disjunctive n.
    dissociated n.
    gaze paretic n.
    jerk n.
    labyrinthine n.

nystagmus (*continued*)
    lateral n.
    oscillating n.
    palatal n.
    paretic nystagmus
    periodic alternating n.
    n. retractorius
    rhythmical n.
    rotatory n.

nystaxis

O

obcecation

obduction

objective
    achromatic objective
    apochromatic objective
    dry objective
    flat field objective
    fluorite objective
    immersion objective
    semiapochromatic
      objective

obliquity
    Litzmann's o.
    Nägele's o.

obliteration
    cortical obliteration

obnubilation

obstipation

obstruent

obtundation

obtundent

obturation

occlusal

occult
    o. blood
    o. carcinoma

ochronosis

ochronosus

ochronotic

oculomandibulodyscephaly

oculomycosis

oculopathy

odaxesmus

odaxetic

odditis

odontalgia

odontalgic

odontoblast

odontoclast

odontogenesis
    o. imperfecta

odontolith

odontolithiasis

odontolysis

odontoma
    fibrous o.

odontopathic

odontopathy

odontoschism

odontoseisis

odontotripsis

odynacusis

odynophagia

oil
    anise o.
    bergamot o.
    bhilawanol o.
    cedar o.
    chenopodium o.
    flaxseed o.
    o. embolism
    o. immersion
    o. of cedar wood
    santal o.
    o.-water ratio

oleogranuloma

oleoma

oligakisuria

oligemia

oligoamnios

oligoanuria

oligoarthritis

oligoblast

oligochromasia

oligocystic

oligodendria

oligodendrocyte

oligodendroglia

oligodipsia

oligodontia

oligogalactia

oligoglia

oligohydramnios

oligohydruria

oligohypermenorrhea

oligohypomenorrhea

oligomeganephronia

oligomeganephronic

oligomenorrhea

oligonecrospermia

oligophosphaturia

oligopnea

oligospermatism

oligospermia

oligotrophia

oligotrophic

oligotrophy

oligozoospermatism

oligozoospermia

oliguresis

oliguria

oliguric

olisthe

olisthetic

olisthy

omagra

omalgia

omarthritis

omentovolvulus

omitis

omodynia

omphalelcosis

omphalitis

omphalocele

omphalophlebitis

omphalorrhagia

omphalorrhea

omphalorrhexis

OncoChek immunoassay

oncoides

oncotic

One Touch II hospital blood glucose monitoring system

One Touch Basic and One Touch Profile

One Touch Fast Take blood glucose monitor/strips

onkinocele

onyalai

onychatrophia

onychatrophy

onychauxis

onychia

onychitis

onychoclasis

onychocryptosis

onychodystrophy

onychogryphosis

onychogryposis

onychoheterotopia

onycholysis

onychomadesis

onychomalacia

onychomycosis
    dermatophytic o.

onycho-osteodysplasia

onychopathic

onychopathy

onychoptosis

onychorrhexis

onychoschizia

onychosis

onyxis

ooblast

oocyesis

oocyte

oolemma

oophoralgia

oophoritis
    o. parotidea

oophorocystosis

oophoropathy

oophorosalpingitis

oophorrhagia

ooplasm

oosperm

ootid

opacification

opacity

opalgia

ophiasis

ophryosis

ophthalmagra

ophthalmalgia

ophthalmatrophia

ophthalmia
    actinic ray o.
    catarrhal o.
    o. eczematosa
    Egyptian o.
    flash o.
    gonorrheal o.
    granular o.
    hepatic o.
    metastatic o.
    migratory o.
    mucous o.
    o. neonatorum
    neuroparalytic o.
    o. nivialis
    o. nodosa
    phlyctenular o.
    purulent o.
    scrofulous o.
    strumous o.
    ultraviolet ray o.

ophthalmiac

ophthalmitic

ophthalmitis

ophthalmoblennorrhea

ophthalmocele

ophthalmocopia

ophthalmodesmitis

ophthalmodonesis

ophthalmodynia

ophthalmolith

ophthalmomalacia

ophthalmomycosis

ophthalmomyiasis

ophthalmomyitis

ophthalmomyositis

ophthalmoneuritis

ophthalmoneuromyelitis

ophthalmopathy
  dysthyroid o.
  external o.
  Graves' o.
  infiltrative o.
  internal o.

ophthalmophthisis

ophthalmoplegia
  basal o.
  exophthalmic o.
  fascicular o.
  internuclear o.
  orbital o.
  Parinaud's o.
  o. totalis

ophthalmoplegic

ophthalmoptosis

ophthalmorrhagia

ophthalmorrhea

ophthalmorrhexis

ophthalmosteresis

ophthalmosynchysis

ophthalmoxerosis

opisthogenia

opisthoporeia

opisthorchiasis

opisthotonoid

opisthotonos

opisthotonus

oppositipolar

opsialgia

opsiuria

opsoclonia

opsoclonus

OraTest

orange
  acid o. 10
  acridine o.
  o. G
  wool o.

orangeophil

orbitopathy
  dysthyroid orbitopathy
  Graves' orbitopathy

orcein

orchella

orchialgia

orchichorea

orchidalgia

orchiditis

orchidopathy

orchidoptosis

orchiepididymitis

orchilytic

orchioblastoma

orchiocele

orchiodynia

orchioneuralgia

orchiopathy

orchioscheocele

orchioscirrhus

orchitic

orchitis
  spermatogenic
    granulomatous o.
  traumatic o.

orchitolytic

orcin

orcinol

organ
    cell o.
    end o.
    Golgi tendon o.
    gustatory o.
    neurotendinous o.
    Ruffini's o.
    tendon o.

organella

organellae

organelle

organizer
    nucleolar o.
    nucleolus o.
    procentriole o.

organomegaly

organopathy

organophilic

organophilism

organotaxis

organotrope

organotropic

organotropism

organotropy

ornithine carbamoyltransferase
  (OCT) deficiency

ornithinemia

ornithosis

oromeningitis

orosomucoid

oroticaciduria

orrhomeningitis

orthochorea

orthochromatic

orthochromophil

orthodentin

orthodeoxia

ortholidine

orthoneutrophil

orthorrhachic

orthotonos

orthotonus

os
    o. naviculare pedis
      retardatum
    o. odontoideum

osazone

oscillopsia

osmiophilic

osmiophobic

osmolality

osmolar

osmolarity

osmoregulation

osmoregulatory

osmotaxis

ossein

osseomucin

osseomucoid

ossification
    ectopic o.
    heterotopic o.
    metaplastic o.

ossifluence

ostalgia

ostarthritis

ostealgia

osteanabrosis

ostearthritis

osteectopia

osteectopy

ostein

osteite

osteitis
    acute o.
    o. albuminosa
    alveolar o.
    carious o.
    o. carnosa
    caseous o.
    central o.
    chronic o.
    chronic nonsuppurative o.
    o. condensans
    o. condensans generalisata
    o. condensans ilii
    condensing o.
    cortical o.
    o. deformans
    o. fibrosa cystica
    o. fibrosa cystica
      generalisata
    o. fibrosa disseminata
    o. fibrosa localisata
    o. fibrosa osteoplastica
    formative o.
    o. fragilitans
    o. fungosa
    Garré's o.
    o. granulosa
    gummatous o.
    necrotic o.
    o. ossificans
    parathyroid o.
    o. pubis
    secondary hyperplastic o.

ostempyesis

osteoaneurysm

osteoarthritic

osteoarthritis
    o. deformans endemica
    hyperplastic o.
    interphalangeal o.

osteoarthropathy
    familial o. of fingers
    idiopathic hypertrophic o.
    primary hypertrophic o.
    hypertrophic pulmonary o.
    pulmonary o.
    secondary hypertrophic o.

osteoarthrosis
    o. juvenilis

osteoblast

osteoblastic

osteocachectic

osteocachexia

osteocalcin

osteocampsia

osteocampsis

osteocarcinoma

osteocartilaginous exostosis

osteocele

osteochondral

osteochondritis
    calcaneal o.
    o. deformans juvenilis
    o. deformans juvenilis dorsi
    o. dissecans
    o. ischiopubica
    juvenile deforming
      metatarsophalangeal o.
    o. necroticans
    o. ossis metacarpi et
      metatarsi
    syphilitic o.

osteochondrodysplasia

osteochondrodystrophia
    o. deformans

osteochondrodystrophy
   familial o.

osteochondrolysis

osteochondromatosis
   synovial o.

osteochondropathy

osteochondrosarcoma

osteochondrosis
   o. deformans tibiae

osteoclasia

osteoclast

osteoclastic
   o. giant cells
   o. resorption

osteocope

osteocopic

osteocystoma

osteocyte

osteodentinoma

osteodiastasis

osteodynia

osteodysplasty
   o. of Melnick and Needles

osteodystrophia
   o. cystica
   o. fibrosa

osteodystrophy
   Albright's hereditary o.
   renal o.

osteoectasia
   familial o.

osteofibromatosis
   cystic o.

osteogen

osteogenesis
   o. imperfecta
   o. imperfecta congenita

osteogenesis (*continued*)
   o. imperfecta cystica
   o. imperfecta tarda

osteohalisteresis

osteoid

osteolysis

osteolytic

osteomalacia
   antacid-induced o.
   anticonvulsant o.
   familial hypophosphatemic
     o.
   hepatic o.
   oncogenous o.
   puerperal o.
   renal tubular o.
   senile o.

osteomalacic

osteomalacosis

osteomiosis

osteomyelitic

osteomyelitis
   acute hematogenous o.
   diffuse sclerosing o.
   focal sclerosing o.
   Garré's o.
   salmonella o.
   sclerosing nonsuppurative
     o.

osteomyelodysplasia

osteon

osteone

osteonecrosis

osteoneuralgia

osteonosus

osteo-odontoma

osteo-onychodysplasia
   hereditary o.

osteopathia
- o. condensans
- o. condensans disseminata
- o. condensans generalisata
- o. hemorrhagica infantum
- o. hyperostotica congenita
- o. hyperostotica multiplex infantilis
- o. striata

osteopathic

osteopathology

osteopathy
- alimentary o.
- disseminated condensing o.
- hunger o.
- myelogenic o.

osteopecilia

osteopenia

osteopenic

osteoperiostitis

osteopetrosis

osteophage

osteophagia

osteophlebitis

osteophyma

osteophyte

osteophytosis

osteoplaque

osteoplast

osteoplastica

osteopoikilosis

osteopoikilotic

osteopontin

osteoporosis
- o. circumscripta cranii
- o. of disuse
- involutional o.

osteoporosis (*continued*)
- postmenopausal o.
- post-traumatic o.
- senile o.

osteoporotic

osteopsathyrosis

osteorrhagia

osteosarcoma
- gnathic o.
- o. of jaw

osteosclerosis
- o. congenita
- o. fragilis
- o. fragilis generalisata
- o. myelofibrosis

osteosclerotic

osteosis
- o. eburnisans monomelica
- parathyroid o.

osteosynovitis

osteotabes

osteothrombophlebitis

osteothrombosis

ostitis

ostium
- o. primum, persistent

ostracosis

otalgia
- o. dentalis
- geniculate o.
- o. intermittens
- reflex o.
- secondary o.
- tabetic o.

otalgic

otitic

otitis
- aviation o.
- o. desquamativa

otitis (*continued*)
 o. externa
 o. externa, acute bacterial
 o. externa, acute fungal
 o. externa, circumscribed
 o. externa, diffuse
 o. externa, fungal
 o. externa, furuncular
 o. externa, malignant
 o. externa, necrotizing
 external o.
 furuncular o.
 o. interna
 o. media
 o. media, adhesive
 o. media, atelectatic
 o. media, catarrhal
 o. media, mucoid
 o. media, purulent
 o. media, secretory
 o. media, serous
 o. media, suppurative

otocerebritis

otoconia

otoconite

otoconium

otodynia

otoencephalitis

otolite

otolith

otomastoiditis

otomucormycosis

otomycosis
 o. aspergillina
 Aspergillus o.

otomyiasis

otoneuralgia

otopyorrhea

otorrhea
 cerebrospinal fluid o.

otosclerosis

otosclerotic

otosis

otospongiosis

ototoxic

ototoxicity

ovalocytary

ovalocyte

ovalocytosis

ovarialgia

ovariocele

ovariocyesis

ovariodysneuria

ovariopathy

ovariorrhexis

ovariotestis

ovaritis

ovary
 oyster o.
 polycystic o.

overhydration

overinflation
 congenital lobar o.
 nonobstructive pulmonary
  o.
 obstructive pulmonary o.

overload
 iron o.

overstain

overstress

overtoe

ovigerm

ovium

ovocyte

ovoid
    myelin o.

ovoplasm

ovotestis

ovular

ovulation
    amenstrual o.

ovule
    primitive o.
    primordial o.

oxalate
    balanced o.

oxalated

oxalation

oxalemia

oxalic acid

oxalosis

oxaluria

oxidosis

5-oxoprolinuria

oxyacoia

oxybutyria

oxybutyricacidemia

oxycephalia

oxycephalic

oxycephalous

oxycephaly

oxychromatic

oxycinesia

oxyecoia

oxyhydrocephalus

oxyhyperglycemia

oxyntic

oxyosis

oxyparaplastin

oxyphil

oxyphilic

oxyphilous

oxyplasm

oxytalan

oxytropism

ozena

ozenous

ozonophore

ozostomia

P

pacemaker
    atrioventricular junctional p.
    ectopic p.
    escape p.
    junctional p.
    latent p.
    secondary p.
    ventricular p.
    wandering atrial p.

pachyblepharon

pachyblepharosis

pachycephalia

pachycephalic

pachycephalous

pachycephaly

pachycheilia

pachydactylia

pachydactyly

pachyderma

pachydermatous

pachydermic

pachydermoperiostosis

pachyglossia

pachygyria

pachyleptomeningitis

pachymeningitis
    cerebral p.
    circumscribed p.
    external p.
    hypertrophic cervical p.
    hypertrophic spinal p.
    internal p.
    p. intralamellaris
    purulent p.
    spinal p.
    syphilitic p.

pachymeningopathy

pachynema

pachynsis

pachyntic

pachyonychia
    p. congenita

pachyperiostitis

pachyperitonitis

pachypleuritis

pachysalpingitis

pachysalpingo-ovaritis

pachytene

pachyvaginalitis

pachyvaginitis
    cystic p.

PadKit (sample collection
    system)

pagetic

pagetoid

pagophagia

pagoplexia

pain
    fulgurant p.
    heterotopic p.
    homotopic p.
    intermenstrual p.
    jumping p.
    lancinating p.
    osteocopic p.
    phantom limb p.
    postprandial p.
    referred p.
    rest p.
    terebrant p.
    terebrating p.
    wandering p.

pairing
    somatic p.

palatitis

palatognathous

palatoplegia

palatoschisis

palatum
   p. fissum

paleopathology

palicinesia

palikinesia

palilalia

palindromia

palindromic

palingraphia

palinopsia

palinphrasia

paliphrasia

palisade

pallanesthesia

palpebritis

palsy
   Bell's p.
   birth p.
   brachial p.
   cerebral p.
   crossed leg p.
   divers' p.
   Erb's p.
   Erb-Duchenne p.
   facial p.
   ischemic p.
   Klumpke's p.
   maternal obstetric p.
   progressive bulbar p.
   progressive supranuclear p.
   pseudobulbar p.
   Saturday night p.
   scriveners' p.
   shaking p.
   spastic bulbar p.

palsy (*continued*)
   tardy median p.
   tardy ulnar p.
   wasting p.

panacinar

panangiitis
   diffuse necrotizing p.

panarteritis
   p. nodosa

panarthritis

panatrophy

panbronchiolitis

pancarditis

panchromia

pancolitis
   necrotizing amebic p.

pancrealgia

pancreas
   aberrant p.
   annular p.
   p. divisum

pancreatalgia

pancreatitis
   acute p.
   acute hemorrhagic p.
   calcareous p.
   centrilobar p.
   chronic p.
   chronic relapsing p.
   interstitial p.
   perilobar p.
   purulent p.

pancreatolith

pancreatolithiasis

pancreatolysis

pancreatolytic

pancreatopathy

pancreolysis

pancreolytic

pancreopathy

pancreoprivic

pancystitis

pancytopenia
    congenital p.
    Fanconi's p.

panencephalitis
    Pette-Döring p.
    subacute sclerosing p.

panhematopenia

panhypogammaglobulinemia

panhypogonadism

panhypopituitarism
    prepubertal p.

panmural

panmyelopathia

panmyelopathy
    constitutional infantile p.
    Fanconi's p.

panmyelophthisis

panniculalgia

panniculitis
    cytophagic histiocytic p.
    LE p.
    lobular p.
    lupus p.
    nodular nonsuppurative p.
    relapsing febrile nodular
      nonsuppurative p.
    subacute nodular migratory
      p.
    Weber-Christian p.

panniculus
    p. adiposus

pannus
    degenerative p.
    p. degenerativus
    glaucomatous p.

pannus (*continued*)
    phlyctenular p.
    p. siccus
    p. trachomatosus

panophthalmia

panophthalmitis

panoptic

panosteitis

panostitis

panotitis

pansclerosis

pansinuitis

pansinusitis

pantachromatic

pantalgia

pantankyloblepharon

pantatrophia

pantatrophy

panting

pantotropic

pantropic

panus

panuveitis

paper
    alkannin p.
    aniline acetate p.
    azolitmin p.
    biuret p.
    blue litmus p.
    p. capacitor
    p. chromotography
    Congo red p.
    filter p.
    litmus p.
    p. radioimmunoassay test
    red litmus p.
    test p.
    turmeric p.

papilla
    Bergmeister's p.
    nerve p.
    tactile p.

papilledema

papillitis
    necrotizing p.
    necrotizing renal p.

papilloma
    p. accuminatum
    basal cell p.
    choroiod plexus p.
    cockscomb p.
    cutaneous p.
    hyperkeratotic p.
    o. inguinale tropicum
    intracanalicular p.
    intracytic p.
    keratotic p.
    Shope p.
    villous p.

papillomatosis
    confluent and reticulate pa.
    florid oral p.
    juvenile laryngeal p.
    laryngeal p.
    recurrent respiratory p.
    subareolar duct p.

papilloretinitis

papular

papulation

papule
    Gottron's p.
    moist p.
    mucous p.
    painful piezogenic pedal p.;
    piezogenic p.
    prurigo p.
    split p.

papuloerythematous

papuloid

papulopustular

papulosis

papulosquamous

papulovesicular

paracarmine

parachromatin

parachromatism

parachromatopsia

paracinesia

paracinesis

paraclinical

paracolitis

paracolpitis

paracousis

paracoxalgia

paracusis
    p. of Willis

paracystitis

paracytic

paradimethylamino-
    benzaldehyde

paradipsia

paraeccrisis

paraepilepsy

paraffinoma

parafunction

parafunctional

parageusia

parageusic

paragnosis

paragonimiasis

paragonimosis

paragraphia

parahemophilia

parahepatitis

parakeratosis
  p. ostracea
  p. scutularis

parakinesia

parakinetic

paralexia

paralexic

paralgesia

paralgesic

paralgia

paralinin

parallagma

paralyses

paralysis
  abducens p.
  acute atrophic p.
  p. of accommodation
  acute ascending spinal p.
  p. agitans
  alternate p.
  ambiguo-accessorius p.
  ambiguohypoglossal p.
  ambiguospinothalamic p.
  ascending p.
  Avellis' p.
  Bell's p.
  brachial plexus p.
  brachial plexus p., lower
  brachial plexus p., upper
  brachiofacial p.
  Brown-Séquard's p.
  bulbar p.
  centrocapsular p.
  cerebral p.
  compression p.
  congenital abducens-facial
    p.
  congenital oculofacial p.
  conjugate p.
  cruciate p.
  crural p.

paralysis (*continued*)
  Cruveilhier's p.
  Dejerine-Klumpke p.
  diaphragmatic p.
  diphtheric p.
  diphtheritic p.
  divers' p.
  Duchenne's p.
  Erb's p.
  flaccid p.
  functional p.
  p. of gaze
  glossolabial p.
  glossopharyngolabial p.
  Gubler's p.
  hereditary cerebrospinal p.
  hyperkalemic periodic p.
  hypoglossal p.
  hypokalemic periodic p.
  infantile p.
  infectious bulbar p.
  ischemic p.
  Jamaica ginger p.
  juvenile p.
  juvenile p. agitans
  Klumpke's p.
  Klumpke-Dejerine p.
  Kussmaul's p.
  Kussmaul-Landry p.
  labial p.
  labioglossolaryngeal p.
  labioglossopharyngeal p.
  Landry's p.
  laryngeal p.
  lingual p.
  Lissauer's p.
  masticatory p.
  Millard-Gubler p.
  mimetic p.
  myogenic p.
  myopathic p.
  normokalemic periodic p.
  ocular p.
  oculomotor p.
  peripheral p.
  peroneal p.
  phonetic p.
  postdormital p.

paralysis (*continued*)
    postepileptic p.
    posthemiplegic p.
    postical p.
    Pott's p.
    predormital p.
    progressive bulbar p.
    pseudobulbar p.
    pseudohypertrophic
     muscular p.
    Ramsay Hunt p.
    Remak's p.
    rucksack p.
    sensory p.
    spinomuscular p.
    supranuclear p.
    tegmental mesencephalic
     p.
    Todd's p.
    trigeminal p.
    vasomotor p.
    vocal cord p.
    Volkmann's ischemic p.
    Weber's p.
    writers' p.

paralytic

paralyzant

paramastitis

paramenia

parameniscitis

parametritic

parametritis
    posterior p.

paramidoacetophenone

paramitome

paramnesia

paramolar

paramucin

paramusia

paramyloidosis

paramyoclonus
    p. multiplex

paramyotonia
    p. congenita

paranalgesia

paranephritis

paranesthesia

paranomia

paranuclear

paranucleolus

paranucleus

paraosmia

paraparesis
    tropical spastic p.

parapedesis

paraphasia
    central p.
    literal p.

paraphasic

paraphemia

paraphia

paraphimosis

paraphrasia

paraphrenia

paraphrenitis

paraplasm

paraplasmic

paraplastic

paraplastin

paraplectic

paraplegia
    alcoholic p.
    ataxic p.
    cerebral p
    flaccid p.

paraplegia (*continued*)
   peripheral p.
   Pott's p.
   senile p.
   spastic p.
   congenital spastic p.
   Erb's spastic p.
   Erb's syphilitic spastic p.
   hereditary spastic p.
   infantile spastic p.
   tropical spastic p.
   p. superior
   syphilitic p.
   tetanoid p.
   toxic p.

paraplegic

paraplegiform

paraproctitis

paraprostatitis

paraproteinemia

parapsia

parapsis

parapsoriasis
   guttate p.
   p. lichenoides
   p. en plaques
   small plaque p.
   p. varioliformis acuta
   p. varioliformis chronica

parapyknomorphous

parareflexia

pararosaniline

pararrhythmia

parasalpingitis

parascarlatina

parasoma

parastruma

parasympathicotonia

parasynapsis

parasyndesis

parasynovitis

parasystole
   ventricular p.

paratenic host

paratonia

paratrachoma

paratrophic

paratyphlitis

paratyphoid

paravaginitis

paraxon

parazone

parectasia

parectasis

parencephalocele

parenchymatitis

paresis
   general p.

paresthesia
   Bernhardt's p.

paresthetic

paretic

parfocal

parietitis

parkinsonian

paronychia
   herpetic p.
   p. tendinosa

paronychial

paroophoritis

parophthalmia

paropsis

parorchidium

parosmia

parosteitis

parosteosis

parostitis

parostosis

parotiditis

parotidoscirrhus

parotitis
p. phlegmonosa
postoperative p.

parovaritis

pars
p. amorpha
p. compacta
p. fibrosa
p. functionalis
p. granulosa
p. recta tubuli renalis

pars planitis

particle
attraction p.
elementary p. of
mitochondria
nuclear p.

parulis

paruria

passage
false p.

patch
ash-leaf p.
Bitot's p.
cotton-wool p.
Hutchinson's p.
lance-ovate p.
MacCallum's p.
mucous p.
Peyer's p.
salmon p.
shagreen p.
smokers' p.
soldiers' p.

pathema

pathogenesis

pathogenetic

pathogenic

pathogenicity

pathogeny

pathology
anatomic p.
cellular p.
clinical p.
comparative p.
dental p.
experimental p.
functional p.
general p.
medical p.
molecular p.
surgical p.

pathomorphism

pathonomia

pathonomy

pathopoiesis

pathovar

pathway
alternative complement p.
biosynthetic p.
coagulation p.
Embden-Meyerhof p.
extrinsic p.
intrinsic p.
metabolic p.
pentose phosphate p.
reentrant p.

pattern
gel electrophoresis p.
indeterminate p.
lobular p.
male sex chromatin p.
mosaic p.
polyclonal p.
trabecular p.
XX/XY sex chromosome p.

Paul-Bunnell test

PB
  protein binding.

PCR

pearl
  enamel p.
  gouty p.
  keratin p.
  Laënnec p.

peau
  p. de chagrin
  p. d'orange

pechyagra

pectenitis

pectenosis

pectinate

pectoralgia

pectorophony

pectus
  p. carinatum
  p. excavatum
  p. gallinatum
  p. recurvatum

pedarthrocace

pedatrophia

pederin

pedialgia

pedicel

pedicellate

pedicellation

pediculate

pediculation

pediculi

pediculosis

pedionalgia

peduncle

peduncular

pedunculated

peg
  rete p.

PEI
  phosphate excretion index

pelade

peliosis
  bacillary p.
  p. hepatis

pellagra

pellagragenic

pellagral

pellagrin

pellagroid

pellagrose

pellagrosis

pellagrous

pellicle

pelviperitonitis

pelvis (pl. pelves)
  beaked p.
  caoutchouc p.
  coxalgic p.
  frozen p.
  kyphoscoliotic p.
  kyphotic p.
  lordotic p.
  Nagele p.
  p. nana
  p. obtecta
  osteomalacic p.
  Otto p.
  p. plana
  Prague p.
  pseudo-osteomalacic p.
  pseudospider p.
  rachitic p.
  Rokitansky's p.
  rostrate p.

pelvis (pl. pelves) (*continued*)
    scoliotic p.
    spider p.
    spondylolisthetic p.

pelvospondylitis
    p. ossificans

pemphigoid
    benign mucosal p.
    bullous p.
    cicatricial p.
    p. gestationis
    localized chronic p.

pemphigus
    p. antibodies
    benign familial p.
    benign mucus membrane
        p.
    Brazilian p.
    p. erythematosus
    p. foliaceus
    ocular p.
    paraneoplastic p.
    p. vegetans
    p. vulgaris

penischisis

pentachromic

pentagastrin

pentalogy
    Cantrell's p.
    p. of Fallot

pentamer

pentasomy

pentdyopent

pentosazone

pentosemia

pentosuria

pentosuric

penumbra
    ischemic p.

pepsinuria

peptonuria
    enterogenous p.
    hepatogenous p.
    nephrogenic p.
    puerperal p.
    pyogenic p.

peracute

percolate

perencephaly

perforation
    Bezold's p.
    inflammatory p.
    pathologic p.
    root p.

perforatorium

perfrigeration

perfusion

periadenitis
    p. mucosa necrotica
        recurrens

periangiitis

periangiocholitis

periaortitis

periappendicitis
    p. decidualis

periarteritis
    p. gummosa
    p. nodosa
    syphilitic p.

periarthritis
    p. of shoulder

periarticular

periaxonal

peribronchiolitis

peribronchitis

pericardiomediastinitis

pericarditic

pericarditis
    acute benign p.
    acute idiopathic p.
    acute nonspecific p.
    adhesive p.
    amebic p.
    bacterial p.
    bread-and-butter p.
    carcinomatous p.
    cholesterol p.
    chronic constrictive p.
    constrictive p.
    dry p.
    p. with effusion
    effusive constrictive p.
    external p.
    fibrinous p.
    fungal p.
    hemorrhagic p.
    idiopathic p.
    localized p.
    neoplastic p.
    p. obliterans
    obliterating p.
    postcardiotomy p.
    postinfarction p.
    post-irradiation p.
    purulent p.
    radiation p.
    rheumatic p.
    serofibrinous p.
    serous p.
    p. sicca
    suppurative p.
    tuberculous p.
    uremic p.
    viral p.

pericardium
    adherent p.
    bread-and-butter p.
    calcified p.
    shaggy p.

pericaryon

pericecitis

pericentriolar

pericholangitis

pericholecystitis
    gaseous p.

perichondrial

perichondritis

perichord

pericolitis
    p. dextra
    membranous p.
    p. sinistra

pericolonitis

pericolpitis

periconchitis

pericoxitis

pericranitis

pericystic

pericystitis

pericystium

pericyte

perideferentitis

peridendritic

peridens

periderm

peridermal

peridesmitis

perididymitis

peridiverticular

peridiverticulitis

periduodenitis

periencephalitis

perienteritis

periesophagitis

perifistular

perifolliculitis
p. capitis abscedens et
suffodiens
superficial pustular p.

perigangliitis

perigastritis

periglandulitis

periglial

periglossitis

perihepatitis
p. chronica hyperplastica
gonococcal p.

perihernial

periimplantitis

peri-islet

perijejunitis

perikarya

perikaryon

perilabyrinthitis

perilesional

perilobulitis

perilymphadenitis

perilymphangitis

perimastitis

perimeningitis

perimetritic

perimetritis

perimetrosalpingitis
encapsulating p.

perimolysis

perimyelitis

perimylolysis

perimyocarditis

perimyoendocarditis

perimyositis

perimysitis

perimysium
external p.
p. externum
internal p.
p. internum

perineocele

perinephritic

perinephritis

perineuritic

perineuritis

perinuclear

period
G1 p.
G2 p.
M p.
reaction p.
S p.
silent p.
Wenckebach p.

perionychia

perioophoritis

perioophorosalpingitis

perioothecitis

periophthalmia

periophthalmitis

periorbititis

periorchitis
p. adhaesiva
p. purulenta

periorchium

periosteitis

periosteodema

periosteoedema

periosteoma

periosteomedullitis

periosteomyelitis

periosteophyte

periosteosis

periostitis
  p. albuminosa
  albuminous p.
  diffuse p.
  hemorrhagic p.
  p. hyperplastica
  p. interna cranii

periostoma

periostomedullitis

periostosis
  hyperplastic p.

periostosteitis

periovaritis

peripancreatitis

periphacitis

periphakitis

peripheraphose

peripherophose

periphlebitic

periphlebitis
  sclerosing p.

periphoria

periphrenitis

peripleuritis

periporitis

periproctitis

periprostatitis

peripylephlebitis

perirectitis

perisalpingitis

perisalpingo-ovaritis

periscleritis

periscopic

perisigmoiditis

perisinusitis

perispermatitis
  p. serosa

perisplanchnitis

perisplenitis
  p. cartilaginea

perispondylitis
  Gibney's p.

peristalsis
  retrograde p.
  reversed p.

peristrumitis

peristrumous

perisyringitis

peritendinitis
  p. calcarea
  p. crepitans
  p. serosa

peritenonitis

peritenontitis

perithelium
  Eberth's p.

perithyroiditis

peritonealgia

peritoneopathy

peritonism

peritonitis
  adhesive p.
  bacterial p.
  benign paroxysmal p.
  biliary p.
  Candida p.
  chemical p.
  p. chronica fibrosa
    encapsulans

peritonitis (*continued*)
    p. deformans
    diaphragmatic p.
    p. encapsulans
    encysted p.
    fibrocaseous p.
    fungal p.
    gas p.
    hemorrhagic p.
    meconium p.
    perforative p.
    puerperal p.
    purulent p.
    sclerosing encapsulating p.
    septic p.
    serous p.
    spontaneous bacterial p.
    traumatic p.
    tuberculous p.

peritonsillitis

perityphlitis
    p. actinomycotica

periureteritis

periurethritis

perivaginitis

perivascularity

perivasculitis

perivesiculitis

perivisceritis

perlèche

permease

permeation

perniciosiform

pernicious

pernio

perseveration

persistence
    hereditary p. of fetal
      hemoglobin

pertussis

pes (pl pedes)
    p. abductus
    p. adductus
    p. calcaneocavus
    p. cavovarus
    p. cavus
    p. equinovalgus
    p. equinovarus
    p. gigas
    p. planovalgus
    p. planus
    p. valgus
    p. valgus, congenital
      convex
    p. varus

petechia (pl. petechiae)
    calcaneal p.

petechial

petrifaction

petrositis

petrousitis

phacitis

phacoanaphylaxis

phacocele

phacocystitis

phacoglaucoma

phacohymenitis

phacoiditis

phacoma

phacomalacia

phacometachoresis

phacometecesis

phacoplanesis

phacosclerosis

phacoscotasmus

phagedena

phagedenic

phagocyte
    alveolar p.

phakitis

phakoma

phakomatosis

phalangette
    drop p.

phalangitis

phalangosis

phallalgia

phallanastrophe

phallaneurysm

phallitis

phallocampsis

phallodynia

phallorrhagia

phaneroplasm

phanerosis
    fat p.

phantasm

phantogeusia

phantom

phantosmia

pharyngalgia

pharyngectasia

pharyngism

pharyngismus

pharyngitic

pharyngitid

pharyngitis
    aphthous p.
    atrophic p.
    diphtheritic p.

pharyngitis (*continued*)
    gangrenous p.
    p. herpetica
    hypertrophic p.
    membranous p.
    p. sicca
    streptococcal p.
    ulcerative p.
    p. ulcerosa
    vesicular p.

pharyngocele

pharyngoceratosis

pharyngodynia

pharyngokeratosis

pharyngolaryngitis

pharyngolith

pharyngolysis

pharyngomycosis

pharyngoparalysis

pharyngopathy

pharyngoplegia

pharyngorrhagia

pharyngosalpingitis

pharyngoscleroma

pharyngospasm

pharyngostenosis

pharyngotonsillitis

pharyngoxerosis

phase
    G1 p
    G2 p
    M p
    m p
    meiotic p
    postmeiotic p.
    premeiotic p.
    prereduction p.
    reduction p.

phase (*continued*)
    resting p.
    S p.
    s p.
    synaptic p.

phenacetolin

o-phenanthroline

phenolemia

phenoluria

phenomenon (pl. phenomena)
    adhesion p.
    anarchic p.
    Arias-Stella p.
    arm p.
    Arthus p.
    Ashman's p.
    atavistic p.
    Babinski's p.
    Becker's p.
    Bell's p.
    Bordet-Gengou p.
    cheek p.
    clasp-knife p.
    cogwheel p.
    Cushing's p.
    Danysz p.
    Debré p.
    Denys-Leclef p.
    d'Herelle p.
    doll's head p.
    Donath-Lansteiner p.
    Duckworth's p.
    Ehrlich's p.
    Erben's p.
    erythrocyte adherence p.
    facialis p.
    Felton p.
    finger p.
    generalized Schwartzman p.
    Gengou p.
    Goldblatt p.
    Gowers' p.
    Grasset's p
    Grasset-Gaussel p.
    Gunn's p.

phenomenon (*continued*)
    Gunn's pupillary p.
    halisteresis p.
    Hamburger p.
    Hering's p.
    Hertwig-Magendie p.
    hip-flexion p.
    Hochsinger's p.
    Hoffmann's p.
    Holmes' p.
    Holmes-Stewart p.
    Houssay p.
    Huebener-Thomsen-
      Friedenreich p.
    Hunt's paradoxical p.
    immune adherence p.
    jaw-winking p.
    Jod-Basedow p.
    Kanagawa p.
    Kienböck's p.
    Koebner's p.
    Koch's p.
    LE p.
    Leichtenstern's p.
    Lucio's p.
    Lust's p.
    Marcus Gunn's pupillary p.
    mucus extravasation p.
    Negro's p.
    no-reflow p.
    paradoxical diaphragm p.
    paradoxical p. of
      dystonia
    paradoxical pupillary p.
    peroneal nerve p.
    Pfeiffer p.
    Pool's p.
    prozone p.
    Queckenstedt's p.
    quellung p.
    Raynaud's p.
    rebound p.
    red cell adherence p.
    release p.
    Rust's p.
    Sanarelli p.
    Sanarelli-Schwartzman p.
    Schlesinger's p.

phenomenon (*continued*)
    Schramm's p.
    Schultz-Charlton p.
    second set p.
    Sherrington's p.
    Somogyi p.
    Souques' p.
    Splendore-Hoeppli p.
    springlike p.
    Strümpell's p.
    Theobald Smith p.
    Trousseau's p.
    Tullio's p.
    Twort p.
    Twort-d'Herelle p.
    Wenckebach p.
    Westphal's p.

phenotype

phenotyping
    alpha-1 p.

phentolamine test

phenylacetic acid

phenylalanine
    p. agar
    p. assay
    p. hydroxylase
      deficiency
    p. tolerance index

phenylalanine-4-
  monooxegenase

phenylalanyl

phenyalamine

phenylhydrazine

phenylketonuria
    atypical p.
    classic p.
    maternal p.
    transient p.

phenyllactic acid

phenylethal alcohol blood sugar

phenylketonuria test (PKU)

phenylpyruvic acid

phenytoin assay

pheochrome
    p. cell

pheochromoblast

pheochromocyte

phialospore

phimosis

phlebalgia

phlebangioma

phlebarteriectasia

phlebectasia
    p. laryngis

phlebectasis

phlebectopia

phlebectopy

phlebemphraxis

phlebismus

phlebitic

phlebitis
    adhesive p
    blue p
    p migrans
    migrating p
    obliterating p
    obstructive p
    plastic p
    productive p
    proliferative p
    puerperal p
    septic p
    sinus p
    suppurative p.

phlebofibrosis

phlebolith

phlebolithiasis

phlebometritis

phleborrhexis

phlebosclerosis

phlebosis

phlebostenosis

phlebothrombosis

phlebotomus
  p. fever

phlegm

phlegmasia
  p. alba dolens
  cellulitic p.
  p. cerulea dolens
  p. malabaria
  thrombotic p.

phlegmon
  emphysematous p.
  pancreatic p.
  periurethral p.

phlegmonous

phlogistic

phlogogen

phlogogenic

phlogogenous

phlogotic

phlorhizin

phlorhizinize

phloridzin

phloridzinize

phlorizin

phloroglucin

phloroglucinol

phlorrhizin

phloxine
  p. B

phlycten

phlyctena

phlyctenar

phlyctenoid

phlyctenula

phlyctenular

phlyctenule

phlyctenulosis
  allergic p.
  tuberculous p.

phonasthenia

phonomyoclonus

phoria

phorocytosis

phose

phosis

phosphatase
  acid p.
  alkaline p.
  bisphosphoglycerate p.
  curpic ion-inhibited acid p.
  leukocyte alkaline p.
  polyclonal anti-placental
    alkaline p.
  prostatic acid p.
  serum p.

phosphate
  acid p.
  p. assay
  q. buffer
  carbamyl p.
  dibasic potassium p.
  Krebs-Ringer p.
  organic p.
  primaquine p.
  stellar p.
  triple p.

3-phosphate

4-phosphate

5-phosphate

6-phosphate

phosphatemia

phosphatidosis

phosphatoptosis

phosphaturia

phosphide
    zinc p.

phosphine

phosphoadenosine
  diphosphosulfate

phosphoethanolamine

phospholipase

phospholipid
    p. assay
    p. staining

phosphomolybdic acid

phosphonecrosis

phosphopenia

phosphorescence

phosphorpenia

phosphoruria

phosphorylase
    hepatic p. deficiency
    muscle p. deficiency

phosphorylase b kinase
  deficiency

phosphotungstate

phosphotungstic acid

phosphuresis

phosphuretic

phosphuria

photalgia

photaugiaphobia

photerythrous

photesthesis

photoaging

photocutaneous

photodermatitis

photodermatosis

photodynia

photodysphoria

photoerythema

photolysis

photometer
    double-beam p.
    filter p.
    flame p.

photomicrography

photomicroscope

photomicroscopy

photoncia

photo-onycholysis

photopathy

photophobia

photophobic

photophthalmia
    flash p.

photoprotection

photopsia

photopsy

photoreactivation

photoretinitis

photoreversal

photosensitive

photosensitivity

photosensitization

photosensitize

phototoxic

phototoxicity

photuria

phragmoplast

phrenalgia

phrenitis

phrenodynia

phrenopericarditis

phrenoplegia

phrenoptosis

phrenospasm

phrynoderma

phthalein
    alpha-naphthol p.
    orthocresol p.

phthalic acid

phthalin

phthisis
    aneurysmal p.
    p. bulbi
    p. corneae
    ocular p.

phycoerythrin

phyllode
    cystosarcoma p.

phyllolith

phyma

phymata

physalides

physaliferous

physaliform

physaliphorous

physalis

physiochemical

physiochemistry

physiology
    morbid p.
    pathologic p.

physiolysis

physiopathologic

physiopathology

physocele

physohematometra

physohydrometra

physometra

physopyosalpinx

phytanate

phytanic acid

phytobezoar

phytonosis

phytophotodermatitis

phytosterolemia

phytotrichobezoar

phytoxylin

piarachnitis

piastrinemia

picric acid

picrocarmine
    p. stain

picroformol
    p. fixative

picro-Mallory trichrome stain

picrogeusia

picronigrosin

picrotoxin

piebald

piebaldism

piedra
    black p.
    p. nostras
    white p.

pigment
    accumulation of p.
    anthrocotic p.
    bile p.
    ceroid p.
    cirrhosis p.
    endogenous p.
    exogenous p.
    formalin p.
    hematogenous p.
    hepatogenous p.
    malarial p.
    melanotic p.

pigmentation
    arsenic p.
    bismuth p.
    hematin p.
    hematoidin p.
    lipochrome p.
    melanin p.
    porphyrin p.

pigmentolysin

pigmentophage

pigmentosa
    retinitis p.

pilar
    p. cyst

piliferous cyst

pilimictio

pilimiction

pillar
    p. of Corti's organ

pilobezoar

pilonidal
    p. cyst
    p. sinus

pilus (pl. pili)
    p. annulati
    p. canaliculi
    p. cuniculati
    p. incarnati
    p. incarnati recurvi
    p. multigemini
    p. torti
    p. trianguli et canaliculi

pimelitis

pimelopterygium

pimelorthopnea

pimelosis

pimeluria

pinacyanole

Pindborg tumor

pinealism

pinealoblastoma

pinealocyte

pinealocytoma

pinealoma
    ectopic p.
    extrapineal p.

pinealopathy

pineoblastoma

pineocytoma

pinguecula

pinguicula

pinkeye

Pinkus disease

pinocyte

pinocytic

pinocytosis

pinocytotic

pinosome

piorthopnea

pipecolic acid

pit
    basilar p.
    coated p.
    Gaul's p.
    Herbert's p.
    Mantoux p.
    preauricular p.

pituicyte

pituitarism

pityriasis
    p. alba
    lichenoid p.
    p. linguae
    p. maculata
    p. nigra
    p. rosea
    p. rotunda
    p. rubra (Hebra)
    p. rubra pilaris
    p. sicca
    p. simplex
    p. versicolor

pityroid

placenta
    p. accreta
    battledore p.
    p. circummarginata
    duplex p.
    p. fenestrata
    incarcerated p
    p. increta
    q. membranacea
    multilobate p.
    p. percreta
    premature separation of the
        p.
    p. previa
    p. spuria
    retained p.
    trilobate p.

placentae
    ablatio p.

placentitis

placentoma

plague
    black p.
    bubonic p.
    hemorrhagic p.
    pneumonic p.
    pulmonic p.
    septicemic p.

plakoglobin

planimetry

planocyte

plantalgia

planuria

plaque
    argyrophil p.
    atheromatous p.
    bacterial p.
    dental p.
    fibrofatty p.
    fibrolipid p.
    fibromyelinic p.
    fibrous p.
    Hollenhorst p.
    Hutchinson's p.
    p. jaunes
    Lichtheim p.
    MacCallum's p.
    neuritic p.
    pleural p.
    Randall's p.
    Redlich-Fisher miliary p.
    senile p.
    talc p.

plasma
    p. activation
    antihemophilic p.
    p. bicarbonate
    blood p.
    p. cell hepatitis
    p. clearance
    p. clotting factor
    p. factor X

plasma (*continued*)
    fresh frozen p.
    p. hemoglobin test
    p. layer
    platelet-poor p.
    p. volume expander

plasmacytoma
    multiple p. of bone

plasmacytosis

plasmagel

plasmahaut

plasmalemma

plasmarrhexis

plasmatogamy

plasmatorrhexis

plasmocytoma

plasmogamy

plasmogen

plasmoid

plasmolysis

plasmolytic

plasmolyzability

plasmolyzable

plasmolyze

plasmoma

plasmorrhexis

plasmoschisis

plasmosin

plasmotomy

plasson

plastin

plastochondria

plastogamy

plastosome

plate
    Abbe test p.
    blood agar p.
    cell p.
    Covalink MicroElisa culture
      p.
    cuticular p.
    end p.
    epiphyseal p.
    equatorial p.
    Hospidex microtiter p.
    Kühne's terminal p.
    metaphase p.
    notochordal p.
    p. culture
    reticular p.
    spread p.
    Strasburger's cell p.
    subgerminal p.

platelet
    p. agglutinin
    p. adhesion
    q. antibody
    p. autoantibody
    p. cofactor
    p. cofactor I, II, V
    p. count
    p. factor
    giant p.
    gray p.
    in vivo adhesive p. (IVAP)
    p. membrane glycoprotein
    p. thrombosis
    p. tissue factor
    plateletpheresis
    platelet-aggregating factor
      (PAF)
    platelet-free plasma
    platelet-poor

platycnemia

platycnemic

platycoria

platyglossal

platyknemia

platymeria

platymeric

platymorphia

platymorphic

platypnea

platypodia

platyspondylia

platyspondylisis

pleiades

pleiochloruria

pleocaryocyte

pleocytosis

pleokaryocyte

pleomorphic
    p. carcinoma
    p. leiomyosarcoma
    p. rhabdomyosarcoma

pleomorphism

pleonosteosis
    Léri p.

pleuralgia

pleurisy
    adhesive p.
    blocked p.
    cholesterol p.
    chylous p.
    circumscribed p.
    costal p.
    diaphragmatic p.
    diffuse p.
    dry p.
    p. with effusion
    encysted p.
    exudative p.
    fibrinous p.
    hemorrhagic p.
    indurative p.
    interlobular p.
    mediastinal p.

pleurisy (*continued*)
    plastic p.
    proliferating p.
    pulmonary p.
    purulent p.
    sacculated p.
    serofibrinous p.
    serous p.
    suppurative p.
    visceral p.
    wet p.

pleuritic

pleuritis
    fibrinous p.
    fibrosing p.
    lupus p.
    rheumatoid p.
    tuberculous p.
    uremic p.

pleuritogenous

pleurobronchitis

pleurocele

pleurocholecystitis

pleurodynia
    epidemic p.

pleurogenic

pleurogenous

pleurohepatitis

pleurolith

pleuropericarditis

pleuropneumonia

pleurothotonos

pleurothotonus

pleurotyphoid

PLEVA
    pityiasis lichenoides et
      varioliformis acuta

plexitis

plexopathy
    brachial p.
    lumbar p.
    lumbosacral p.
    sacral p.

plexosarcoma

plexus
    Exner's p.
    molecular p.
    p. of Raschkow
    solar p.
    supraradial p.

plug
    Dittrich's p.
    Ecker's p.
    epithelial p.
    mucous p.
    Traube's p.

plurilocular

plurimenorrhea

plurinuclear

pluripotent

pluripotential

pluripotentiality

pneumarthrosis

pneumatinuria

pneumatocardia

pneumatocele
    p. cranii
    extracranial p.
    intracranial p.
    parotid p.

pneumatocephalus

pneumatosis
    p. coli
    p. cystoides intestinalis
    p. cystoides intestinorum
    intestinal p.
    p. intestinalis

pneumaturia

pneumoamnios

pneumobilia

pneumocele

pneumocephalus

pneumocholecystitis

pneumococcosis

pneumococcosuria

pneumoconiosis
    antimony p.
    bauxite p.
    coal workers' p.
    collagenous p.
    fuller's earth p.
    graphite p.
    hematite p.
    kaolin p.
    mica p.
    mixed dust p.
    noncollagenous p.
    polyvinyl chloride p.
    rheumatoid p.
    p. siderotica
    talc p.
    titanium dioxide p.

pneumocrania

pneumocranium

pneumocystiasis

pneumocystosis

pneumocyte

pneumoderma

pneumoempyema

pneumoencephalocele

pneumoencephalos

pneumoenteritis

pneumogalactocele

pneumohemia

pneumohemopericardium

pneumohemothorax

pneumohydrometra

pneumohydropericardium

pneumohydrothorax

pneumokidney

pneumokoniosis

pneumolith

pneumolithiasis

pneumology

pneumomalacia

pneumomediastinum

pneumomelanosis

pneumonectasia

pneumonectasis

pneumonia
    Acinetobacter
        calcoaceticus p.
    acute gelatinous p.
    adenovirus p.
    p. alba
    alcoholic p.
    amebic p.
    anaerobic p.
    anthrax p.
    apex p.
    apical p.
    Aspergillus p.
    aspiration p.
    atypical p.
    bacterial p.
    bronchial p.
    Candida p.
    caseous p.
    central p.
    Chlamydia pneumoniae p.
    coccidioidal p.
    cold agglutinin p.
    confluent p.
    contusion p.
    core p.
    cryptogenic organizing p.

pneumonia (*continued*)
    cytomegalovirus p.
    deglutition p.
    desquamative interstitial p.
    diffuse interstitial p
    p. dissecans
    double p.
    Eaton agent p.
    embolic p.
    Enterobacter p.
    eosinophilic p.
    Escherichia coli p.
    fibrous p.
    Friedländer's bacillus p.
    fungal p.
    gangrenous p.
    giant cell p.
    glanders p.
    Haemophilus influenzae p.
    Hecht's p.
    herpes simplex virus p.
    hypostatic p.
    influenza virus p.
    inhalation p
    p interlobularis purulenta
    interstitial p.
    interstitial p., acute
    intrauterine p.
    Klebsiella p.
    Legionella p.
    lipid p.
    lobar p.
    lobular p.
    Löffler's p.
    Louisiana p.
    p. malleosa
    measles virus p.
    meningococcal p.
    metastatic p.
    migratory p.
    Moraxella p.
    Moraxella catarrhalis p.
    Mycoplasma p.
    mycoplasmal p.
    necrotizing p.
    Neisseria meningitidis p.
    Nocardia p.
    obstructive p.

pneumonia (*continued*)
oil-aspiration p.
organizing p.
parainfluenza virus p.
paratuberculous p.
Pasteurella multocida p.
Pittsburgh p.
plague p.
plasma cell p.
pleuritic p.
pneumococcal p.
pneumocystis p.
Pneumocystis carinii p.
primary atypical p.
Proteus p.
Pseudomonas aeruginosa p.
purulent p.
Q fever p.
respiratory syncytial virus p.
rheumatic p.
Rhodococcus equi p.
secondary p.
Serratia p.
staphylococcal p.
streptococcal p.
suppurative p.
terminal p.
traumatic p.
tuberculous p.
tularemic p.
typhoid p.
unresolved p.
varicella p.
Varicella zoster p.
ventilator-associated p.
viral p.
wandering p.
white p.
woolsorter's p.

pneumonitis
acute lupus p.
Ascaris p.
aspiration p.
chemical p.
cholesterol p.
granulomatous p.
hypersensitivity p.

pneumonitis (*continued*)
interstitial p., lymphocytic
malarial p.
manganese p.
mercury p.
pneumocystis p.
radiation p.
trimellitic anhydride p.
uremic p.

pneumonocele

pneumonoconiosis

pneumonocyte
granular p.
membranous p.

pneumonoenteritis

pneumonokoniosis

pneumonolipidosis

pneumonomoniliasis

pneumonomycosis

pneumonopathy
eosinophilic p.

pneumonopleuritis

pneumonorrhagia

pneumonosis

pneumopathy

pneumopericardium

pneumoperitoneal

pneumoperitoneum

pneumoperitonitis

pneumopleuritis

pneumoprecordium

pneumopreperitoneum

pneumopyopericardium

pneumopyothorax

pneumorachis

pneumoretroperitoneum

pneumorrhagia

pneumoserothorax

pneumosilicosis

pneumosinus dilatans

pneumothorax
    catamenial p.
    clicking p.
    pressure p.
    spontaneous p.
    tension p.
    traumatic p.
    valvular p.

pneumouria

pneumoventricle

pneumoventriculi

pocket
    p. dosimeter
    endocardial p.
    p. of Zahn

podagra

podagral

podagric

podagrous

podalgia

podarthritis

podedema

podocyte

pododynia

pogoniasis

poikiloblast

poikilocyte

poikilocythemia

poikilocytosis

poikiloderma
    p. atrophicans vasculare
    p. of Civatte
    p. congenitale

poikilothrombocyte

point
    Boas' p.
    Brewer's p.
    cold rigor p.
    Cova's p.
    dorsal p.
    eye p.
    isoelectric p.
    isoionic p.
    Krafft p.
    McBurney's p.
    McEwen's p.
    Mackenzie's p.
    Pauly's p.
    phrenic-pressure p.
    Ramond's p.
    retromandibular tender p.
    Robson's p.
    supraorbital p.

poisoning
    arsenic p.
    beryllium p.
    blood p.
    carbon disulfide p.
    carbon monoxide p.
    chloroform p.
    cyanide p.
    ethyl alcohol p.
    food p.
    heavy-metal p.
    manganese p.
    mercury p.
    methyl alcohol p.
    naphthol p.
    oxygen p.
    parathyroid p.
    salmonella p.
    sombroid p.
    systemic p.
    thallium p.
    zinc p.

polarization

polarogram

polarographic

polarography

pole
    vascular p. of renal
        corpuscle
    vascular p. of renal
        glomerulus

poliencephalitis

poliencephalomyelitis

polio

poliodystrophia
    p. cerebri
    p. cerebri progressiva
    p. cerebri progressiva
        infantilis

poliodystrophy
    progressive cerebral p.
    progressive infantile p.

polioencephalitis

polioencephalomeningomyelitis

polioencephalomyelitis

polioencephalopathy

poliomeningitis
    nonparalytic p.

poliomyelencephalitis

poliomyelitis
    abortive p.
    acute anterior p.
    acute lateral p.
    bulbar p.
    cerebral p.
    endemic p.
    epidemic p.
    p. I, II, III titer
    p. immune globulin
        (human)
    mmunization reaction p.
    nonparalytic p
    paralytic p
    post-tonsillectomy p.
    spinal paralytic p.

poliomyeloencephalitis

poliomyelopathy

poliosis

polkissen

pollakidipsia

pollakisuria

pollakiuria

pollenosis

polocytes

polonium

polyadenitis

polyadenopathy

polyadenosis

polyagglutination

polyalveolar

polyamine

polyandry

polyangiitis
    microscopic p.

polyarteritis
    p. nodosa

polyarthritis
    chronic secondary p.
    chronic villous p.
    p. destruens
    epidemic p.
    tuberculous p.

polyavitaminosis

polyaxonic

polyblennia

polychloruria

polycholia

polychondritis
    chronic atrophic p.
    relapsing p.

polychondropathia

polychondropathy

polychromasia

polychromatia

polychromatocyte

polychromatocytosis

polychromatophil

polychromatophilia

polychromatophilic

polychromatosis

polychromemia

polychromophil

polychromophilia

polychylia

polycoria
    p. spuria
    p. vera

polycystic

polycyte

polycythemia
    absolute p
    appropriate p
    benign p
    compensatory p
    hypertonic p
    inappropriate p.
    myelopathic p
    primary p
    relative p
    relative p., chronic
    p. rubra
    p. rubra vera
    secondary p.
    splenomegalic p.
    spurious p.
    stress p.
    p. vera

polydipsia

polydysplasia
    hereditary ectodermal p.

polydysspondylism

polydystrophic

polydystrophy
    pseudo-Hurler p.

polyembryoma

polyendocrinoma

polyendocrinopathy

polyesthesia

polygalactia

polygyny

PolyHeme (blood substitute)

polyhidrosis

polyhydramnios

polyhydruria

polyhypermenorrhea

polyhypomenorrhea

polyidrosis

polykaryocyte

polymenia

polymenorrhea

polymetacarpia

polymetatarsia

polymicrolipomatosis

polymorphic
    p. epithelial mucin
    p. genetic marker
    p. reticulosis

polymorphism

polymorphocytic leukemia

polymorphonuclear
    p. basophil
    p. eosinophil
    p. leukocyte
    p. leukocytic infiltrate
    p. neutrophil

polymorphous

polymyalgia
    p. arteritica
    p. rheumatica

polymyoclonus

polymyopathy

polymyositis

polynesic

polyneuralgia

polyneuritic

polyneuritis
    acute febrile p.
    acute idiopathic p.
    acute infective p.
    anemic p.
    cranial p.
    endemic polyneuritis
    Guillain-Barré p.
    Jamaica ginger p.
    leprous p.

polyneuromyositis

polyneuropathy
    acute postinfectious p.
    amyloid p.
    Andrade-type familial
      amyloid p.
    anemic p.
    arsenic p.
    arsenical p.
    carcinomatous p.
    critical illness p.
    diphtheritic p.
    erythredema p.
    familial amyloid p.
    inflammatory demyelinating
      p.
    Meretoja type familial
      amyloid p.
    nutritional p.
    paraneoplastic p.
    porphyric p.
    symmetrical sensory p
    uremic p.

polyneuropathy (*continued*)
    Van Allen type familial
      amyloid p.

polyneuroradiculitis

polynuclear

polynucleate

polynucleolar

polyodontia

polyonychia

polyopia
    binocular p.
    p. monophthalmica

polyopsia

polyopy

polyorchidism

polyorchis

polyorchism

polyp
    adenomatous p.
    aural p.
    bleeding p.
    cardiac p.
    cellular p.
    cervical p.
    choanal p.
    cholesterol p.
    colorectal p.
    cystic p.
    endocervical p.
    endometrial p.
    fibrinous p.
    fibroepithelial p.
    gastric p.
    gelatinous p.
    granulomatous p.
    gum p.
    hamartomatous p.
    hydatid p.
    hyperplastic p.
    inflammatory p.
    juvenile p.

polyp (*continued*)
  laryngeal p.
  p. of larynx
  lipomatous p.
  lymphoid p.
  metaplastic p.
  mucus p.
  myomatous p.
  nasal p.
  osseus p.
  papillary adenomatous p.
  Peutz-Jegers p.
  placental p.
  regenerative p.
  retention p.
  sessile p.
  villous p.

polypathia

polypeptidemia

polypeptidorrhachia

polyperiostitis
  p. hyperesthetica

polypi

polypiform

polypnea

polypneic

polypoid

polypoidosis

polyposia

polyposis
  p. coli
  familial p.
  familial adenomatous p.
  familial intestinal p.
  juvenile p.
  juvenile intestinal p.
  multiple familial p.

polypous
  p. endocarditis
  p. gastritis

polypus
  p. cysticus
  p. hydatidosus

polyradiculitis

polyradiculoneuritis

polyradiculoneuropathy
  acute inflammatory
    demyelinating p.
  chronic inflammatory p.
  chronic inflammatory
    demyelinating p.
  chronic relapsing p.
  inflammatory demyelinating
    p.

polyradiculopathy

polyrrhea

polyserositis
  periodic p.
  recurrent p.

polysialia

polysinuitis

polysinusitis

polysomatic

polysomaty

polysomic

polysomy

polyspermia

polyspermism

polystichia

polysynovitis

polytendinitis

polytendinobursitis

polytenosynovitis

polytrauma

polytrichia

polytrichosis

polytrophia

polytrophic

polytrophy

polyunguia

polyuria

pompholyhemia

pompholyx

ponceau 3B

pontobulbia

poradenia

poradenitis

porencephalia

porencephalic

porencephalitis

porencephalous

porencephaly
    encephaloclastic p.
    schizencephalic p.

porin

porokeratosis
    actinic p.
    disseminated superficial
      actinic p.
    Mibelli p.
    p. palmaris et plantaris
      disseminata

porokeratotic

porosis (pl. poreses)
    cerebral p.

porosity

porospore

porotic

porphin

porphobilinogenuria
    p. deaminase
    p. synthase
    p. synthase assay

porphyria
    acute intermittent p.
    congenital p.
    p. cutanea tarda
    congenital erythropoietic p.
    congenital photosensitive p.
    cutaneous hepatic p.
    erythrohepatic p.
    erythropoietic p.
    hepatic p.
    hepatoerythropoietic p.
    intermittent acute porphyria
    latent p.
    mixed p.
    photosensitive p.
    South African genetic p.
    Swedish p.
    symptomatic p.
    variegate p.

porphyrin
    p. assay
    p. pigmentation

porphyrinemia

porphyrinuria

porphyrismus

porphyruria

porrigo
    p. favosa
    p. furfurans
    p. lupinosa

portal-systemic encephalopathy

Porter-Silber
    P-S. chromogen test
    P-S reaction

Porteus maze test

Portmann classification

port-wine
    p-w. mark
    p-w. stain

positron

postdiphtheritic

postdysenteric

postgamma proteinuria

posthemorrhagic anemia

posthitis

postholith

postabsorptive state

postductal coarctation of the aorta

postmeiotic

postmiotic

postmitotic

postmortem
    p. hypostasis
    p. sugillation

potassemia

potassium
    p. oxalate
    p. dichromate

pouce
    pouce flottant

pouch
    Blake's p.
    Hartmann's p.
    Physick's p.
    Zenker's p.

pouchitis

pounds per square inch (p.s.i.)

pour plate

pragmatagnosia

pragmatamnesia

prebetalipoproteinemia

precementum

precipitate
    keratitic p.
    keratotic p.

precocious
    p. puberty

precocity

precursor lesion

pregnancy
    aborted ectopic p.
    cornual p.
    ectopic p.
    exochorial p.
    extrauterine p.
    fallopian p.
    heterotopic p.
    hydatid p.
    interstitial p.
    intramural p.
    intraperitoneal p.
    megaloblastic anemia of p.
    membranous p.
    mesenteric p.
    molar p.
    mural p.
    ovarian p.
    ovario-abdominal p.
    post-term p.
    prolonged p.
    sarcofetal p.
    toxemia of p.
    tubal p.
    tuboabdominal p.
    tubo-ovarian p.
    tubouterine p.
    uteroabdominal p.
    uterotubal p.
    voluntary interruption of p.

prehallux

preictal

premature

prematurity

premeiotic

premitotic

prepuce
    redundant p.

presbyacusia

presbycardia

presbyesophagus

presbyopia

presenile spontaneous
  gangrene

PreservCyt fixative

prespermatogonia

prespondylolisthesis

pressor
  p. amine
  p. base

pressure
  barometric p.
  colloidal osmotic p.
  Donders' p.
  osmotic p.
  plasma oncotic p.
  screen filtration p.

priapism

Price precipitation reaction

prion

proboscis
  p. lateralis

procallus

procaryon

procaryosis

procaryote

procedure
  Cherry-Crandall p.
  Chryptosporidium
    diagnostic p.
  Gomori-Takamatsu
    procedure
  helminth identification p.
  hypophysis staining p.

process
  Deiters p.
  dendritic p.
  filiform p.
  p. of nerve cell

process (*continued*)
  styloid p.
  ThinPrep slide p.
  Tomes p.

procidentia

procoagulant

procollagen

proctatresia

proctectasia

proctencleisis

proctitis
  factitial p.
  idiopathic p.
  radiation p.
  ulcerative p.

proctocele

proctocolitis

proctodynia

proctoparalysis

proctoplegia

proctoptosis

proctorrhagia

proctorrhea

proctosigmoiditis

procurvation

product
  advanced glycation end p.
  fibrin breakdown p.
  fibrin breakdown p.
  fission p.
  scalar p.
  spallation p.
  vector p.
  waste p.

proenzyme

profilin

progenitor cell

progeny

progeria

prognostic factor

prokaryote

prokaryotic

prolapse
    mitral valve p.
    Morgagni's p.

prolepsis

prolidase deficiency

proliferans
    retinitis p.

proliferative
    p. bronchiolitis
    p. chronic arthritis
    p. fasciitis
    p. glomerulonephritis
    p. myositis

proliferous cyst

proline
    p. deoxyhydrogenase
    p. hydroxylase
    q. oxidase

prolinemia

prolinuria

prolonged
    p. bleeding time
    p. coagulation time

PROM
    premature rupture of (fetal)
        membranes

promegakaryoblast

promegaloblast

prometaphase

promethium

pronucleus

propagating thrombus

1-propanol

2-propanol

propanoic acid

prophage

prophage

prophase

propidium iodide

propionicacidemia

propria

proptosis

prosodemic

prosopagnosia

prosopoanoschisis

prosoposchisis

prostatalgia

prostatauxe

prostatelcosis

prostatic
    p.acid phosphatase
    p. adenoma
    p. calculus
    p. intraepithelial neoplasia

prostatocystitis

prostatodynia

prostatolith

prostatomegaly

prostatorrhea

prostatovesiculitis

prosternation

protanomalous

protanomaly

protanope

protanopia

✗ *Proteus* ~~zzz~~ *mirabilis*

protanopic

protanopsia

protein
    acute phase p.
    acyl carrier p.
    AL p.
    amyloid A p.
    amyloid light chain p.
    anti-S-100 p.
    Bence Jones p.
    p. binding
    p. buffer
    carrier p.
    C-reactive p.
    conjugated p.
    G protein
    glial fibrillary acidic p.
    GTPase-activating p.
    GTP-binding p.
    HER-2 p.
    HER-2/neu p.
    heterologous p.
    p. deficiency anemia
    p. electrophoresis
    guanyl-nucleotide-binding
      p.
    insoluble p.
    membrane transport p.
    muscle contractile p.
    prion p.
    p. separation method
    proteolipid p.
    reactive p.
    SAA p.
    serum amyloid A p.
    thyroxine binding p.
    total p.
    total serum p.

proteinase

protein-binding

protein-caloric malnutrition

proteinemia

proteinosis
    alveolar p.

proteinosis (continued)
    lipid p.
    pulmonary alveolar p.
    tissue p.

proteinuria
    adventitious p.
    Bence Jones p.
    cardiac p.
    colliquative p.
    digestive p.
    emulsion p.
    enterogenic p.
    globular p.
    gouty p.
    hematogenous p.
    hemic p.
    lordotic p.
    nephrogenous p.
    orthostatic p.
    palpatory p.
    paroxysmal p.
    postrenal p.
    postural p.
    prerenal p.
    pretuberculous p.
    pseudo-p.
    pyogenic p.
    residual p.
    serous p.
    physiologic p.

proteinuric

proteosuria

proteuria

proteuric

✗ prothrombinopenia

protocaryon

protochondral

protochondrium

protocoproporphyria

protoplasm

protoplasmic

protoplast fusion

protoporphyria
    erythropoietic p. (EPP)

protoporphyrin
    erythrocyte p.
    free erythrocyte p.
    p. assay
    zinc p.
    p. test

protoporphyrinuria

prototype

protozoa

protozoologist

protrusio
    p. acetabuli

protrusion

proventriculus

proximoataxia

pruinate

pruriginous

prurigo
    p. agria
    Besnier's p.
    p. chronica multiformis
    p. estivalis
    p. ferox
    p. gestationis
    p. of Hebra
    melanotic p.
    p. mitis
    nodular p.
    p. simplex
    summer p. of Hutchinson

pruritic

pruritogenic

prussiate

prussic acid

psammous

pseudagraphia

pseudalbuminuria

pseudangina

pseudankylosis

pseudaphia

pseudarthrosis

pseudoacanthosis
    p. nigricans

pseudoagglutination

pseudoagraphia

pseudoalbuminuria

pseudoalveolar

pseudoanemia

pseudoaneurysm

pseudoangina

pseudoankylosis

pseudoanodontia

pseudoapoplexy

pseudoarthrosis

pseudoathetosis

pseudoatrophoderma colli

pseudobacillus

pseudobacterium

pseudobasedow

pseudobronchiectasis

pseudobulbar

pseudocartilage

pseudocast

pseudocephalocele

pseudochromidrosis

pseudochromosome

pseudochylothorax

pseudoclonus

pseudocolloid

pseudocoloboma

pseudocoma

pseudo-corpus luteum

pseudocoxalgia

pseudocroup

pseudocyanin

pseudocyesis

pseudocylindroid

pseudocyst

pseudodecidual

pseudodiphtheria

pseudodiverticulum

pseudodysentery

pseudoedema

pseudoemphysema

pseudoendometritis

pseudoerysipelas

pseudoexfoliation

pseudofolliculitis

pseudo-Gaucher cell

pseudoglioma

pseudogout

pseudographia

pseudogynecomastia

pseudohaustration

pseudohemagglutination

pseudohematuria

pseudohemophilia

pseudohemoptysis

pseudohermaphrodism

pseudohermaphrodite

pseudohermaphroditism

pseudohernia

pseudoheterotopia

pseudohydrocephalus

pseudohydronephrosis

pseudohypacusis

pseudohyperkalemia

pseudohypertension

pseudohypertrichosis

pseudohypertriglyceridemia

pseudohypertrophic

pseudohypertrophy

pseudohypoaldosteronism

pseudohyponatremia

pseudohypoparathyroidism

pseudohypophosphatasia

pseudohypothyroidism

pseudoicterus

pseudoinfarction

pseudoisocyanin

pseudojaundice

pseudolamellar

pseudolithiasis

pseudoluxation

pseudomamma

pseudomegacolon

pseudomelanosis

pseudomelia

pseudomeningitis

pseudomethemoglobin

pseudomonilethrix

pseudomucinous

pseudomyiasis

pseudomyxoma
    p. peritonei

pseudoneoplasm

pseudoneuritis

pseudoneuroma

pseudoneuronophagia

pseudo-ochronosis

pseudo-osteomalacia

pseudoparalysis
    Parrot's p.
    syphilitic p.

pseudopelade

pseudopellagra

pseudoperitonitis

pseudophakia
    p. adiposa
    p. fibrosa

pseudoplasm

pseudopneumonia

pseudopodia

pseudopodium

pseudopolycythemia

pseudopolymelia

pseudopolyp

pseudopolyposis

pseudoporphyria

pseudoproteinuria

pseudopterygium

pseudoptosis

pseudoptyalism

pseudoretinitis pigmentosa

pseudorickets

pseudorosette

pseudosclerema

pseudosclerosis
    Jakob-Creutzfeld p.
    Westphal-Strümpell p.

pseudosmallpox

pseudostratified

pseudotabes
    diabetic p.
    pupillotonic p.

pseudotetanus

pseudotrachoma

pseudotrismus

pseudotruncus arteriosus

pseudotubercle

pseudotuberculoma

pseudotumor
    p. cerebri
    inflammatory p.
    orbital p.

pseudouremia

pseudoxanthoma elasticum

psittacosis

psoitis

psorenteritis

psoriasiform

psoriasis
    p. annularis
    p. arthropica
    arthritic p.
    Barber's p.
    buccal p.
    circinate p.
    discoid p.
    exfoliative p.
    figurate p.
    follicular p.
    gyrate p.

psoriasis (*continued*)
    inverse p.
    nummular p.
    ostraceous p.
    p. of palms and soles
    pustular p.
    p. rupioides
    seborrheic p.
    volar p.
    von Zumbusch's p.
    p. vulgaris
    Zumbusch's p.

psoriatic

psorophthalmia

psychroalgia

psychroesthesia

psyllium hydophilic mucilloid

PT
    pneumothorax
    prothrombin time

ptarmic

ptarmus

pterin

pteroic acid

pternalgia

pterygium
    p. colli
    congenital p.

ptosed

ptosis (pl. ptoses)

ptotic

ptyalism

ptyalocele

ptyalogenic

ptyalolithiasis

ptyalorrhea

pubic
    p. louse

Puchtler-Sweat stain

puerperal
    p. eclampsia
    p. septicemia
    p. thrombosis

pulmolith

pulmonale
    cor p.

pulpiform

pulmonary
    p. alveolus
    p. artery hypertension
    p. dysmaturity syndrome
    p. function test
    p. fibrosis
    p. interstitial emphysema
    p. pneumonosis
    p. sarcoidosis
    p. tuberculosis
    p. ventilation scan

pultaceous

punch biopsy

punctate lesion

punctiform

puncture
    Bernard's p.
    diabetic p.
    femoral p.
    lumbar p.
    sternal p.
    transethmoidal p.

pupil
    Adie's p.
    Argyll Robertson p.
    Behr's p.
    Hutchinson's p.
    Marcus Gunn p.
    myotonic p.
    pinhole p.

pupillatonia

pupilloplegia

pupillotonia

pupiparous

puriform

purine bodies test

purinometer

purple
    bromcresol p.

purpura
    anaphylactoid p.
    p. annularis telangiectodes
    autoimmune
      thrombocytopenic p.
    fibrinolytic p.
    Henoch's p.
    Henoch-Schönlein p.
    hyperglobulinemic p.
    idiopathic p.
    immune thrombocytopenic
      p.
    Majocchi's p.
    p. fulminans
    p. nervosa
    p. of newborn
    p. rheumatica
    Schönlein p.
    Schönlein-Henoch p.
    p. simplex
    steroid p.
    thrombocytopenic p.
    Waldenstrom p.

purpuric

purpuric acid

purpurin

purpurine

purpurinuria

puruloid

pus
    anchovy sauce p.
    blue p.
    burrowing p.
    cheesy p.

pus (*continued*)
    curdy pus
    green p.
    ichorouos p.
    laudable p.
    sanious pus

pustula

pustular inflammation

pustulation

pustule
    malignant p.
    multilocular p.
    simple p.
    spongiform p.
    spongiform p. of Kogoj
    unilocular p.

pustulosis
    p. palmaris et plantaris
    palmoplantar p.
    p. vacciniformis acuta
    p. varioliformis acuta

putrefaction

putrescine

PV
    plasma volume
    polycythemia vera

pyarthrosis

pyelectasia

pyelectasis

pyelitic

pyelitis
    calculous p.
    p. cystica
    defloration p.
    p. glandularis
    p. gravidarum
    hematogenous p.
    hemorrhagic p.
    suppurative p.

pyelocaliectasis

pyelocystitis

pyelonephritis
    acute p.
    chronic p
    emphysematous p
    p of pregnancy
    xanthogranulomatous p.

pyelonephrosis

pyelopathy

pyelophlebitis

pyeloureteritis
    p. cystica

pyemesis

pyemia
    arterial p.
    cryptogenic p.
    otogenous p.
    portal p.

pyemic

pyencephalus

pyesis

pygalgia

pyknocyte

pyknocytosis

pyknodysostosis

pyknoepilepsy

pyknometer

pyknometry

pyknomorphic

pyknomorphous

pyknoplasson

pyknosis

pyknotic

pylephlebectasis

pylephlebitis
    adhesive p.
    suppurative p.

pylethrombophlebitis

pylethrombosis

pyloralgia

pyloric stenosis

pyloritis

pyloroduodenitis

pylorospasm
    congenital p.
    reflex p.

pylorostenosis

Pym fever

pyocalix

pyocele

pyocelia

pyocephalus

pyochezia

pyocolpocele

pyocolpos

pyocyanic

pyocyanin

pyocyst

pyocyte

pyoderma
    chancriform p.
    p. chancriforme faciei
    p. faciale
    p. gangrenosum
    malignant p.
    p.vegetans

pyodermia

pyofecia

pyogenesis

pyogenic
    p. bacterium
    p. granuloma
    p. meningitis
    p. salpingitis

pyogenous

pyohemia

pyohemothorax

pyohydronephrosis

pyoid

pyometra

pyometritis

pyometrium

pyonephritis

pyonephrolithiasis

pyonephrosis

pyonephrotic

pyo-ovarium

pyopericarditis

pyopericardium

pyoperitoneum

pyoperitonitis

pyophagia

pyophthalmia

pyophthalmitis

pyophysometra

pyoplania

pyopneumocholecystitis

pyopneumocyst

pyopneumohepatitis

pyopneumopericardium

pyopneumoperitoneum

pyopneumoperitonitis

pyopneumothorax

pyopoiesis

pyopoietic

pyoptysis

pyopyelectasis

pyorubin

pyosalpingitis

pyosalpingo-oophoritis

pyosalpinx

pyosclerosis

pyosepticemia

pyospermia

pyostomatitis
    p. vegetans

PY test (C-14 urea)

pyothorax

pyoumbilicus

pyourachus

pyoureter

pyovesiculosis

pyoxanthine

pyoxanthose

pyrectic

pyrenolysis

pyretic

pyretogen

pyretogenesis

pyretogenetic

pyretogenic

pyretogenous

pyretotyphosis

pyrexia
    Pel-Ebstein p.
    p. of unknown etiology

pyrexial

pyrexiogenic

pyridoxic

pyriform

pyrimethamine assay

pyrimidine base

pyrogen
    bacterial p.

pyrogenetic

pyrogenic

pyrogenous

pyroglobulinemia

pyroglutamicaciduria

pyrolysis

pyronin
    p. B
    p. G
    p. Y

pyronine

pyroninophilia

pyroninophilic

pyropoikilocytosis

pyrosis

pyrroloporphyria

pyruvate kinase (PK) deficiency

pyruvemia

pythogenesis

pythogenic

pythogenous

pyuria
    miliary p.

Q

Q-banding stain

Q-enzyme

QRZ
    wheal reaction time

quadrant

quadrantanopsia

quadrigeminal

quadriparesis

quadrivalent

qualitative analysis

quantitation test

quantum (pl. quanta)
    q. limit

quark

quasidiploid

Queckenstedt test

quellung phenomenon

Quick Screen (at home drug
    test)

Quick Vue Chlamydia test

quinaldine red

quinhydrone

quinidine assay

quinolinic acid

quinsy

quotient
    albumin q.
    circadian q.
    D q.
    permeability q.
    protein q.
    reaction q.

R

Rf

rabbetting

racemose

rachialgia

rachiocampsis

rachiochysis

rachiocyphosis

rachiodynia

rachiokyphosis

rachiomyelitis

rachiopathy

rachioscoliosis

rachischisis
    r. partialis
    r. posterior
    r. totalis

rachitic

rachitis

rachitism

rachitogenic

radiation
    mitogenetic r.
    mitogenic r.
    r. of thalamus

radical
    color r.
    free r.

radiculalgia

radiculitis

radiculoganglionitis

radiculomeningomyelitis

radiculomyelopathy

radiculoneuritis

radiculoneuropathy

radiculopathy
    cervical r.
    spondylotic caudal r.

radiocystitis

radiodermatitis

radioepidermitis

radioepithelitis

radiomutation

radioneuritis

radiopathology

radiothanatology

radiotoxemia

radix
    r. unguis

rale
    amphoric r
    atelectatic r.
    border r.
    bubbling r.
    cavernous r.
    cellophane r.
    clicking r.
    consonating r.
    crackling r.
    crepitant r.
    gurgling r.
    guttural r.
    marginal r.
    metallic r.
    mucous r.
    subcrepitant r.
    tracheal r.
    vesicular r.

ramitis

ramollissement

ranine

ranula
    plunging r.
    pancreatic r.

ranular

rapture of the deep

rate
- sedimentation r.
- protein catabolic r.

ratio
- A-G r.
- albumin-globulin r.
- concentration r.
- extraction r.
- karyoplasmic r.
- nucleocytoplasmic r.
- nucleoplasmic r.
- urea excretion r.
- urea reduction r.

ray
- astral r
- beta r.
- cathode r.
- delta r.
- gamma r.
- grenz r.
- necrobiotic r.
- polar r.

Raynaud
- R. disease
- R. phenomenon

R-banding stain

reactant
- acute phase r.
- limiting r.

reaction
- acetic acid r.
- acid r.
- acrosome r.
- acute hemolytic transfusion r.
- alkaline r.
- alpha-naphthol r.
- anaphylactic r.
- antigen-antibody r.
- Arias-Stella r.
- Arthus r.
- Ascoli r.

reaction (*continued*)
- autoimmune r.
- azo coupling r.
- axon r.
- axonal r.
- Bauer r.
- Bekhterevs (Bechterews) r.
- Bence Jones r.
- Berthelot r.
- Bittorfs r.
- Biuret r.
- blocking antibody r.
- Bonlet and Gengou r.
- Burchard-Lieberman r.
- cadaveric r.
- capsular pigmentation r.
- carbamino r.
- cell mediated r.
- chemical r.
- Christeler r.
- chromaffin r.
- clot r.
- cocarde r.
- colloidal gold r.
- complement-fixation r.
- contrast media r.
- cutaneous r.
- cytotoxic r.
- decidual r.
- delayed hemolytic transfusion r.
- dermotuberculin r.
- desmoplastic r.
- diazo r.
- digitonin r.
- Dold r.
- dopa r.
- Edman r.
- egg yellow r.
- Ehrlichs aldehyde r.
- Ehrlichs diazo r.
- endergonic r.
- exergonic r.
- false-negative r.
- false-positive r.
- febrile nonhemolytic transfusion r.
- Felix-Weil r.

reaction (*continued*)
    Fernandez r.
    Feulgen r.
    fixation r.
    flocculation r.
    foreign body r.
    Forsman antigen-antibody
        r.
    Frei-Hoffman r.
    fuchsinophil r.
    Fujiwara r.
    gel diffusion r.
    Gerhardt r.
    giant cell r.
    glycine-argnine r.
    graft-versus-host r.
    Grimelius argyrophil r.
    hemoclastic r.
    hemolytic transfusion r.
    Henle r.
    Hersheimer r.
    heterophil antigen r.
    hunting r.
    id r.
    immune r.
    Jaffe r.
    Jones-Mote r.
    leukomoid r.
    Liebermann-Burchard r.
    lymphocytic leukomoid r.
    Marchi r.
    Meinicke turbidity r.
    miostagmin r.
    Mitsuda r.
    mixed agglutinin r.
    mixed lymphocyte r.
    Molisch r.
    Nadi r.
    Nagler r.
    Nessler r.
    Neufeld r.
    Nickerson-Kveim test r.
    nnhydrin-Schiff r.
    Oestreicher r.
    oxidase r.
    oxidation-reduction r.
    Pandy r.
    PAS r.

reaction (*continued*)
    Perls r.
    peroxidase r.
    photochemical r.
    plasmal r.
    plasmocytic leukomoid r.
    polymerase chain r.
    precipitin r.
    prozone r.
    reagin r.
    rheumatoid factor r.
    Rivalta r.
    Sakaguchi r.
    Schmorl r.
    Schultz r.
    Schwartzman r.
    Selivanoff (Seliwanow) r.
    serum sickness-like r.
    streptococcal toxin
        immunization r.
    tetanus toxin immunization
        r.
    thermoprecipitin r.
    transferred antigen-cell-
        bound antibody r.
    transferred antigen-
        transferred antibody r.
    tuberculin r.
    vaccinoid r.
    VP r.
    Wasserman r.
    Weil-Felix r.
    wheal-and-erythema r.
    xanthydrol r.
    Yorke autolytic r.

reagent
    amino-acid r.
    arsenic-sulfuric acid r.
    Benedict r.
    Berthelot r.
    Bial r.
    biuret r.
    Bogg r.
    diazo r.
    Ehrlich aldehyde r.
    Ehrlich diazo r.
    Fouchet r.

reagent (*continued*)
    general r.
    Gies' biuret r.
    Lloyd r.
    Millon r.
    Mörner r.
    Nessler r.
    Ninhydrin r.
    Rosenthaler r.
    Schiff r.
    Scott-Wilson r.

receptor
    cell-surface r.
    membrane r.
    nuclear r.
    paciniform r.

recidivation

recidivism

recrudescence

recrudescent

rectalgia

rectitis

rectolabial

rectostenosis

rectourethral

rectouterine

rectovaginal

rectovesical

rectovestibular

rectovulvar

recurvation

red
    alizarin r.
    alizarin r.S
    alizarin water-soluble r.
    aniline r.
    basic r.2
    basic r.9
    bromphenol r.

red (*continued*)
    carmine r.
    cerasine r.
    chlorophenol r.
    Congo r.
    cotton r.
    cotton r. B
    cotton r. C
    cotton r. 4 B
    cresol r.
    dianil r. 4 C
    dianin r. 4 B
    direct r.
    direct r. 4 B
    indigo r.
    indoxyl r.
    magdala r.
    methyl r.
    naphthaline r.
    neutral r.
    oil r.
    oil r. IV
    oil r. O
    scarlet r.
    Sudan r.
    toluylene r.
    tony r.
    trypan r.

reductase
    5α-r.

reflex
    Babinski's r.
    bar r.
    Bechterew's r.
    Bekhterev's r.
    Bekhterev's deep r.
    Bekhterev-Mendel r.
    Brain's r.
    Brudzinski's r.
    bulbomimic r.
    cat's eye r.
    Chaddock's r.
    chin r.
    clasp-knife r.
    corneomandibular r.
    corneopterygoid r.
    cuboidodigital r.

reflex (*continued*)
    digital r.
    dorsocuboidal r.
    Erben's r.
    Escherich's r.
    facial r.
    femoral r.
    flexor r.
    Gordon's r
    grasp r.
    grasping r.
    gustolacrimal r.
    heel-tap r.
    Hoffmann's r.
    inverted radial r.
    jaw r.
    jaw jerk r.
    Joffroy's r.
    Juster r.
    lacrimal r.
    Lust's r.
    Magnus and de Kleijn neck
        r.
    mandibular r.
    mass r.
    Mendel's r.
    Mendel's dorsal r. of foot
    Mendel-Bekhterev r.
    Mondonesi's r.
    myopic r.
    oculovagal r.
    Oppenheim's r.
    paradoxical pupillary r.
    pathologic r.
    peritoneointestinal r.
    Puusepp's r.
    quadrupedal extensor r.
    Remak's r.
    renointestinal r.
    renorenal r.
    retrobulbar pupillary r.
    reversed pupillary r.
    Riddoch's mass r.
    Rossolimo's r.
    Saenger's r.
    Schäffer's r.
    senile r.
    tarsophalangeal r.

reflex (*continued*)
    Throckmorton's r.
    toe r.
    vagus r.
    vesicointestinal r.
    visceromotor r.
    viscerosensory r.
    viscerotrophic r.
    Weiss' r.

reflexophil

reflux
    duodenogastric r.
    duodenogastroesophageal
        r.
    gastroesophageal r.
    intrarenal r.
    valvular r.
    venous r.
    vesicoureteral r.
    vesicoureteric r.
    esophageal r.

regulator
    cystic fibrosis
        transmembrane
        conductance r.

remnant
    acroblastic r.

ren
    r. mobilis
    r. unguliformis

reninism
    primary r.

renopathy

renoprival

resazurin

reserve
    alkali r.

resin
    anion exchange r.
    azure A carbacrylic r.
    cation exchange r.
    ion exchange r.

resistance
    androgen r.
    androgen r., complete
    androgen r., incomplete
    insulin r.

resonance
    amphoric r.
    bandbox r.
    skodaic r.
    vesiculotympanitic r.
    whispering r.
    wooden r.

respiration
    amphoric r.
    asthmoid r.
    Biot's r.
    bronchocavernous r.
    cavernous r.
    cell r.
    Cheyne-Stokes r.
    cogwheel r.
    collateral r.
    controlled diaphragmatic r.
    divided r.
    interrupted r.
    Kussmaul's r.
    Kussmaul-Kien r.
    paradoxical r.
    periodic r.
    puerile r.
    suppressed r.
    vesicular r.
    vesiculocavernous r.
    vicarious r.
    jerky r.

rest
    aberrant r.
    carbon r.
    Walthard's cell r.

rete
    malpighian r.
    r. mirabile

reticula

reticulocytopenia

reticulocytosis

reticuloendotheliosis

reticuloid

reticulonodular

reticulopenia

reticulopituicyte

reticulosis
    familial hemophagocytic r.
    familial histiocytic r
    histiocytic medullary r
    lipomelanotic r

reticulum
    agranular r.
    Chiari's r.
    Ebner's r.
    endoplasmic r.
    granular r.
    sarcoplasmic r.
    stellate r.

retinitis
    actinic r.
    r. albuminurica
    apoplectic r.
    azotemic r.
    central angiospastic r.
    r. circinata
    circinate r.
    Coats' r.
    cytomegalovirus r.
    diabetic r.
    disciform r.
    exudative r.
    gravidic r.
    hypertensive r.
    Jacobson's r.
    Jensen's r.
    leukemic r.
    metastatic r.
    nephritic r.
    r. pigmentosa
    r. pigmentosa sine
        pigmento
    proliferating r.
    r. punctata albescens

retinitis (*continued*)
    renal r.
    r. sclopetaria
    serous r.
    simple r.
    solar r.
    r. stellata
    striate r.
    suppurative r.
    syphilitic r.
    r. syphilitica
    uremic r.

retinochoroiditis
    r. juxtapapillaris
    toxoplasmic r.

retinodialysis

retinomalacia

retinopapillitis

retinopathy
    AIDS-associated r.
    arteriosclerotic r.
    background r.
    background diabetic r.
    bull's eye r.
    central angiospastic r.
    central disk-shaped r.
    central serous r.
    circinate r.
    diabetic r.
    exudative r.
    hemorrhagic r.
    HIV-associated r.
    hypertensive r.
    leukemic r.
    r. of prematurity
    pigmentary r.
    proliferative r.
    proliferative diabetic r.
    Purtscher's angiopathic r.
    renal r.
    stellate r.

retinoschisis

retinosis

retinotoxic

retisolution

retispersion

retrocalcaneobursitis

retrocession

retrochiasmatic

retrocollic

retrocollis

retrocursive

retrodeviation

retrodisplacement

retrograde

retrogression

retroinfection

retrolisthesis

retromorphosis

retroperitonitis

retropharyngitis

retroplasia

retroposed

retroposition

retropulsion

retrospondylolisthesis

retrostalsis

retroversioflexion

retroversion

retroverted

rhabdomyoblast

rhabdomyoblastic

rhabdomyolysis

rhacoma

rhaebocrania

rhaeboscelia

rhaebosis

rhagades

rhagadiform

rhegma

rhegmatogenous

rheostosis

rheum

rheumatalgia

rheumatic

rheumatid

rheumatism
    articular r.
    Besnier's r.
    desert r.
    Heberden's r.
    muscular r.
    palindromic R.
    Poncet's r.
    subacute r.
    tuberculous r.

rheumatismal

rheumatogenic

rheumatoid

rheumatosis

rheumic

rhexis

rhinalgia

rhinedema

rhinoantritis

rhinodynia

rhinoentomophthoromycosis

rhinokyphosis

rhinolaryngitis

rhinolith

rhinolithiasis

rhinomycosis

rhinonecrosis

rhinopathia
    r. vasomotoria

rhinopathy

rhinopharyngitis

rhinopharyngocele

rhinopharyngolith

rhinophyma

rhinopolypus

rhinorrhagia

rhinorrhea
    cerebrospinal fluid r.

rhinosalpingitis

rhinoscleroma

rhinosinusitis

rhinosporidiosis

rhinostenosis

rhinotracheitis

rhizomeningomyelitis

rhodamine
    r. B

rhonchal

rhonchial

rhonchus
    sibilant r.
    sonorous r.
    whistling r.

Rhus

rhytidosis

ribbon
    synaptic r.

ribosome

rickets
    anticonvulsant r.

rickets (*continued*)
 autosomal dominant
  vitamin D-resistant r.
 familial hypophosphatemic
  r.
 hereditary
  hypophosphatemic r. with
  hypercalciuria
 hypophosphatemic r
 pseudodeficiency ri
 pseudovitamin D-deficiency
  r
 scurvy r
 vitamin D-dependent r, type
  I
 vitamin D-dependent r, type
  II
 vitamin D-refractory r
 vitamin D-resistant r

rictal

rictus

ridge
 rete r
 supplemental r
 synaptic r

rigidity
 cadaveric r
 clasp-knife r
 cogwheel r
 decerebrate r
 hemiplegic r
 lead-pipe r
 paratonic r
 postmortem r

rigor
 acid r.
 calcium r.
 heat r.
 r. mortis
 water r.

rimose

rimula

ring
 Bandl's r.

ring (*continued*)
 Cabot's r.
 circumaortic venous r.
 contact r.
 Döllinger's tendinous r.
 esophageal r.
 Fleischer r.
 Fleischer-Strümpell r.
 germ r.
 glaucomatous r.
 Kayser-Fleischer r.
 Liesegang r.
 neonatal r.
 Schatzki's r.
 Schwalbe's r.
 Schwalbe's anterior border
  r.
 Soemmering's r.
 vascular r.
 Vossius' r.

ringworm
 black-dot r.
 gray-patch r.
 honeycomb r.
 Oriental r.
 Tokelau r.

RLP (remnant-like particle)
 cholesterol assay

rod
 Corti's r.
 enamel r.
 muscle r.
 olfactory r.
 retinal r.

rombergism

rootlet
 r. of spinal nerve

rosacea
 granulomatous r.
 lupoid r.
 papular r.

rosacic acid

rosaniline

rosary
    rachitic r.
    scorbutic r.

rose
    r. bengal

rosein

roseola
    r. infantum
    syphilitic r.

rosette
    ependymal r.

rosin

rot
    Barcoo r.
    liver r.

rouleau

rubeola

rubeosis
    r. iridis
    r. retinae

rubiginose

rubiginous

rubin

rupia

rupial

rupioid

rutidosis

S

Sf

saburra

saburral

sac
  aneurysmal s.
  hernial s

saccharephidrosis

saccharimeter

saccharometer

saccharopinemia

saccharopinuria

sacculus
  s. of Beale

sacralgia

sacralization

sacrarthrogenic

sacrocoxalgia

sacrocoxitis

sacrodynia

sacroiliitis

sacrolisthesis

sacrum
  scimitar s.
  tilted s.

sactosalpinx

Safe Step blood collection
  needle

safranin O

safrosin

salicylemia

salicylsulfonic acid

salpingemphraxis

salpingitic

salpingitis
  chronic interstitial s.
  eustachian s.
  hemorrhagic s.
  hypertrophic s.
  s. isthmica nodosa
  mural s.
  nodular s.
  parenchymatous s.
  s. profluens
  pseudofollicular s.
  purulent s.
  tuberculous s.

salpingocele

salpingolithiasis

salpingo-oophoritis

salpingo-oophorocele

salpingo-oothecitis

salpingo-oothecocele

salpingoperitonitis

salt
  bone s.

saluresis

saluretic

sanguine

sanguineous

sanguinolent

sanguinopurulent

sanguinous

sanies

saniopurulent

sanioserous

sanious

sap
  cell s.
  nuclear s.

sarcoblast

sarcocele

sarcogenic

sarcohydrocele

sarcoid
  Boeck's s.
  Darier-Roussy s.
  Schaumann's s.

sarcoidosis
  cardiac s.
  muscular s.

sarcolemma

sarcolemmic

sarcolemmous

sarcomere

sarcopenia

sarcoplasm

sarcoplasmic

sarcoplast

sarcopoietic

sarcosinemia

sarcosinuria

sarcosis

sarcostosis

sarcostyle

sarcotic

sarcotubules

satellite
  centriolar s.
  chromosomal s.

satellitism
  platelet s.

satellitosis

saturation
  transferrin s.

saucerization

scabetic

scabies

scabietic

SCAD deficiency

scale
  hydrometer s.
  adhesive s.

scaphocephalia

scaphocephalic

scaphocephalism

scaphocephalous

scaphocephaly

scaphohydrocephalus

scaphohydrocephaly

scaphoiditis
  tarsal s.

scapulalgia

scapulodynia

scarlatina
  s. anginosa
  puerperal s.

scarlatinella

scarlet
  Biebrich s.
  s. G
  s. R

scatology

scatoma

scelalgia

scelotyrbe

scharlach R

scheroma

schistocystis

schistocyte

schistocytosis

schistorachis

schistosis

schistosomiasis
    cutaneous s.
    hepatic s.
    pulmonary s.

schizaxon

schizencephalic

schizencephaly

schizocyte

schizocytosis

schizogyria

schizonychia

schizotrichia

schwannitis

schwannoma
    acoustic s.

schwannomin

schwannosis

sciatica

scieropia

scirrhophthalmia

scleradenitis

scleratitis

scleratogenous

sclerectasia

sclerectasis

scleredema
    s. adultorum
    Buschke's s.
    s. neonatorum

sclerema
    s. adiposum
    s. adultorum
    s. neonatorum

sclerencephalia

sclerencephaly

scleriasis

scleritis
    annular s.
    anterior s.
    brawny s.
    s. necroticans
    necrotizing s.
    nodular s.
    posterior s.

scleroadipose

sclerochoroiditis
    s. anterior
    s. posterior

scleroconjunctivitis

sclerodactylia

sclerodactyly

scleroderma
    circumscribed s.
    diffuse s.
    linear s.
    localized s.
    systemic s.
    generalized s.

sclerodermatous

sclerodesmia

sclerogenic

sclerogenous

sclerogummatous

scleroid

scleroiritis

sclerokeratitis

sclerokeratoiritis

sclerokeratosis

scleroma
    s. respiratorium

scleromalacia

scleromyxedema

scleronychia

sclero-oophoritis

sclero-oothecitis

sclerophthalmia

sclerosal

sclérose en plaques

sclerosis
- amyotrophic lateral s.
- anterolateral s.
- arterial s.
- arteriocapillary s.
- arteriolar s.
- bone s.
- combined s.
- concentric s.
- dentinal s.
- diaphyseal s.
- diffuse s.
- disseminated s.
- endocardial s.
- Erb's s.
- familial centrolobar s.
- focal s.
- focal glomerular s.
- glomerular s.
- hippocampal s.
- hyperplastic s.
- insular s.
- lateral s.
- lobar s.
- medial calcific s.
- mesial temporal s.
- miliary s.
- Mönckeberg's s.
- multiple s.
- Pelizaeus-Merzbacher s.
- peritoneal s.
- posterior s.
- posterior spinal s.
- posterolateral s.
- primary lateral s.
- progressive systemic s.

sclerosis (*continued*)
- renal arteriolar s.
- subendocardial s.
- systemic s.
- tuberous s.
- unicellular s.
- valvular s.
- vascular s.
- venous s.
- ventrolateral s.

sclerostenosis

scleroticochoroiditis

sclerotitis

sclerous

scoliokyphosis

scoliorachitic

scoliosis
- Brissaud's s.
- cicatricial s.
- coxitic s.
- empyematic s.
- habit s.
- inflammatory s.
- ischiatic s.
- myopathic s.
- ocular s.
- ophthalmic s.
- osteopathic s.
- paralytic s.
- rachitic s.
- rheumatic s.
- sciatic s.
- static s.

scoliotic

scopometer

scopometry

scorbutic

scorbutigenic

scorbutus

scotodinia

scotoma
    absolute s.
    annular s.
    arcuate s.
    aural s.
    s auris.
    Bjerrum's s.
    cecocentral s.
    central s.
    centrocecal s.
    color s.
    flittering s.
    hemianopic s.
    motile s.
    negative s.
    paracentral s.
    peripapillary s.
    peripheral s.
    positive s.
    relative s.
    ring s.
    scintillating s.
    Seidel's s.

scotomata

scotomatous

scrotitis

scrotocele

scutula

scutular

scutulum

scybala

scybalous

scybalum

scythropasmus

SDS

seam
    osteoid s.

sebolith

seborrhea
    s. adiposa

seborrhea (*continued*)
    s. oleosa
    s. sicca

seborrheal

seborrhiasis

secretion
    paralytic s.

sediment
    urinary s.

self-fermentation

semelincident

semiapochromat

semiapochromatic

semiluxation

seminuria

semiplegia

senescence
    dental s.

senopia

sensitization
    autoerythrocyte s.

Sentinel urine HIV-1 test

Sephadex

sepia

sepsis
    oral s.
    intestinal s
    pneumococcal s.
    puerperal s.

septemia

septicemia
    anthrax s.
    cryptogenic s
    meningococcal s.
    metastasizing s.
    phlebitic s.
    puerperal s.
    sputum s.
    typhoid s.

septicemic

septicopyemia
    cryptogenic s.
    spontaneous s.

septicopyemic

septimetritis

septineuritis
    Nicolau's s.

sequester

sequestra

sequestral

sequestration
    s. bronchopulmonary
    bronchopulmonary s.
    s. cyst
    s. dermoid
    disk s.
    extralobar s.
    intralobar s.
    pulmonary s.

sequoiosis

serangitis

seriflux

seroalbuminuria

serocolitis

serocystic

seroenteritis

serofibrinous

seroma

seroperitoneum

seroplastic

seropneumothorax

seropurulent

seropus

serosamucin

serosanguineous

serositis

serosynovitis

serothorax

serpiginous

serumal

serumuria

sexdigitate

shagreen

shakes
    kwaski s.

sheath
    arachnoid s.
    carotid s.
    caudal s.
    chordal s.
    common s. of testis and
      spermatic cord
    dentinal s.
    dural s.
    enamel prism s.
    enamel rod s.
    external s. of optic nerve
    fibrous s. of optic nerve
    fibrous s. of spermatozoon
    giant cell tumor of tendon s.
    s. of Henle
    Hertwig s.
    internal s. of optic nerve
    s. of Key and Retzius
    lamellar s.
    Mauthner's s.
    medullary s.
    mitochondrial s.
    myelin s.
    nerve s.
    Neumann s.
    neurilemmal s.
    notochordal s.
    s. of optic nerve
    pial s.
    prism s.
    rod s.
    root s.

sheath (*continued*)
    Scarpa's s.
    Schwann s.
    Schweigger-Seidel s.
    spiral s.
    tendon s.

shock
    anaphylactic s
    s. antigen
    s. artifact
    cardiogenic s.
    hematogenic s.
    hemoclastic s.
    hemorrhagic s.
    histamine s.
    hypoglycemic s.
    hypovolemic s.
    insulin s.
    neurogenic s.
    oligemic s.
    osmotic s.
    pleural s.
    thyrotoxin s.
    vasogenic s.

shotty
    s. breast
    s. node

sialadenitis

sialadenopathy
    benign lymphoepithelial s.

sialadenosis

sialidosis

sialism

sialismus

sialitis

sialoadenitis

sialoangiitis

sialoangitis

sialocele

sialodochitis

sialoductitis

sialolith

sialolithiasis

sialometaplasia
    necrotizing s.

sialorrhea

sialoschesis

sialosis

sialostenosis

sialosyrinx

sibilant

sicklemia

sickling

siderinuria

sideroblast
    ringed s.

sideroderma

siderofibrosis

sideropenia

sideropenic

siderosilicosis

siderosis
    Bantu s.
    s.bulbi
    s. conjunctivae

siderotic

sieve
    molecular s.

sievert

sigmoiditis

sigmoidovesical fistula

sign
    Abadie's s.
    Allis' s.
    Amoss' s.

sign (*continued*)
André Thomas s.
anterior tibial s.
Argyll Robertson pupil s.
Arroyo's s.
Auenbrugger's s.
Auspitz s.
Babinski's s.
Baccelli's s.
Baillarger's s.
Ballet's s.
Bamberger's s.
Barré's s.
Barré's pyramidal s.
Bastian-Bruns' s.
Battle's s.
Becker's s.
Beevor's s.
Bekhterev's s.
Bell's s.
Berger's s.
Bezold's s.
Biernacki's s.
Biot's s.
Bird's s.
Bjerrum's s.
Blumberg's s.
Boas' s.
Bonnet's s.
Bordier-Fränkel s.
Boston's s.
Bouillaud's s.
Bragard's s.
Branham's s.
Braunwald s.
Broadbent's s.
Broadbent's inverted s.
Brockenbrough's s.
Brodie's s.
broken straw s.
Brown's s.
Brown-Séquard's s.
Brudzinski's s.
Brunati's s.
Bruns' s.
Bryant's s.
Bryce's s.
cardinal s.

sign (*continued*)
Chaddock's s.
Charcot's s.
Cheyne-Stokes s.
Chvostek's s.
Chvostek-Weiss s.
Claude's hyperkinesis s.
Cleeman's s.
cogwheel s.
Comolli's s.
complementary opposition s.
contralateral s.
Coopernail's s.
Cope's s.
Corrigan's s.
coughing s.
Courvoisier's s.
Cowen's s.
crescent s.
Crichton-Browne's s.
Cullen's s.
Dalrymple's s.
D'Amato's s.
Darier's s.
Dejerine's s.
Delbet's s.
Demarquay's s.
Demianoff's s.
de Musset's s.
Dennie's s.
Desault's s.
dimple s.
Dixon Mann's s.
Dorendorf's s.
Drummond's s.
DTP s.
Dubois' s.
Duchenne's s.
Duckworth's s.
Dupuytren's s.
echo s.
Elliot's s.
Enroth's s.
Erben's s.
Escherich's s.
Ewing s.
external malleolar s.

sign (*continued*)
- facial s.
- Fajersztajn's crossed sciatic s.
- forearm s.
- formication s.
- Fränkel's s.
- Friedreich's s.
- Froment's paper s.
- Galeazzi s.
- Gilbert's s.
- Goldstein's s.
- Goldthwait's s.
- Gordon's s.
- Gorlin's s.
- Gottron's s.
- Gowers' s.
- Graefe's s.
- Grancher's s.
- Grasset's s.
- Grasset-Bychowski s.
- Grasset-Gaussel-Hoover s.
- Grey Turner's s.
- Griesinger's s.
- Griffith's s.
- Guilland's s.
- Gunn's s.
- Hahn's s.
- Hall's s.
- Hamman's s.
- harlequin s.
- Hawkins s.
- Heberden's s.
- Heilbronner's s.
- Heim-Kreysig s.
- Helbing's s.
- Hennebert's s.
- Hennings' s.
- Higoumenakia s.
- Hill's s.
- Hitzelberger's s.
- Hochsinger's s.
- Hoehne's s.
- Hoffmann's s.
- Holmes' s.
- Hoover's s.
- Hope's s.
- Horn's s.

sign (*continued*)
- Horsley's s.
- Howship-Romberg s.
- Huntington's s.
- Hutchinson's s.
- hyperkinesis s.
- interossei s.
- Jendrassik's s.
- jugular s.
- Keen's s.
- Kehr's s.
- Kernig's s.
- Kerr's s.
- Kleist's s.
- Klippel-Weil s.
- Knies' s.
- Kocher's s.
- Kreysig's s.
- Krisovski's (Krisowski's) s.
- Krisowski's s.
- Kussmaul's s.
- Küstner's s.
- Lafora's s.
- Langoria's s.
- Lasègue's s.
- Laugier's s.
- Leichtenstern's s.
- Lennhoff's s.
- Léri's s.
- Lhermitte's s.
- Linder's s.
- Livierato's s.
- Lucas' s.
- Ludloff's s.
- Lust's s.
- McBurney's s.
- Macewen's s.
- Magendie's s.
- Magendie-Hertwig s.
- Maisonneuve's s.
- Mann's s.
- Marcus Gunn's pupillary s.
- Marie's s.
- Marie-Foix s.
- Marinesco's s.
- Mean's s.
- Mendel-Bekhterev s.
- Minor's s.

sign (*continued*)
- Mirchamp's s.
- Möbius' s.
- Moebius' s.
- Mosler's s.
- Munson's s.
- Musset's s.
- Myerson's s.
- neck s.
- Negro's s.
- Neri's s.
- Nicoladoni's s.
- Nikolsky's s.
- Oppenheim's s.
- orbicularis s.
- Ortolani's s.
- Osler's s.
- Parkinson's s.
- Parrot's s.
- Pende's s.
- peroneal s.
- Pitres' s.
- Plummer's s.
- Pool-Schlesinger s.
- Prévost's s.
- pronation s.
- pseudo-Graefe's s.
- psoas s.
- pyramid s.
- pyramidal s.
- Quant's s.
- Queckenstedt's s.
- Quincke's s.
- radialis s.
- Ramond's s.
- Raynaud's s.
- Remak's s.
- reservoir s.
- Revilliod's s.
- Riesman's s.
- Romana's s.
- Romberg's s.
- Rosenbach's s.
- Rossolimo's s.
- Rust's s.
- Saenger's s.
- Schick's s.
- scimitar s.

sign (*continued*)
- Schlesinger's s.
- Schultze's s.
- Schultze-Chvostek s.
- Schwartze's s.
- Séguin's s.
- Seidel's s.
- setting-sun s.
- Siegert's s.
- Silex' s.
- Simon's s.
- Sisto's s.
- Skoda's s.
- Snellen's s.
- Souques' s.
- spinal s.
- stairs s.
- Stellwag's s.
- Sternberg's s.
- Stewart-Holmes s.
- Strauss' s.
- Strümpell's s.
- Suker's s.
- swinging flashlight s.
- Tay's s.
- Thomas' s.
- Thornton's s.
- Throckmorton's s.
- tibialis s.
- Tinel's s.
- toe s.
- Trousseau's s.
- Turner's s.
- Turyn's s.
- Unschuld's s.
- Vanzetti's s.
- vein s.
- Vierra's s.
- vital s.
- von Graefe's s.
- Wartenberg's s.
- Weber's s.
- Wegner's s.
- Weill's s.
- Westphal's s.
- Wilder's s.

silicatosis

silicoanthracosis

silicoproteinosis

silicosiderosis

silicosis
　　infective s.

silicotic

silicotuberculosis

siliquose

silver
　　methenamine s.

simultagnosia

simultanagnosia

singultation

singultous

singultus

sinistrocardia

sinistrotorsion

sinobronchitis

sinospiral

sinus (pl. sinuses)
　　Aschoff-Rokitansky s.
　　coccygeal s.
　　dermal s.
　　s. histiocytosis
　　s. phlebitis
　　pilonidal s.
　　rhomboidal s.
　　Rokitansky-Aschoff s.
　　sacrococcygeal s.
　　traumatic s.
　　s. venous remnant

sinusal

sinusoid

Sipple syndrome

sirenomelia

Sirius red

sissorexia

sitosterolemia

site
　　antibody combinging s.
　　immunologically privileged
　　　s.
　　receptor s.

skein cell

skeinoid fiber

skelasthenia

skeletal muscle antibody

skeinitis, skenitis

skew

skewed distribution

skin
　　alligator skin
　　s. biiospy
　　collodion skin
　　deciduous skin
　　elastic skin
　　farmers' skin
　　fish skin
　　s. fungus culture
　　glabrous s.
　　India rubber skin
　　s. Mycobacteria culture
　　parchment s.
　　piebald s.
　　porcupine s.
　　sailors' s.
　　shagreen s.

skin puncture test

skin-sensitizing antibody

skull
　　cloverleaf s.
　　hot cross bun s.
　　natiform s.
　　steeple s.
　　tower s.

SKY (spectral karyotyping)
　　technology

sludging
    s. of blood

slyke

SMA
    sequential multichannel
      autoanalyzer
    SMA antibody

SMA 6/60

SMA 12/60

SMAC

SMAF
    specific macrophage
      arming factor

smear
    AFB s.
    Bethesda Pap s.
    Breed s.
    buccal s.
    cervical s.
    colonic s.
    cytologic s.
    Diff-Quik s.
    endocervical s.
    FGT (female genital tract)
      cytologic s.
    Papanicolaou s.
    peripheral blood s.
    Tzanck s.

smegma

smegmalith

smudge cell

SNB
    scalene node biopsy

socioacusis

sodium
    fractional excretion of s.
    s. alizarinsulfonate
    s. dodecyl sulfate
    s. metabisulfate
    s. nitroferricyanide
    s. sulfite
    s. nitroprusside

softening
    colliquative s.
    hemorrhagic s.
    mucoid s.
    pyriform s.

solanoid

solenonychia

solferino

solution
    Alsever's s.
    ammoniacil silver s.
    anisotonic solution
    aqueous s.
    azeotropic s.
    Balamuth buffer s.
    balanced salt s.
    Benedict's solution
    Bouin's solution
    buffered saline s.
    Burow s.
    Cajal formol ammonium
      bromide s.
    carmine solution
    Carnoy's solution
    cochineal solution
    Cytyc CytoLyt s.
    Cytyc Preservcyt
      preservative s.
    Dakin s.
    DAKO target retrieval s.
    Delafield fixative s.
    Diaphane s.
    Dragendorff s.
    Earle s.
    Fehling's solution
    fixative solution
    Flemming's solution
    Fonio s.
    formaldehyde s.
    formalin s.
    formol-Zenker solution
    Fowler s.
    FU-48 Zenker fixatiave s.
    Gallego differentiating s.
    Gilson's solution
    Gowers s.

solution (*continued*)
    Hank's s.
    Hartmann's s.
    Histoclear slide processing
      s.
    s. hybridization s.
    hydrogen peroxide s.
    isotonic sodium
      chloride s.
    Lang's solution
    Locke-Ringer s.
    Lugol's solution
    Lumi-Phos s.
    Nessler's s.
    nonideal s.
    Orth s.
    Perenyi's s.
    physiological saline s. (PSS)
    propidium iodide
    ribonuclease s.
    Ringer lactate s.
    Ruge s.
    saline s.
    Seyderhelm's s.
    Shallibaum s.
    susa s.
    TAC's s.
    test s.
    Toison s.
    Tyrode's s.
    volumetric s.
    Weigert iodine s.
    Zamboni s.
    Zenker's solution
    Ziehl's solution

soma

somaplasm

somasthenia

somatalgia

somatasthenia

somatochrome

somatoderm

somatomegaly

somatoplasm

somatotopagnosia

somatotrope

somatotroph

sopor

soporous

sordes
    sordes gastricae

sound
    adventitious s.
    discontinuous s.

space
    apical s.
    Blessig's s.
    Bowman's s.
    capsomer capsular s.
    chyle s.
    circumlental s.
    corneal s.
    Czermak's s.
    s. in dentin
    Disse s.
    episcleral s.
    female genital s.
    fetal s.
    Fontana's s.
    gastrointestinal s.
    globular s. of Czermak
    haversian s.
    Held's s.
    His's s.
    iliocostal s.
    intercristal s.
    interfascial s.
    intervaginal s.
    intervillous s.
    intramembranous s.
    s. of iridocorneal angle
    medullary s.
    meningeal s.
    mitochondrial membrane s.
    periaxial s.
    perichoroidal s.
    perineuronal s.

space (*continued*)
    perinuclear s.
    perisinusoidal s.
    Poiseuille s.
    retrobulbar s.
    Schwalbe's s.
    Tenon's s.
    zonular s.
    urinary tract s.
    Virchow-Robin s.

spacer

spasm
    s. of accommodation
    athetoid s.
    Bell's s.
    bronchial s.
    cadaveric s.
    carpopedal s.
    clonic s.
    dancing s.
    diffuse esophageal s.
    esophageal s.
    facial s.
    fixed s.
    glottic s.
    habit s.
    hemifacial s.
    histrionic s.
    infantile s.
    infantile massive s.
    inspiratory s.
    intention s.
    jackknife s.
    lock s.
    malleatory s.
    massive s.
    mixed s.
    mobile s.
    myopathic s
    nictitating s
    nodding s
    phonatory s
    progressive torsion s
    respiratory s
    retrocollic s
    Romberg's s
    rotatory s

spasm (*continued*)
    salaam s
    saltatory s
    tonoclonic s
    torsion s
    toxic s
    winking s
    writers' s

spasmogen

spasmogenic

spasmolygmus

spasmophile

spasmophilic

spasmus
    s. nutans

spasticity
    clasp-knife s.

spatium
    s. interfasciale [Tenoni]
    s. intervaginale

specimen
    anaerobic urine s.
    bacteriologic s.
    blood specimen
    clinical bacteriologic s.
    cytologic s.

speckled leukoplakia

spectral resolution

spectrometer
    gamma s.
    mass s.

spectrometry
    gas chromotography-mass
        s.
    isotope dilution-mass s.

spectrophotometer
    atomic absorption s.

spectrophotometry
    atomic absorption s.
    diode array s.

spectrophotometry (*continued*)
    double beam s.
    flame emission
    infrared s.
    ultraviolet/visible s.

spectrum
    fortification spectrum

sperm
    s. crystal
    s. duct ectasia
    muzzled sperm
    s. count

spermatid stalk

spermatoblast

spermatocele

spermatocyst

spermatocytal

spermatocyte

spermatogonium (pl.
    spermatogonia)

spermatospore

spermatozoon (pl.
    spermatozoa)

spermatozoid

spermiocyte

spermiogonium

spermoblast

spermolith

spermoneuralgia

spermophlebectasia

spermoplasm

spermosphere

spermospore

sphacelate

sphacelation

sphacelism

sphacelous

sphacelus

sphenoiditis

sphere
    attraction s.
    embryonic s.
    Morgagni's s.
    prelytic s.
    segmentation s.
    vitreline s.

spherocyte

spherocytic
    s. anemia
    s. jaundice

spherocytosis
    hereditary s.

spherophakia

spheroplast

spherospermia

spherule
    s. of Fulci
    rod s.

spherulin

sphincteral achalasia

sphincteralgia

sphincterismus

sphincteritis

sphincterotomy

sphinganine

sphingogalactoside

sphingoin

sphingolipidosis
    cerebral
        sphingolipidosis

sphingolipodystrophy

sphingomyelinosis

spider
    s. angioma
    arterial s.
    s. cell rhabdomyoblast
    s. nevus
    s. talengiectasia
    vascular s.

spina (pl. spinae)
    spina bifida

spin-cool filter method

spindle
    achromatic s.
    Axenfeld-Krukenberg s.
    barbiturate s.
    bipolar s.
    Bütschli's nuclear s.
    central s.
    cleavage s.
    enamel s.
    Krukenberg's s.
    mitotic s.
    muscle s.
    neuromuscular s.
    neurotendinous s.
    nuclear s.
    s. cell carcinoma
    tendon s.
    urine s.

spindling

spindly squamoid cell

spine
    anterior inferior iliac s.
    anterior superior iliac s.
    bamboo s.
    cleft s.
    dendritic s.
    ischial s.
    posterior inferior iliac s.
    posterior superior iliac s.
    typhoid spine

spinnbarkeit

spinner method

spinocellular

spintherism

spintheropia

spiral
    Curschmann's s.
    Herxheimer's s.
    s. lamina
    s. plica

spiramycin

spireme

spirilla

Spirillaceae

spirillosis

spirochetosis
    bronchopulmonary s.

splanchnectopia

splanchnocele

splanchnoderm

splanchnodiastasis

splanchnolith

splanchnomegalia

splanchnomegaly

splanchnomicria

splanchnopathy

splanchnopleural

splanchnopleure

splanchnosclerosis

splayfoot

spleen
    Banti's s.
    flecked s. of Feitis
    floating spleen
    Gandy-Gamna spleen
    lardaceous spleen
    porphyry spleen
    sago spleen
    scrotal s.
    waxy s.

splenalgia

splenatrophy

splenauxe

splenceratosis

splenectasis

splenectopia

splenectopy

splenelcosis

splenemia

splenemphraxis

splenic
    s. corpuscle
    s. leukemia
    s. lymphatic follicle
    s. mycosin
    s. trabeculae

splenicterus

spleniform

splenitis
    spodogenous s.

splenoblast

splenocele

splenoceratosis

splenocyte

splenodynia

splenogram

splenohepatomegalia

splenohepatomegaly

splenoid

splenokeratosis

splenolysis

splenomalacia

splenomegalia

splenomegaly
    congestive s.
    Egyptian s.
    Gaucher's s.
    hemolytic s.
    infectious s.
    myelophthisic s.
    siderotic s.
    spodogenous s.
    thrombophlebitic s.

splenomyelomalacia

splenonephroptosis

splenoparectasis

splenopathy

splenoptosia

splenoptosis

splenorrhagia

splenosis

splenotoxin

spodogenous

spondylalgia

spondylarthritis
    s. ankylopoietica

spondylarthrocace

spondylarthropathy

spondylexarthrosis

spondylitic

spondylitis
    s. ankylopoietica
    ankylosing s.
    Bekhterev's (Bechterew's) s.
    s. deformans
    hypertrophic s.
    s. infectiosa
    Kümmell's s.
    Marie-Strümpell s.
    muscular s.
    post-traumatic s.
    rheumatoid s.

spondylitis (*continued*)
    rhizomelic s.
    traumatic s.
    tuberculous s.
    s. typhosa

spondylizema

spondyloarthropathy
    seronegative s.

spondylocace

spondylodynia

spondylolisthesis
    congenital s.
    degenerative s.
    dysplastic s.
    isthmic s.
    pathological s.
    traumatic s.

spondylolisthetic

spondylolysis

spondylomalacia
    s. traumatica

spondylopathy
    traumatic s.

spondyloptosis

spondylopyosis

spondyloschisis

spondylosis
    cervical s.
    s. chronica ankylopoietica
    s. deformans
    hyperostotic s.
    lumbar s.
    rhizomelic s.
    s. uncovertebralis

spondylotic

spongeitis

spongiform

spongiitis

spongioblast

spongiocyte

spongioid

spongioplasm

spongiosis

spongiositis

spongiotic

spot
    ash-leaf s
    Bitot's s
    blood s.
    blue s
    Brushfield's s
    café au lait s
    Carleton's s
    Cayenne pepper s
    cherry-red s
    Christopher's s
    cotton-wool s
    De Morgan's s
    epigastric s
    flame s
    Fordyce's s
    germinal s
    Koplik s
    lance-ovate s
    liver s
    Maurer's s
    milk s
    mongolian s
    Roth's s
    sacral s
    shin s
    soldier's s
    Stephen's s
    Tardieu's s
    Tay's s
    tendinous s
    Trousseau's s
    s. test for infectious
      mononucleosis

sprue
    celiac s
    collagenous s
    hypogammaglobulinemic s

sprue (*continued*)
    nontropical s
    refractory s
    tropical s

spur cell

sputum
    s. aeroginosum
    albuminoid s.
    s. cruentum
    s. cytology
    s. fungus culture
    globular s.
    green s.
    icteric s.
    s. mycobacteria culture
    nummular s.
    prune juice s.
    rusty s.

squama
    s. alveolaris

squamatization

stactometer

stage
    algid s.
    Arneth s.
    cold s.
    defervescent s.
    eruptive s.
    s. of fervescence
    hot s.
    incubative s.
    latent s.
    knäuel s.
    mechanical s.
    prodromal s.
    pyretogenic s.
    pyrogenetic s.
    Ranke's s.
    Tanner s.
    resting s.
    transitional pulp s.
    vegetative s.

stain
    Abbott s. for spores

stain (*continued*)
    aceto-orcein s.
    acid s.
    Achúcarro's s.
    acid-fast s.
    acid fuchsin s.
    Albert's diphtheria s.
    alum-carmine s.
    Alzheimer s.
    ammonium silver
        carbonate s.
    amyloid s.
    Anthony capsule s.
    argentaffin s.
    ATPase s.
    auramine O fluoroscent s.
    auramine-rhodamine s.
    azan s.
    azure-eosin s.
    B72.3 s.
    basic s.
    basic fuchsin-methylene
        blue s.
    Belke-Kleihauer s.
    Benda's s.
    Bensley's neutral gentian
        orange G s.
    Berg s.
    Best's carmine s.
    Bethe's s.
    Betke s.
    Bielschowsky's s.
    Biondi-Heidenhain s.
    Bodian s.
    Bowie s.
    Brown-Hopp tissue gram s.
    butyrate esterase s.
    Cajal s.
    Cajal's double s.
    carbolfuchsin s.
    carbol-gentian violet s.
    Castaneda's s.
    C-banding s.
    CEA M s.
    CEA-P s.
    centromere banding s.
    chromotrypsin s.
    Ciaccio's s.

stain (*continued*)
  colloidal iron s.
  contrast s.
  counter s.
  Cox's modification of
    Golgi's corrosive
    sublimate s.
  cresyl blue brilliant s.
  Da Fano s.
  Dane and Herman keratin s.
  DAPI s.
  Davenport's s.
  Delafield's hematoxylin
  Del Rio Hortega s.
  Dieterle's s.
  differential s.
  direct fluorescent antibody s.
  DOPA s.
  D-PAS s.
  DU-PAN-2 s.
  Ehrlich's acid hematoxylin
  Ehrlich's neutral s.
  Ehrlich's triacid s.
  elastic fiber s.
  electron s.
  eosin s.
  F s.
  ferric amonium sulfate s.
  Feulgen s.
  Field rapid s.
  Fite's s.
  Fontana's s.
  Fontana-Masson s.
  G- banding s.
  gentian orange s.
  gentian violet s.
  Giemsa s.
  Gimenez s.
  glycogen s.
  glycolipid s.
  Golgi's mixed s.
  Gomori's s.
  Gomori-Takamatsu s.
  Gomori-Wheatley s.
  Gomori's methenamine
    silver s.
  Goodpasture's s.
  Gordon and Sweet s.

stain (*continued*)
  Grimelius' argyrophil s.
  Grocott-Gomori
    methenamine-silver
    nitrate s.
  Hale's colloidal iron s.
  Hansel s.
  Harris' hematoxylin.
  Harris' s.
  heavy-metal s.
  Heidenhain's iron
    hematoxylin s.
  hemalum s.
  hematoxylin-eosin s.
  hematoxylin-eosin-azure II.
  Hiss capsule s.
  histochemical s.
  Hortega s.
  Hucker-Conn s.
  India ink capsule s.
  iron hematoxylin s.
  Jenner's s.
  Jenner-Giemsa s.
  Kinyoun carbolfuchsin s.
  Kluver-Barrera Luxol fast
    blue s.
  Kossa s.
  LAP s.
  lead hydroxide s.
  Leifson flagella s.
  Leishman's s.
  Lendrum inclusion body s.
  Levaditi's s.
  Lillie azure-eosin s.
  lipoid s.
  Lison-Dunn s.
  lithium-carmine s.
  Löffler's alkaline methylene
    blue s.
  Lorrain Smith s.
  Lugol's iodine s.
  Luxol fast blue s.
  Macchiavello's s.
  Mallory's acid fuchsin,
    orange G, and aniline blue
    s.
  Mallory's phloxine-
    methylene blue s.

stain (*continued*)

Mallory's phosphotungstic acid-hematoxylin s.

Mallory's triple s.

Mancini iodine s.

Marchi's s.

Masson s.

Maximow's.

May's spore s.

May-Grünwald s.

Mayer's hemalum s.

Mayer's mucihematein s.

M-DES s.

meconium s.

metachromatic s.

methenamine silver s.

methyl green-pyronin s.

methyl violet s.

Michaelis' s.

Milligan's trichrome s.

Movat pentrachrome s.

Musto s.

Nakanishi s.

Nauta s.

neutral s.

Neisser s.

Nile blue fat s.

Nissl's s.

Noble s.

NSE s.

nuclear s.

oligodendroglia s.

orcein s.

Orth s.

oxalic acid s.

Pal's modification of Weigert's myelin sheath s.

Papanicolaou's s.

PAPI s.

Pappenheim's s.

paracarmine s.

PAS s.

Perdrau's s.

periodic acid-Schiff (PAS) s.

Perls' s.

phosphotungstic acid-hematoxylin s.

picric s.

stain (*continued*)

plasmatic s.

plasmic s.

polychrome methylene blue.

port-wine s.

potassium metabisulfate s.

Protargol s.

protoplasmic s.

Prussian blue s.

PTA s.

PTAH s.

pyrol blue s.

Q-banding s.

quinacrine chromosome banding s.

quinacrine fluorescent s.

Rambourg chromic acid-chromic methamine-silver s.

Ranson's pyridine silver s.

resorcin-fuchsin s.

reticulin s.

reverse Giemsa s.

Romanovsky's (Romanowsky's) blood s.

Schiff s.

selective s.

Seller's s.

Snook reticulum s.

Sternheimer-Malbin s.

Sudan black B fat s.

T s.

Taenzer-Unna s.

Takayama s.

tetrachrome s.

thiozine s.

Tizzoni s.

trichrome s.

Truant auramine-rhodamine s.

trypsin G-banding s.

Turnbull blue s.

Unna-Pappenheim s.

uranyl acetate s.

urate crystals s.

stain (*continued*)
 van Gieson's solution of trinitrophenol and acid fuchsin s.
 Verhoeff's s.
 Verhoeff-van Gieson s.
 von Kossa's s.
 Warthin-Starry silver s.
 Wayson s.
 Weigert's fibrin s.
 Weigert's iron hematoxylin s.
 Weigert's myelin sheath method s.
 Weigert's neuroglia fiber s.
 Weigert's resorcin-fuchsin s.
 Weil's myelin s.
 Williams s.
 Wirtz-Conklin spore s.
 Wright's s.
 Ziehl-Neelsen s acid-fast s.
 Ziehl-Neelsen carbolfuchsin s.

stained urinary sediment

staining
 acid phosphatase s.
 amyloid s.
 astroycte s.
 bipolar s.
 chondroitin sulfate s.
 differential s.
 double s.
 fibrin s.
 fluorescent s.
 fungi s.
 glycogen s.
 glycolipid s.
 glycoprotein s.
 H and E s.
 hemosiderin s.
 immunohistochemical s.
 intravital s.
 keratin s.
 mast cell s.
 multiple s.
 negative s.

staining (*continued*)
 phospholipid s.
 polar s.
 postvital s.
 preagonal s.
 relief s.
 reticulum s.
 simple s.
 substantive s.
 supravital s.
 telomeric s.
 terminal s.
 triple s.
 vital s.

stannosis

stannous
 s. chloride

staphyledema

staphylitis

Staphylococcal protein A immunoabsorption (Prosorba column) pheresis

staphyloderma

staphyloedema

staphyloma

staphylomatous

staphyloncus

staphyloptosia

staphyloptosis

staphyloschisis

stasimorphia

stasimorphy

stasis
 bile s.
 s. dermatitis
 intestinal s.
 urinary s.
 venous s.

state
    absorptive s.
    complement deficiency s.
    de-efferented s
    dreamy s
    hypercoagulable s
    immunity deficiency s.
    oxidation s.
    transition s.

stathmokinesis

statolith

Stat Simple (H. pylori test)

status
    absence s.
    s. asthmaticus
    s. calcifames
    s. choreicus
    complex partial s.
    s. convulsivus
    s. cribalis
    s. cribrosus
    s. criticus
    s. dysmyelinatus
    s. dysmyelinisatus
    s. epilepticus
    s. hemicranicus
    s. lacunaris
    s. lacunosus
    s. lymphaticus
    s. marmoratus
    s. migrainosus
    petit mal s.
    psychomotor s.
    simple partial s.
    s. thymicolymphaticus
    s. thymicus
    s. verrucosus
    s. vertiginosus

stauroplegia

staxis

stearrhea

steatitis

steatocele

steatocystoma
    s. multiplex

steatohepatitis
    nonalcoholic s.

steatoma

steatomatosis

steatonecrosis

steatopygia

steatopygous

steatorrhea
    idiopathic s.

steatosis
    s cardiaca

stegnosis

stegnotic

stenochoria

stenosal

stenosis (pl. stenoses)
    aortic s.
    buttonhole s.
    caroticovertebral s.
    congenital pyloric s.
    discrete subaortic s.
    hypertrophic pyloric s.
    infundibular s.
    mitral s.
    nodular calcific aortic s.
    postdiphtheritic s.
    pulmonary s.
    pyloric s.
    renal artery s.
    spinal s.
    subaortic s.
    subglottic s.
    subvalvar s.
    tricuspid s.
    valvular s.

stenothorax

stenotic

step
    Rönne's nasal s.

stercolith

stercorolith

stercoroma

stereoagnosis

stereoanesthesia

stereocilium

stereometer

stereometry

stereophotomicrograph

stereoplasm

sternalgia

Sterneedle tuberculin test

sternodynia

sternutation

sternzellen

stertor

stethalgia

stethomyitis

stethomyositis

stethoparalysis

stethospasm

stigma
    Giuffrida-Ruggieri s.

stimulus
    heterotopic s.

stippling
    malarial s.
    Maurer's s.
    Schüffner's s.

stomacace

stomach
    aberrant umbilical s.
    bilocular s.
    hourglass s.
    thoracic s.

stomach (*continued*)
    trifid s.
    upside-down s.
    waterfall s.
    watermelon s.

stomachalgia

stomachodynia

stomalgia

stomatalgia

stomatitides

stomatitis
    allergic s.
    angular s.
    aphthous s.
    arsenic s.
    bismuth s.
    bovine popular s.
    catarrhal s.
    contact s.
    denture s.
    erythematopultaceous s.
    fusospirochetal s.
    gangrenous s.
    gonococcal s.
    gonorrheal s.
    herpetic s.
    infectious s.
    lead s.
    membranous s.
    mercurial s.
    mercury s.
    mycotic s.
    primary hepatic s.
    nonspecific s.
    s. scarlatina
    syphilitic s.
    tropical s.
    ulcerative s.
    uremic s.
    vesicular s.
    Vincent's s.

stomatocace

stomatocyte

stomatocytosis

stomatodynia

stomatodysodia

stomatoglossitis

stomatomalacia

stomatomenia

stomatomycosis

stomatopathy

stomatorrhagia
    s. gingivarum

stomatoschisis

stool
    bilious s.
    fatty s.
    lienteric s.
    melanotic s.
    mucous s.
    ribbon s.
    rice-water s.
    sago-grain s.
    tarry s.

storiform

strabismal

strabismic

strabismus

strain
    cell strain

strand
    lateral enamel s.

strangalesthesia

stranguria

strangury

stratum

streak
    angioid s.
    culture s.
    fatty s

streak (*continued*)
    germinal s
    gonadal s.
    Knapp's s
    meningitic s
    primitive s.

streaming
    cytoplasmic s.
    protoplasmic s.

streblomicrodactyly

strephenopodia

strephexopodia

strephopodia

strephosymbolia

streptomicrodactyly

stress
    oxidative s.

stria (pl. striae)
    s. albicantes
    s. of Amici
    s. atrophicae
    s. ciliares
    s. distensae
    s. gravidarum
    Kaes' s.
    Kaes-Bekhterev s.
    Knapp's s.
    Langhans' s.
    meningitic s.
    Nitabuch's s.
    Retzius' parallel s.
    Rohr's s.
    Wickham's s.

stricture
    annular s.
    bridle s.
    false s.
    functional s.
    Hunner's s.
    organic s.
    spasmodic s.
    spastic s.

stricturization

stripe
    s. of Retzius
    Vicq d'Azyr's s.

stroma
    hyalinized s.
    mucinous s.
    Rollet s.
    s. of cornea

stromatolysis

stromatosis

strongyloidiasis
    intestinal s.
    pulmonary s.

strophulus

structure
    analagous s.
    dipolar s.
    fine s.
    homologous s.
    quaternary s.
    tubuloreticular s.

struma (pl. strumae)
    s. aberrata
    s. colloides
    s. follicularis
    Hashimoto's s.
    ligneous s.
    s. lymphomatosa
    s. maligna
    s. nodosa
    Riedel's s.

strumitis

struvite

stye
    meibomian s.
    zeisian s.

styloiditis

stylosteophyte

stymatosis

subalimentation

subcalcareous

subcrepitant

subcrepitation

subendocardium

subepicardium

suberosis

subglossitis

subgrondation

subicteric

subintimal

subintrance

subintrant

subinvolution

sublinguitis

subluxate

subluxation

sublymphemia

submaxillaritis

submicroscopic

subnucleus

subpapillary

subpapular

subperichondrial

subplasmalemmal

subscaphocephaly

subsclerotic

subsibilant

substance
    alpha s.
    antidiuretic s.
    β-substance
    beta substance
    blood group specific s.

substance (*continued*)
    chromidial s.
    chromophil s.
    colloid s.
    hemolytic s.
    interfibrillar s. of Flemming
    interfilar s.
    interprismatic s.
    interspongioplastic s.
    Nissl's s.
    onychogenic s.
    prelipid s.
    renal pressor s.
    Rollett's secondary s.
    sarcous s.
    tigroid s.
    tumor polysaccharide s.

subtetanic

succinate
    s. semialdehyde

succinic semialdehyde
  dehydrogenase deficiency

succinylacetoacetate

succinylacetone

succorrhea

sucrase-isomaltase deficiency

sucrosemia

sucrosuria

sudamen

sudaminal

Sudan
    S IV
    S black B fat stain
    S brown
    S red III
    S yellow

sudanophil

sudanophilia

sudanophilic

sudanophilous

suffocation

suffusion

suggillation

sulcus
    Harrison's s.

sulfanilate

sulfanilic acid

sulfatase
    multiple s. deficiency

sulfate
    conjugated s.
    ethereal s.
    mineral s.
    preformed s.

sulfatemia

sulfhemoglobin

sulfhemoglobinemia

sulfmethemoglobin

sulfoconjugation

sulfosalicylate

sulfosalicylic acid

superacid

superacidity

superantigen

superdistention

superinduce

superinfection

superlethal

supermotility

supernumerary
    s. kidney
    s.organ

SuperQuant HCV assay

supersaturated

suppression
    bone marrow s.

suppuration

suppurative

suprarenalism

suprarenalopathy

suprarenopathy

supravital

Supreme II blood glucose meter

suspenopsia

suspensiometer

SUTI (sperm-ubiquitin tag
   immunoassay)

sutika

svedberg

sweat
   fetid s.
   phosphorescent s.

sweating
   gustatory s.

swelling
   blennorrhagic swelling
   Soemmering's crystalline
    swelling

sychnuria

sycosiform

sycosis
   s. barbae
   lupoid s.
   s. vulgaris

symbion

symblepharon

sympatheticotonia

sympathetoblast

sympathicoblast

sympathicopathy

sympathicotonia

sympathicotonic

sympathoblast

sympathogone

sympathogonia

sympathogonium

sympectothiene

sympectothion

sympexion

symphalangia

symphalangism

symphysic

symphysiolysis

synalgia

synaphymenitis

synapsis

synaptene

synaptic

synaptosome

synarthrophysis

synathresis

synathroisis

syncanthus

syncaryon

synchesis

synchiria

synchrony

synchysis

syncopal

syncretio

syncytioma

syncytiotrophoblast

syncytiotrophoblastic

syndactylia

syndactylism

syndactylous

syndactylus

syndactyly

syndesis

syndesmectopia

syndesmitis

syndesmophyte

syndrome
   Aarskog syndrome
   Aarskog-Scott syndrome
   Aase s.
   Aberchrombie s.
   abdominal muscle
    deficiency syndrome
   achalasia-addisonian
    syndrome
   Achard syndrome
   Achard-Thiers syndrome
   Achenbach s.
   acquired
    immunodeficiency s.
    (AIDS)
   acrofacial s.
   acute chest syndrome
   acute nephritic syndrome
   acute respiratory distress
    syndrome
   acute retinal necrosis
    syndrome
   Adair-Dighton syndrome
   Adams-Stokes syndrome
   addisonian syndrome
   addisonian-achalasia
    syndrome
   Adie syndrome
   adiposogenital syndrome
   adremal feminizing s.
   adrenal gland virilizing s.
   adrenogenital syndrome
   adult respiratory distress
    syndrome (ARDS)

syndrome (*continued*)
   AEC syndrome
   Ahumada-Del Castillo
    syndrome
   Aicardi syndrome
   akinetic-rigid
    syndrome
   Alagille syndrome
   Alajouanine syndrome
   Albright syndrome
   Albright-McCune-Sternberg
    syndrome
   Aldrich s.
   Alezzandrini s.
   Allemann's s.
   Allen-Masters s.
   Allgrove s.
   Alport syndrome
   Alström syndrome
   amenorrhea-galactorrhea s.
   amniotic infection
    syndrome of Blane
   Amsterdam s.
   amyostatic syndrome
   Andersen's syndrome
   Andrade's syndrome
   androgen insensitivity
    syndrome
   Angelman's syndrome
   Angelucci syndrome
   angio-osteohypertrophy s.
   angular gyrus syndrome
   ankyloblepharon-
    ectodermal dysplasia-
    clefting s.
   anorexia-cachexia
    syndrome
   anterior abdominal wall
    syndrome
   anterior chamber cleavage
    syndrome
   anterior cord syndrome
   anterior cornual
    syndrome
   anterior interosseous
    syndrome
   anterior spinal artery
    syndrome

syndrome (*continued*)

anterior tibial compartment s.

antibody deficiency s.

anticholinergic syndrome

antiphospholipid-antibody s.

Anton syndrome

Anton-Babinski syndrome

aortic arch syndrome

apallic s.

Apert's syndrome

aplastic anemia s.

Arnold-Chiari syndrome

Arnold's nerve reflex cough syndrome

arthritis-dermatitis s.

arthropathy-camptodactyly syndrome

Ascher syndrome

Asherman syndrome

Asherson syndrome

asplenia syndrome

ataxia telangiectasia syndrome

auriculotemporal syndrome

autoerythrocyte sensitization syndrome

autoimmune polyendocrine-candidiasis syndrome

Avellis' syndrome

Axenfeld's syndrome

Ayerza's syndrome

Baastrup's syndrome

Babinski's syndrome

Babinski-Fröhlich syndrome

Babinski-Nageotte syndrome

Babinski-Vaquez syndrome

bacterial overgrowth syndrome

BADS syndrome

Bäfverstedt s.

Balint's syndrome

Baller-Gerold syndrome

ballooning mitral valve syndrome

syndrome (*continued*)

ballooning posterior leaflet syndrome

Bamberger-Marie s.

Bannayan-Zonana s.

Banti s.

Bardet-Biedl syndrome

bare lymphocyte s.

Barlow's syndrome

Barraquer-Simons' syndrome

Barré-Guillain syndrome

Barrett's syndrome

Bart syndrome

Bartter syndrome

basal cell nevus s.

basilar artery syndrome

Bassen-Kornzweig syndrome

Bateman s.

Batten-Mayou s.

battered-child syndrome

Bazex s.

Beals' syndrome

Bearn-Kunkel syndrome

Bearn-Kunkel-Slater syndrome

Beau s.

Beckwith's syndrome

Beckwith-Wiedemann syndrome

Behçet's syndrome

Benedikt's syndrome

benign hypermobility syndrome

Berardinelli-Seip syndrome

Bernard's syndrome

Bernard-Horner syndrome

Bernard-Sergent syndrome

Bernard-Soulier syndrome

Bernhardt-Roth s.

Bernheim s.

Bertolotti s.

Besnier-Boeck-Schaumann s.

Bianchi s.

Biemond s., II

syndrome (*continued*)
    bile salt deficiency s.
    billowing mitral valve
        syndrome
    billowing posterior leaflet
        syndrome
    Bing-Neel syndrome
    Birt-Hogg-Dubé syndrome
    Björnstad's syndrome
    Blackfan-Diamond
        syndrome
    Blatin s.
    blind loop s.
    Bloch-Sulzberger syndrome
    Bloom syndrome
    blue diaper s.
    blue rubber bleb nevus
        syndrome
    blue toe syndrome
    Blum s.
    body of Luys syndrome
    Boerhaave syndrome
    Bonnet-Dechaume-Blanc s.
    Bonnevie-Ullrich s.
    Böök syndrome
    BOR syndrome
    Börjeson syndrome
    Börjeson-Forssman-
      Lehmann syndrome
    Bouillaud's syndrome
    Bourneville-Pringle
        syndrome
    Bouveret's syndrome
    bowel bypass syndrome
    brachial syndrome
    Brachmann-de Lange
        syndrome
    Bradbury-Eggleston
        syndrome
    bradycardia-tachycardia
        syndrome
    brady-tachy syndrome
    brain death s.
    branchio-oto-renal s
    Brennemann s
    Briquet s.
    Brissaud-Marie s.

syndrome (*continued*)
    Brissaud-Sicard s
    Bristowe s
    brittle bones s
    brittle cornea s
    Brock s
    bronchiolitis obliterans s.
    Brown vertical retraction s
    Brown-Séquard s
    Brown-Vialetto-van Laere
    Brueghel's s
    Brugsch s.
    Brun s
    Brunsting s
    Brushfield-Wyatt s
    Buckley s
    Budd s.
    Budd-Chiari s
    bulbar s
    Bürger-Grütz
    Burnett s
    burning feet s
    Buschke-Ollendorff
        syndrome
    Bywaters syndrome
    Cacchi-Ricci s.
    Caffey syndrome
    Caffey-Silverman syndrome
    camptomelic s.
    Canada-Cronkhite
        syndrome
    capillary leak syndrome
    Capgras s.
    Caplan syndrome
    carcinoid s.
    Carney syndrome
    carotid sinus syndrome
    carpal tunnel syndrome
    Carpenter syndrome
    cat cry s.
    cat's eye syndrome
    cauda equina syndrome
    caudal dysplasia syndrome
    caudal regression
        syndrome
    cavernous sinus syndrome
    Ceelen-Gellerstadt s.

syndrome (*continued*)
 celiac syndrome
 cellular immunity
  deficiency s. (CIDS)
 central alveolar
  hypoventilation s
 central cord s
 central sleep apnea s
 centroposterior s
 cerebellar s
 cerebellopontine angle s
 cerebellomedullary
  malformation s.
 cerebrocostomandibular s
 cerebrohepatorenal s
 cervical s
 cervical disk s
 cervical rib s
 cervicobrachial s
 Cestan s
 Cestan-Chenais s
 Cestan-Raymond s
 chancriform s.
 Charcot's s
 Charcot-Marie s
 Charcot-Weiss-Baker s
 CHARGE s
 Charlin's s
 Chauffard s.
 Chauffard-Still s.
 Chédiak-Higashi s
 Chédiak-Steinbrinck-
  Higashi s.
 Cheney s.
 Chiari's s
 Chiari-Arnold s
 Chiari-Budd s.
 Chiari-Frommel s
 Chiari II s.
 chiasma s
 chiasmatic s
 Chilaiditi s
 CHILD s
 childhood hemolytic
  uremic s.
 Chinese restaraunt s. (CRS)
 Chotzen's s

syndrome (*continued*)
 Christian's s
 Christ-Siemens s.
 Christ-Siemens-Touraine s
 chromosomal breakage s.
 chromosomal malformation
  s.
 chronic brain s.
 chronic fatigue s
 Churg-Strauss s
 chylomicronemia s
 Citelli's s
 Clarke-Hadfield
  syndrome
 Claude's syndrome
 Claude Bernard-Horner
  syndrome
 click syndrome
 click-murmur syndrome
 closed head syndrome
 Clough-Richter s.
 Clouston's syndrome
 cloverleaf skull syndrome
 Cockayne's syndrome
 Coffin-Lowry syndrome
 Coffin-Siris syndrome
 Cogan's syndrome
 cold agglutinin syndrome
 Collet's syndrome
 Collet-Sicard syndrome
 combined
  immunodeficiency s.
 common variable
  immunodefiency s.
 compartment syndrome
 compartmental syndrome
 compression syndrome
 concussion syndrome
 congenital rubella
  syndrome
 Conn syndrome
 Conradi's syndrome
 Conradi-Hünermann
  syndrome
 contiguous gene syndrome
 continuous muscle activity
  syndrome

syndrome (*continued*)

    continuous muscle fiber
      activity syndrome

    Cornelia de Lange
      syndrome

    syndrome of corpus
      striatum

    Costen syndrome

    costoclavicular syndrome

    Cotard s.

    Courvoisier-Terrier s.

    Crandall s.

    craniosynostosis-radial
      aplasia syndrome

    CREST syndrome

    Creutzfeldt-Jakob s.

    cricopharyngeal achalasia s

    cri du chat s

    Crigler-Najjar s

    s of crocodile tears

    Cronkhite-Canada s

    Cross s

    Cross-McKusick-Breen s

    Crouzon s.

    Crow-Fukase s

    CRST s

    crush s

    Cruveilhier-Baumgarten s

    cryptopathic hemolytic s.

    cryptophthalmos s

    cubital tunnel s

    Currarino-Silverman s

    Curschmann-Batten-
      Steinert s

    Curtius' s

    Curtis-Fitz-Hugh s.

    Cushing's s

    Cushing's s, iatrogenic

    Cushing's s
      medicamentosus

    cutaneomucouveal s.

    Cyriax's s

    DaCosta s.

    Danbolt-Closs s

    Dandy-Walker s

    Danlos' s

    Debré-Sémélaigne s

syndrome (*continued*)

    de Clerambault s.

    defibrination s

    Degos s.

    Dejean's s

    Dejerine's s

    Dejerine-Klumpke s

    Dejerine-Roussy s

    Dejerine-Sottas s.

    Dejerine-Thomas s

    de Lange's s

    del Castillo's s

    de Morsier's s

    dengue shock s.

    Dennie-Marfan s

    Denny-Brown's s

    Denys-Drash s

    De Sanctis-Cacchione s

    De Toni-Fanconi s

    dialysis dysequilibrium
      syndrome

    Diamond-Blackfan
      syndrome

    diarrheogenic syndrome

    DIDMOAD syndrome

    diencephalic syndrome

    DiGeorge syndrome

    Di Guglielmo's syndrome

    disconnection syndrome

    disseminated intravascular
      coagulation syndrome

    Donohue's syndrome

    DOOR syndrome

    Down syndrome

    Drash syndrome

    Dresbach syndrome

    Dressler syndrome

    Duane syndrome

    Dubin-Johnson syndrome

    Dubin-Sprinz syndrome

    Dubreuil-Chambardel
      syndrome

    Duchenne syndrome

    Duchenne-Erb syndrome

    dumping s.

    Duncan syndrome

    Dyggve-Melchior-Clausen s.

syndrome (*continued*)
Dyke-Davidoff-Masson
syndrome
dyskinetic cilia syndrome
dysmaturity syndrome
dismyelopoiectic s.
dysplasia
oculodentodigitalis
syndrome
dysplastic nevus s.
dysuria-pyuria s.
Eagle-Barrett syndrome
Eagle s.
ectopic ACTH syndrome
ectopic corticotropin-
releasing hormone
syndrome
ectrodactyly-ectodermal
dysplasia-clefting
syndrome
Eddowe syndrome
Edwards syndrome
Edwards-Patau s.
EEC syndrome
egg-white syndrome
Ehlers-Danlos syndrome
Eisenmenger syndrome
Ekbom syndrome
Ekman syndrome
Ekman-Lobstein syndrome
elfin facies syndrome
Ellis-van Creveld syndrome
embryonic testicular
regression syndrome
EMG syndrome
empty sella syndrome
encephalotrigeminal
vascular syndrome
endocrine polyglandular s.
eosinophilia-myalgia
syndrome
epiphyseal syndrome
Epstein syndrome
Erb s.
erythrocyte
autosensitization
syndrome

syndrome (*continued*)
erythrodysesthesia s.
Escobar syndrome
euthyroid sick syndrome
Evans syndrome
excited skin s.
exomphalos-macroglossia-
gigantism syndrome
extrapyramidal syndrome
Faber syndrome
faciodigitogenital
syndrome
Fallot s.
Fanconi syndrome
Fanconi-Zinsser s.
Farber syndrome
Farber-Uzman syndrome
Favre-Racouchot syndrome
Felty syndrome
feminizing testes syndrome
fertile eunuch syndrome
fetal alcohol syndrome
fetal face syndrome
fetal hydantoin syndrome
fetal trimethadione s.
Feuerstein-Mims s.
Fèvre-Languepin syndrome
FG syndrome
fibrinogen-fibrin conversion
s.
Fiessinger-Leroy-Reiter
syndrome
Figuiera s.
Fisher syndrome
first arch s.
Fitz-Hugh-Curtis syndrome
Fleischner s.
floppy infant syndrome
floppy valve syndrome
Flynn-Aird syndrome
Foix syndrome
Foix-Alajouanine syndrome
folded lung syndrome
Forbes-Albright syndrome
Forney s.
Forsius-Eriksson syndrome
Förster syndrome

syndrome (*continued*)
    Förster atonic-astatic
      syndrome
    Foster Kennedy syndrome
    Foville syndrome
    fragile X syndrome
    Fraley s.
    Franceschetti syndrome
    Franceschetti-Jadassohn
      syndrome
    François syndrome
    Fraser syndrome
    Freeman-Sheldon
      syndrome
    Frenkel anterior ocular
      traumatic s.
    Frey syndrome
    Friderichsen-Waterhouse
      syndrome
    Friedmann vasomotor
      syndrome
    Fröhlich syndrome
    Froin syndrome
    Frommel-Chiari syndrome
    Fuchs syndrome
    Fukuhara syndrome
    Fukuyama's syndrome
    functional prepubertal
      castrate syndrome
    Furst-Ostrum s.
    G syndrome
    Gailliard syndrome
    Gaisböck s.
    galactorrhea-amenorrhea
      syndrome
    Gamstorp s.
    Ganser s.
    Garcin syndrome
    Gardner syndrome
    Gardner-Diamond
      syndrome
    Gasser syndrome
    gay lymph node s.
    Gee-Herter-Heubner
      syndrome
    Gélineau syndrome
    Gerstmann syndrome

syndrome (*continued*)
    Gerstmann-Sträussler
      syndrome
    Gerstmann-Sträussler-
      Scheinker syndrome
    Gianotti-Crosti syndrome
    giant platelet syndrome
    Gilbert syndrome
    Gilles de la Tourette
      syndrome
    Gillespie syndrome
    Gitelman syndrome
    Glanzmann-Riniker s.
    glioma-polyposis
      syndrome
    glomangiomatous osseous
      malformation s.
    glucagonoma syndrome
    Goldberg syndrome
    Goldenhar syndrome
    Goldz-Gorlin s.
    Goltz syndrome
    Good syndrome
    Goodman syndrome
    Goodpasture syndrome
    Gopalan syndrome
    Gordon's syndrome
    Gorlin s.
    Gorlin-Chaudhry-Moss s.
    Gorlin-Goltz s.
    Gorlin-Psaume s.
    Gorman s.
    Gougerot-Blum syndrome
    Gougerot-Carteaud
      syndrome
    Gougerot-Nulock-Houwer
      syndrome
    Gowers syndrome
    gracilis s.
    Gradenigo syndrome
    Graham Little syndrome
    gray syndrome
    gray platelet syndrome
    Gregg s.
    Greig syndrome
    Griscelli syndrome
    Grisel syndrome

syndrome (*continued*)
  Grönblad-Strandberg
    syndrome
  Gruber syndrome
  Grublere s.
  Guillain-Barré syndrome
  Gulf War s.
  Gull-Sutton s.
  Gunn syndrome
  gustatory sweating
    syndrome
  Haber s.
  Hadfield-Clarke syndrome
  Hakim syndrome
  half base syndrome
  Hallermann-Streiff
    syndrome
  Hallermann-Streiff-François
    syndrome
  Hamman syndrome
  Hamman-Rich syndrome
  hand-arm vibration
    syndrome
  hand-foot-and-mouth
    syndrome
  hand-foot s.
  hand-foot-uterus
    syndrome
  Hand-Schüller-Christian
    syndrome
  hand-shoulder syndrome
  Hanhart syndrome
  Hanot-Chauffard syndrome
  Hantavirus pulmonary
    syndrome
  happy puppet syndrome
  Harada syndrome
  HARD syndrome
  Hare s.
  Harris syndrome
  Hartnup syndrome
  Hassin s.
  Hay-Wells syndrome
  Hayem-Widal syndrome
  heart-hand syndrome
  Hecht syndrome
  Hecht-Beals syndrome

syndrome (*continued*)
  Hecht-Beals-Wilson
    syndrome
  Heerfordt syndrome
  Hegglin s.
  Heidenhain syndrome
  HELLP syndrome
  Helweg-Larsen syndrome
  hemangioma-
    thrombocytopenia s.
  hemohistioblastic
    syndrome
  hemolytic uremic
    syndrome
  hemolytic-uremic s. (HUS)
  hemophagocytic syndrome
  hemopleuropneumonic
    syndrome
  Hench-Rosenberg
    syndrome
  Henoch-Schönlein
    syndrome
  hepatorenal syndrome
  hereditary benign
    intraepithelial dyskeratosis
    s.
  Herlitz s.
  Hermansky-Pudlak
    syndrome
  herniated disk s.
  Herrmann syndrome
  HHH syndrome
  Hick's syndrome
  Hines-Bannick syndrome
  Hinman syndrome
  Hirschowitz s.
  Hoffmann-Werdnig
    syndrome
  holiday heart syndrome
  Holmes-Adie syndrome
  Holt-Oram syndrome
  Homén syndrome
  Horner syndrome
  Horner-Bernard syndrome
  Horton syndrome
  Houssay s.
  Howel-Evans' syndrome

syndrome (*continued*)
  Hughes-Stovin syndrome
  hungry bone syndrome
  Hunt syndrome
  Hunter syndrome
  Hunter-Hurler s.
  Hurler syndrome
  Hurler-Scheie syndrome
  Hutchinson syndrome
  Hutchinson-Gilford
    syndrome
  17-hydroxylase deficiency
    syndrome
  hyperabduction syndrome
  hypercalcemia syndrome
  hypereosinophilic
    syndrome
  hyper-IgE s.
  hyperimmunoglobulin E
    syndrome
  hyperimmunoglobulin M s.
  hyperkinetic heart
    syndrome
  hyperlucent lung syndrome
  hyperornithinemia-
    hyperammonemia-
    homocitrullinuria s.
  hypersomnia-bulimia
    syndrome
  hypertelorism-hypospadias
    syndrome
  hyperventilation syndrome
  hyperviscosity syndrome
  hypophysial s.
  hypophyso-sphenoidal s.
  hypoplastic left heart
    syndrome
  hypothenar hammer
    syndrome
  hypotonic syndromes
  idiopathic nephrotic s.
    (INS)
  idiopathic postprandial
    syndrome
  idiopathic respiratory
    distress s. (IRDS)
  Imerslund syndrome

syndrome (*continued*)
  Imerslund-Graesbeck
    syndrome
  immotile cilia syndrome
  immunodeficiency s.
  impingement syndrome
  syndrome of inappropriate
    antidiuretic hormone
  inferior syndrome of red
    nucleus
  inspissated bile syndrome
  intrauterine parabiotic
    syndrome
  irritable bowel syndrome
  irritable colon syndrome
  Irvine s.
  Isaacs syndrome
  Isaacs-Mertens syndrome
  Ivemark syndrome
  IVIC syndrome
  Jaccoud syndrome
  Jackson syndrome
  Jacod syndrome
  Jadassohn-Lewandowski
    syndrome
  Jahnke syndrome
  Janz syndrome
  Jarcho-Levin syndrome
  jaw-winking syndrome
  Jefferson's syndrome
  Jeghers-Peutz s.
  Jervell and Lange-Nielsen
    syndrome
  Jeune syndrome
  Job syndrome
  Johnson-Dubin s.
  Joseph s.
  Joubert's syndrome
  jugular foramen syndrome
  juvenile polyposis
    syndrome
  Kabuki make-up syndrome
  Kallmann syndrome
  Kandindkii-Clerambault s.
  Kanner s.
  Kartagener syndrome
  Kasabach-Merritt syndrome

syndrome (*continued*)
Kast s.
Kaufman-McKusick
syndrome
Kearns-Sayre syndrome
Kearns s.
Kennedy syndrome
keratitis-ichthyosis-deafness
syndrome
KID syndrome
Kiloh-Nevin syndrome
Kimmelstiel-Wilson
syndrome
King syndrome
Kinsbourne syndrome
kleeblattschädel syndrome
Kleine-Levin s.
Klein-Waardenburg
syndrome
Klinefelter syndrome
Klippel-Feil syndrome
Klippel-Trénaunay
syndrome
Klippel-Trénaunay-Weber
syndrome
Klumpke-Dejerine
syndrome
Klüver-Bucy syndrome
Kneist s.
Kocher-Debré-Sémélaigne
syndrome
Koenig s.
Koerber-Salus-Elschnig
syndrome
Königs syndrome
Korsakoff s.
Kostmann's syndrome
Krabbe s.
Krause syndrome
Kugelberg-Welander
syndrome
Kunkel syndrome
Kuskokwin s.
Ladd s.
LADD s.
LAMB syndrome
Lambert-Eaton s.

syndrome (*continued*)
Landau-Kleffner syndrome
Landry syndrome
Landry-Guillain-Barré s.
Langer-Giedion syndrome
Lannois-Gradenigo
syndrome
Laron syndrome
Larsen syndrome
lateral medullary syndrome
Laubry-Soulle syndrome
Launois syndrome
Launois-Bensaude s.
Launois-Cléret s.
Laurence-Biedl s.
Laurence-Moon syndrome
Laurence-Moon-Bardet-
Biedl s.
Laurence-Moon-Biedl s.
Lawford s.
Lawrence-Seip syndrome
lazy leukocyte syndrome
Legg-Calvé-Perthes
syndrome
Lemierre syndrome
Lemieux-Neemeh
syndrome
Lennox syndrome
Lennox-Gastaut syndrome
Lenz syndrome
LEOPARD syndrome
Leredde syndrome
Leriche syndrome
Leri-Weill s.
Lermoyez syndrome
Lesch-Nyhan syndrome
lethal multiple pterygium
syndrome
levator syndrome
Levy-Hollister s.
Lévy-Roussy syndrome
Leyden-Möbius syndrome
Lhermite_mcAlpine s.
Libman-Sacks s.
Lichtheim syndrome
Liddle's syndrome
Li-Fraumeni cancer s.

syndrome (*continued*)
Lightwood syndrome
Lignac syndrome
Lignac-Fanconi syndrome
linear sebaceous nevus s.
lissencephaly syndrome
liver-kidney syndrome
Lobstein's syndrome
locked-in syndrome
loculation syndrome
Löffler's syndrome
Löfgren's syndrome
long QT syndrome
Looser-Milkman syndrome
Lorain-Lévi syndrome
Louis-Bar's syndrome
low cardiac output
   syndrome
Lowe syndrome
Lowe-Terrey-MacLachlan
   syndrome
lower radicular syndrome
Lown-Ganong-Levine
   syndrome
Lucey-Driscoll syndrome
lupus-like syndrome
Lutembacher's syndrome
Lyell's syndrome
lymphadenopathy s.
lymphoproliferative
   syndromes
lymphoreticular syndromes
Mackenzie's syndrome
Macleod s.
Maffucci s.
McCune-Albright syndrome
McKusick-Kaufman
   syndrome
McLeod syndrome
Macleod's syndrome
malabsorption syndrome
male Turner s.
malignant carcinoid s.
Mallory-Weiss syndrome
mandibulofacial dysotosis
   s.
mandibulo-oculofacial s.

syndrome (*continued*)
Marañón s.
Marchesani's syndrome
Marchiafava-Micheli
   syndrome
Marcus Gunn's syndrome
Marfan syndrome
Marie-Bamberger syndrome
Marie-Robinson s.
Marinesco-Garland s.
Marinesco-Sjögren
   syndrome
Maroteaux-Lamy syndrome
Marshall s.
Martin-Bell syndrome
Martorell's syndrome
mastocytosis syndrome
maternal deprivation
   syndrome
Mauriac syndrome
May-White syndrome
Mayer-Rokitansky-Küster-
   Hauser syndrome
Meckel's syndrome
Meckel-Gruber syndrome
meconium aspiration
   syndrome
meconium plug syndrome
median cleft facial
   syndrome
megacystic s.
megacystis-megaureter
   syndrome
megacystis-microcolon-
   intestinal hypoperistalsis
   syndrome
Meig syndrome
MELAS syndrome
Melchior s.
Melkersson's syndrome
Melkersson-Rosenthal
   syndrome
Melnick-Fraser syndrome
Melnick-Needles s.
MEN s.
Ménétrier s.
Mendelson's syndrome

syndrome (*continued*)
    Mengert's shock syndrome
    Ménière's syndrome
    Menkes' syndrome
    menopausal s.
    Meretoja's syndrome
    MERRF syndrome
    metameric syndrome
    metatastic carcinoid s.
    methionine malabsorption
      syndrome
    Meyenburg-Altherr-
      Uchlinger s.
    Meyer-Betz s.
    Meyer-Schwickerath and
      Weyers syndrome
    middle lobe syndrome
    midsystolic click-late
      systolic murmur
      syndrome
    Miescher s.
    Mikulicz's syndrome
    milk alkali syndrome
    Milkman's syndrome
    Millard-Gubler syndrome
    Miller syndrome
    Miller-Dieker syndrome
    Miller Fisher syndrome
    minimal change nephrotic
      syndrome
    Minkowski-Chauffard
      syndrome
    Minot-von Willebrand
      syndrome
    Mirizzi s.
    mitral valve prolapse
      syndrome
    mixed cryoglobulin s.
    Möbius' syndrome
    Mohr syndrome
    Monakow's syndrome
    monosomy 9p- syndrome
    Moore's syndrome
    Morel's syndrome
    Morgagni s.
    Morgagni-Adams-Stokes
      syndrome

syndrome (*continued*)
    Morgagni-Stewart s.
    morning glory syndrome
    Morquio's syndrome
    Morquio-Brailsford s.
    Morquio-Ullrich s.
    Morris syndrome
    Morton's syndrome
    Morvan's syndrome
    Mosse's syndrome
    Mounier-Kuhn's syndrome
    Mount's syndrome
    Mount-Reback syndrome
    Moynahan's syndrome
    Mucha-Habermann s.
    Muckle-Wells syndrome
    mucocutaneous lymph
      node syndrome
    mucosal neuroma
      syndrome
    Muir-Torre s.
    multiple endocrine
      deficiency syndrome
    multiple glandular
      deficiency syndrome
    multiple hamartoma
      syndrome
    multiple lentigines
      syndrome
    multiple pterygium
      syndrome
    Münchausen syndrome
    Murchison-Sandreson s.
    MVP syndrome
    myelodysplastic s.
    myelofibrosis-osteosclerosis
      syndrome
    myeloproliferative
      syndromes
    Naegeli syndrome
    Naffziger's syndrome
    Nager's syndrome
    Nager-de Reynier syndrome
    nail-patella syndrome
    NAME syndrome
    neck-tongue syndrome
    Negri-Jacod syndrome

syndrome (*continued*)
Nélaton's syndrome
Nelson's syndrome
nephritic s.
nephrotic syndrome
nerve compression
syndrome
Netherton's syndrome
neurocutaneous syndrome
neuroleptic malignant
syndrome
newborn respiratory s.
Nezelof syndrome
Noack's syndrome
Nonne-Milroy-Meige
syndrome
nonstaphylococcal scalded
skin syndrome
Noonan's syndrome
Nothnagel's syndrome
Nyssen-van Bogaert
syndrome
OAV syndrome
obesity-hypoventilation
syndrome
obstructive sleep apnea
syndrome
occipital horn syndrome
ocular-mucous membrane
s.
oculobuccogential s.
oculocerebral-
hypopigmentation
syndrome
oculocerebrorenal
syndrome
oculodentodigital syndrome
oculodento-osseous
syndrome
oculomandibulodyscephaly
-hypotrichosis syndrome
oculomandibulofacial
syndrome
oculo-oto-radial syndrome
oculopharyngeal syndrome
oculovertebral s.
ODD syndrome

syndrome (*continued*)
OFD syndrome
orofacialdigital s.
Ogilvie's syndrome
Oldfield's syndrome
Omenn's syndrome
OMM syndrome
one-and-a-half syndrome
Opitz syndrome
Opitz-Frias syndrome
Oppenheim s.
orbital apex syndrome
orbital floor syndrome
organic brain s. (OBS)
organic dust toxic
syndrome
orofaciodigital (OFD)
syndrome
Ortner's syndrome
osteomyelofibrotic s.
Ostrum-Furst syndrome
otomandibular s.
outlet syndrome
ovarian hyperstimulation
syndrome
ovarian-remnant syndrome
ovarian vein syndrome
overlap syndrome
overwear syndrome
pacemaker syndrome
Paget-Schroetter syndrome
Paget-von Schroetter
syndrome
painful arc syndrome
painful bruising syndrome
paleostriatal syndrome
pallidal syndrome
Pancoast's syndrome
pancreatic cholera
syndrome
pancreaticohepatic
syndrome
pancytopenia-dysmelia
syndrome
papillary muscle s.
Pappilon-Léage and
Psaume s.

syndrome (*continued*)
Papillon-Lefèvre syndrome
paraneoplastic s.
paratrigeminal syndrome
Parinaud's syndrome
Parinaud's oculoglandular
   syndrome
Parkes Weber syndrome
parkinsonian syndrome
parotitis s.
Parry-Romberg syndrome
Patau's syndrome
Paterson's syndrome
Paterson-Brown Kelly
   syndrome
Paterson-Kelly syndrome
Pearson's syndrome
Pellegrini-Stieda syndrome
Pellizzi's syndrome
Pendred's syndrome
PEP syndrome
Pepper s.
pericolic membrane
   syndrome
periodic s.
Perlman syndrome
Persian Gulf s.
persistent müllerian duct
   syndrome
pertussis syndrome
pertussis-like syndrome
petrosphenoid syndrome
Peutz s.
Peutz-Jeghers syndrome
Pfaundler-Hurler s.
Pfeiffer's syndrome
pharyngeal pouch
   syndrome
PHC syndrome
Picchini's syndrome
pickwickian syndrome
PIE syndrome
Pierre Robin syndrome
pineal syndrome
placental dysfunction
   syndrome
plica syndrome

syndrome (*continued*)
Plummer-Vinson syndrome
POEMS syndrome
Poland's syndrome
Polhemus-Schafer-Ivemark
   syndrome
polyangiitis overlap
   syndrome
polycystic ovary syndrome
polyglandular autoimmune
   syndromes
polysplenia syndrome
pontine syndrome
popliteal pterygium
   syndrome
popliteal web syndrome
Porak-Durante syndrome
post-cardiac injury
   syndrome
postcardiotomy syndrome
postconcussion syndrome
postconcussional syndrome
posterior column syndrome
posterior cord syndrome
posterior inferior cerebellar
   artery syndrome
postmaturity syndrome
postmenopausal s.
post-myocardial infarction
   syndrome
postphlebitic syndrome
postpump s. (PPS)
postrubella s.
post-thrombotic syndrome
post-traumatic syndrome
post-traumatic brain
   syndrome
Potter's syndrome
Prader-Willi syndrome
preexcitation syndrome
premature senility s.
premenstrual syndrome
premotor syndrome
primary fibromyalgia s.
Profichet's syndrome
prolonged QT interval
   syndrome

syndrome (*continued*)

    pronator syndrome
    pronator teres syndrome
    Proteus syndrome
    prune belly syndrome
    pseudo-Cushing's
      syndrome
    pseudothalidomide s.
    pseudo-Turner s.
    pterygium s.
    pulmonary acid aspiration
      syndrome
    pulmonary dysmaturity
      syndrome
    pulmonary sling
      syndrome
    Purtilo's syndrome
    Putnam-Dana syndrome
    Rabson-Mendenhall
      syndrome
    radial aplasia-
      thrombocytopenia s.
    radicular syndrome
    Raeder's syndrome
    Raeder's paratrigeminal
      syndrome
    Ramsay Hunt syndrome
    Rapp-Hodgkin syndrome
    Raymond-Cestan syndrome
    reactive airways
      dysfunction syndrome
    Recklinghausen-
      Applebaum s.
    red cell fragmentation s.
    redundant supraglottic
      mucosa syndrome
    Refetoff s.
    Reichel's syndrome
    Reichmann's syndrome
    Reifenstein's syndrome
    Reiter's syndrome
    REM s.
    Rendu-Osler-Weber
      syndrome
    Renpenning s.
    respiratory distress
      syndrome

syndrome (*continued*)

    respiratory distress
      syndrome of the newborn
    restless legs syndrome
    retraction syndrome
    syndrome of retroparotid
      space
    Rett syndrome
    Reye's syndrome
    Reye-Johnson syndrome
    Rh null syndrome
    Richards-Rundle syndrome
    Richner-Hanhart syndrome
    Richter s.
    Rieger's syndrome
    right ovarian vein s.
    Riley-Day syndrome
    Riley-Smith syndrome
    Roaf s.
    Roberts syndrome
    Robin syndrome
    Robinow's syndrome
    Rochon-Duvigneaud's
      syndrome
    Roger's syndrome
    Rokitansky-Küster-Hauser
      syndrome
    rolandic vein syndrome
    Rollet's syndrome
    Romano-Ward s.
    Romberg s.
    Rosenbach s.
    Rosenberg-Bergstrom
      syndrome
    Rosenberg-Chutorian
      syndrome
    Rosenthal syndrome
    Rosenthal-Kloepfer
      syndrome
    Rosewater syndrome
    Roth (Rot) s.
    Roth-Bernhardt (Rot-
      Bernhardt) syndrome
    Rothmann-Makai syndrome
    Rothmund-Thomson
      syndrome
    Rotor s.

syndrome (*continued*)
Rotter s.
Roussy-Dejerine syndrome
Roussy-Lévy syndrome
Rovsing syndrome
rubella syndrome
Rubinstein syndrome
Rubinstein-Taybi syndrome
rubrospinal cerebellar
  peduncle s.
Rud syndrome
rudimentary testis s.
Rukavina syndrome
Rundles-Falls syndrome
runting syndrome
Russell syndrome
Russell-Silver syndrome
Rust syndrome
Ruvalcaba syndrome
Sabin-Feldman syndrome
Saethre-Chotzen syndrome
Sakati-Nyhan syndrome
salt-depletion syndrome
salt-losing syndrome
Sanchez Salorio s.
Sandifer syndrome
Sanfilippo syndrome
Santavuori syndrome
Santavuori-Haltia
  syndrome
scalded skin s.
scalenus syndrome
scalenus anterior syndrome
scalenus anticus s.
scapulocostal s.
Schäfer s.
Schanz s.
Schaumann s.
Scheie s.
Schirmer s.
Schmid-Fraccaro s.
Schmidt s.
Schönlein-Henoch
  syndrome
Schridde s.
Schroeder s.
Schüller syndrome

syndrome (*continued*)
Schüller-Christian
  syndrome
Schultz syndrome
Schwartz-Jampel syndrome
Schwartz-Jampel-Aberfeld
  syndrome
scimitar syndrome
sea-blue histiocyte
  syndrome
Seabright bantam
  syndrome
Seckel syndrome
Secretan s.
segmentary syndrome
Selye syndrome
Senear-Usher syndrome
Senior-Loken syndrome
s. of sensory dissociation
  with brachial amyotrophy
Senter syndrome
Sertoli-cell-only syndrome
serum sickness-like
  syndrome
Sever s.
Sézary s.
Sheehan s.
short-bowel syndrome
short-gut syndrome
shoulder-hand syndrome
Shprintzen syndrome
Shulman syndrome
Shwachman syndrome
Shwachman-Diamond
  syndrome
Shy-Drager syndrome
Shy-Magee syndrome
Sicard syndrome
sicca syndrome
sick building s.
sick sinus syndrome
Silfverskiöld syndrome
Silver syndrome
Silver-Russell syndrome
Silverman syndrome
Silvestrini-Corda syndrome
Simmonds syndrome

syndrome (*continued*)
    Sipple syndrome
    Sjögren syndrome
    Sjögren-Larsson syndrome
    sleep apnea syndrome
    SLE-like syndrome
    slipping rib syndrome
    Sluder syndrome
    Sly syndrome
    Smith-Lemli-Opitz
      syndrome
    Sneddon syndrome
    SO syndrome
    Sohval-Soffer syndrome
    somnolence syndrome
    Sorsby syndrome
    Sotos syndrome
    Sotos syndrome of cerebral
      gigantism
    Spanish toxic oil syndrome
    Spens syndrome
    sphenoidal fissure-optic
      canal syndrome
    spherophakia-
      brachymorphia syndrome
    splenic flexure syndrome
    split-brain syndrome
    Sprinz-Dubin syndrome
    Sprinz-Nelson syndrome
    sprue-like s.
    spun glass hair syndrome
    Spurway syndrome
    stagnant loop syndrome
    staphylococcal scalded skin
      syndrome
    stasis syndrome
    Steele-Richardson-
      Olszewski syndrome
    Steiner s.
    Stein-Leventhal syndrome
    Steinbrocker's syndrome
    Steiner syndrome
    Stevens-Johnson syndrome
    Stickler syndrome
    stiff heart syndrome
    Still-Chauffard s.
    Stilling syndrome

syndrome (*continued*)
    Stilling-Türk-Duane
      syndrome
    Stokes syndrome
    Stokes-Adams syndrome
    Stokvis-Talma syndrome
    Strachan syndrome
    Strachan-Scott syndrome
    straight back syndrome
    stroke syndrome
    Stryker-Halbeisen s.
    Sturge syndrome
    Sturge-Kalischer-Weber
      syndrome
    Sturge-Weber syndrome
    subclavian steal syndrome
    sudden infant death
      syndrome
    sudden unexplained death
      syndrome
    Sudeck-Leriche syndrome
    Sulzberger-Garbe
      syndrome
    superior mesenteric artery
      syndrome
    superior orbital fissure
      syndrome
    superior vena cava
      syndrome
    supraspinatus syndrome
    supravalvular aortic
      stenosis syndrome
    sweat retention syndrome
    Sweet's syndrome
    Swyer syndrome
    Swyer-James syndrome
    sylvian syndrome
    sylvian aqueduct syndrome
    syringomyelic syndrome
    systolic click-murmur
      syndrome
    Takayasu syndrome
    Tapia syndrome
    TAR syndrome
    tarsal tunnel syndrome
    Taussig-Bing syndrome
    tegmental syndrome

syndrome (*continued*)
- temporomandibular dysfunction syndrome
- temporomandibular joint syndrome
- Terry syndrome
- Terson syndrome
- testicular feminization syndrome
- testicular regression s.
- tethered cord syndrome
- thalamic syndrome
- thalamic pain syndrome
- Thévenard syndrome
- Thibierge-Weissenbach syndrome
- Thiele syndrome
- Thiemann's syndrome
- third and fourth phalangeal pouch s.
- thoracic outlet syndrome
- Thorn syndrome
- thrombocytopenia-absent radius syndrome
- thromboembolic syndrome
- Tietze syndrome
- Timme s.
- Tolosa-Hunt s.
- TORCH syndrome
- Tornwaldt s.
- Torre s.
- Touraine-Solente-Golé syndrome
- Tourette syndrome
- Townes syndrome
- toxic oil syndrome
- toxic shock syndrome
- translocation Down syndrome
- Treacher Collins syndrome
- Treacher Collins-Franceschetti s.
- triad s.
- trichorhinophalangeal syndrome
- triple-A syndrome

syndrome (*continued*)
- trismus-pseudocamptodactyly syndrome
- trisomy 8 s.
- trisomy 11q s.
- trisomy 13 s.
- trisomy 13-15 s.
- trisomy 16-18 s.
- trisomy 18 s.
- trisomy 20 s.
- trisomy 21 syndrome
- trisomy 22 syndrome
- trisomy C syndrome
- trisomy D syndrome
- trisomy E syndrome
- Troisier s.
- tropical splenomegaly s.
- Trousseau s.
- tryptophan malabsorption s.
- tumor lysis s.
- Turcot syndrome
- Turner syndrome
- twiddler syndrome
- twin transfusion syndrome
- twin-twin transfusion syndrome
- Uehlinger s.
- Ullrich-Feichtiger syndrome
- Ullrich-Turner syndrome
- Ulysses s.
- uncombable hair syndrome
- unilateral nevoid telangiectasia syndrome
- Unna-Thost syndrome
- upper airway resistance syndrome
- urethral syndrome
- urogenital s.
- Usher syndrome
- uveo-encephalitic
- vagoaccessory syndrome
- vagoaccessory-hypoglossal syndrome
- Vail syndrome
- Van Allen syndrome

syndrome (*continued*)

van Bogaert-Nyssen syndrome
van Buchem syndrome
van der Hoeve syndrome
Van der Woude syndrome
vanishing testes syndrome
vanishing twin syndrome
vascular syndrome
vascular leak syndrome
vasulocardiac s.
VCF syndrome
velocardiofacial syndrome
Verner-Morrison syndrome
Vernet syndrome
vertebrobasilar syndrome
Villaret syndrome
Vinson syndrome
Virchow-Seckel syndrome
virilizing s.
Vogt syndrome
Vogt-Koyanagi syndrome
Vogt-Koyanagi-Harada syndrome
Vohwinkel syndrome
Volkmann syndrome
Waardenburg syndrome
WAGR syndrome
Walker-Warburg syndrome
Wallenberg syndrome
Warburg syndrome
Ward-Romano syndrome
Waterhouse-Friderichsen syndrome
WDHA syndrome
WDHH syndrome
Weber syndrome
Weber-Christian syndrome
Weber-Cockayne syndrome
Weber-Gubler syndrome
Weber-Leyden syndrome
Wegener syndrome
Weill-Marchesani syndrome
Welander syndrome
Wells s.
Wermer syndrome
Werner syndrome

syndrome (*continued*)

Wernicke syndrome
Wernicke-Korsakoff syndrome
West syndrome
Weyers oligodactyly syndrome
whiplash shake syndrome
whistling face syndrome
Widal syndrome
Wildervanck s.
Willebrand syndrome
Williams syndrome
Williams-Beuren s
Williams-Campbell s
Wilson-Mikity s
Winchester s
Winter s
Wiskott-Aldrich s
Wohlfart-Kugelberg-Welander s
Wolf-Hirschhorn s
Wolff-Parkinson-White s
Wolfram s
WPW s
Wright s
Wyburn-Mason's s
s. X
X-linked lymphoproliferative s.
XO s.
XXY s.
XYZ s.
yellow nail s
Young s
Zahorsky s
Zellweger s
Zieve s.
Zinsser-Cole-Engman s.
Zollinger-Ellison s.

syndromic

synechia (pl. synechiae)
annular s.
s. pericardii
posterior s.
s. vulvae

synencephalocele

synergenesis

synesthesia

synesthesialgia

synezesis

syngnathia

syngraft

synizesis

synkaryon

synonychia

synophridia

synophrys

synorchidism

synorchism

synoscheos

synosteosis

synosteotic

synostosis
    radioulnar s.
    sagittal s.
    tarsal s.
    tribasilar s.

synostotic

synovioblast

synoviocyte

synovitis
    acute serous s.
    bursal s.
    dendritic s.
    fungous s.
    localized nodular s.
    pigmented villonodular s.
    serous s.
    s. sicca
    simple s.
    tendinous s.
    vaginal s.

synovitis (*continued*)
    vibration s.
    villonodular s.

synphalangism

synpneumonic

syntectic

syntexis

syntripsis

syphilid
    annular s.
    corymbose s
    follicular s.
    gummatous s.
    lenticular s.
    macular s.
    nodular s.
    palmar s.
    papular s.
    plantar s.

syphilide

syphilis
    cardiovascular s
    cerebrospinal s
    congenital s
    hemagglutinin treponemal
      test for s.
    meningovascular s
    parenchymatous s
    quaternary s.

syrigmus

syringitis

syringobulbia

syringocele

syringoencephalia

syringoencephalomyelia

syringohydromyelia

syringoid

syringomyelia

syringomyelus

syrinx

system
      10-20 s
      AEC detection s.
      accessory portal system of
         Sappey
      Bactalert s.
      BACTEC blood culture s.
      Bethesda System
      bicarbonate buffer s.
      buffer system
      cell-free s.
      centimeter-gram-second s.
      CGS s.
      CRYO-VAC-A cryostat
         vacuum s.
      Cyto-Rich cervical cytology
         monolayer s.
      dichroic filer s.

system (*continued*)
      Difco ESP testing s.
      Edumondson tumor
         grading s.
      Halon s.
      haversian system
      interstitial system
      keratinizing system
      malpighian system
      melanocyte system
      pigmentary system
      T system
      triad system

systremma

Syva EMIT II assay

syzgial

Szent-Gyorgi reaction

T

T-1824

tabacosis

tabes
  diabetic t.
  t. dorsalis
  Friedreich's t.
  t. mesenterica
  t. spinalis

tabescent

tabetic

tabetiform

tabic

tabid

tabification

taboparalysis

taboparesis

tache
  t. blanche
  t. bleuâtres
  t. cérébrale
  t. méningéale
  t. motrice
  t. noire
  t. spinale

tachyarrhythmia

tachyauxesis

tachycardiac

tachycardic

tachydysrhythmia

tachypnea

tachyrhythmia

tactoid

Takayama stain

talalgia

talcosis

taliped

talipedic

talipomanus

talon
  t. noir

tamponade
  cardiac t.

Tanner stage

tanycyte

tarsalgia

tarsitis

tarsomalacia

tarsomegaly

tarsoptosis

taurocholemia

TBW

technique
  Brown-Brenn t.
  Carey-Ranvier t.
  Cattoretti t.
  DGGE t.
  dilution-filtration t.
  enzyme-assisted
    immunoassay t.
  extracorporeal
    phosphoresis t.
  Ficoll-Hypaque t.
  fluorescent antibody t.
  hanging drop t.
  immunofluorescence t.
  immunoperoxidase t.
  Kato thick smear t.
  McMaster t.
  membrane-filter t.
  Northern blot t.
  PAP t.
  scintillation t.
  sedimentation t.
  Seldinger t.
  titration t.

tectocephalic

tectocephaly

teichopsia

tela
    t. submucosa tubae
        uterinae

telalgia

telangiectasia
    generalized essential t
    hereditary hemorrhagic t
    t lymphatica
    spider t
    unilateral nevoid t

telangiectasis

telangiectatic

telangiectodes

telangiitis

telangiosis

telecanthus

teleneurite

teleneuron

teleomitosis

teleopsia

telepathology

telodendron

teloglia

telokinesis

telolecithal

telophase

telophragma

telosynapsis

temperature
    absolute t.
    ambient t.
    t. coefficient
    critical t.

temperature (*continued*)
    eutectic t.
    flash-point t.
    ignition t.
    maximal growth t.
    normal body t.
    optimal growth t.

TEN
    toxic epidermal necrolysis

tenalgia

tenesmic

tenesmus
    rectal t.
    vesical t.

tenifugal

tenodynia

tenofibril

tenonitis

tenonostosis

tenosynovitis
    t. crepitans
    villous t.

tenontagra

tenontitis
    t. prolifera calcarea

tenontodynia

tenontolemmitis

tenontophyma

tenophyte

tenositis

tenostosis

teratoma
    sacrococcygeal t.

teratospermia

terebrant

terebrating

terebration

test
- AAN t.
- Abrams's t.
- acetowhite t.
- acid challenge t.
- acid perfusion t.
- acid phosphatase t.
- ACPA t.
- ACTH stimulation t.
- activated partial thromboplastinc substitution t.
- Adamkiewicz t.
- Addis t.
- Adler t.
- adrenal function t.
- adrenocorticotrophic hormone stimulation t.
- agglutinin t.
- A/G ratio t.
- ALA t.
- AlaSTAT latex allergy t.
- aldosterone stimulation t.
- aldosterone suppression t.
- alizarin t.
- alkaline phosphatase t.
- ammonium chloride loading
- antitoxoplasma antibody t.
- antitrypsin t.
- Apt t.
- APTT t.
- arginine t.
- Ascheim-Zondek t.
- Ascoli t.
- ASO t.
- Aspergillus antibody t.
- AST t.
- Astra profile t.
- atropine suppression t.
- Benedict's t.
- bentonite flocculation t.
- benzidine t
- Bial's t
- bicarbonate titration t.
- bile esculin hydrolysis t.
- bilirubin t.
- Binz t.

test (*continued*)
- biuret t
- blood urea nitrogen t. (BUN)
- blot t.
- Blount t.
- Boas' t
- Bonanno t.
- breath hydrogen t
- bromocriptine suppression t.
- brucella agglutinin t.
- BSP excretion t.
- Burchard-Liebermann t
- butyric acid t
- calcium oxylate t.
- Calmette t.
- CAMP t.
- candida precipitin t.
- capillary fragility t.
- carbohydrate fermentation t.
- carbohydrate utilizaton t.
- carbon dioxide combining power t.
- carbon monoxide t.
- CA15-3 RIA t.
- catalase t.
- catecholamine t.
- cephalin-cholesterol flocculation t.
- cercarien-hullen reaktion t.
- ceruloplasmin t.
- cetylpyridium chloride t.
- CFF t.
- Chagas disease serological t.
- Chediak t.
- chemiluminescence t.
- Chemstrip BG t.
- Chen t.
- chi-squared t.
- Chlamydiazyme t.
- chlormerodrin accumulation t.
- cholesterol t.
- cholinesterase t.
- chorionic gonadotropin t.

test (*continued*)

- chromaffin reaction t.
- chromogenic
  cephalosporin t.
- C lactose t.
- Clauberg t.
- Clinitest stool t.
- clomiphene t.
- CLOtest t.
- coagulase t.
- colchicine t.
- cold agglutinin t.
- cold hemolysin t.
- colloidal gold t.
- concentration t.
- Coomb's t.
- copper binding protein t.
- copper reduction t.
- corpoporphyrin t.
- Corner-Allen t.
- C-peptide t.
- C reactive protein t.
- creatinine clearance t
- CSF glutamine t.
- cutaneous tuberculin t.
- cyanide ascorbate t.
- cysteine t.
- cystine urea t.
- cytosine t.
- D-dimer t.
- deoxyuridine suppression t
- dextrose t.
- DFA-TP t.
    - direct fluorescent
      antibody t.
- DHEA t.
- diabetes t
- diacetyl t.
- Diagnex blue t.
- diazepam breath t.
- direct agglutinin pregnancy
  t. (DAPT)
- direct antiglobulin t.
  (DAGT)
- direct bilirubin t.
- direct Coomb's t.
- direct fluorescent antibody
  t.

test (*continued*)

- Dnase t.
- double diffusion t.
- double glucagon t.
- Duke bleeding time t.
- dye exclusion t.
- dye excretion t.
- Ehrlich's t.
- electrophoresis t.
- Elek t.
- Emmen S/L t.
- enzyme linked antibody t.
- EP t.
- E-rosette t.
- erythrocyte protoporphyrin
  t.
- estradiol t.
- Exac-Tech blood glucose
  meter t.
- FANA t.
- Farber t.
- fat absorption t.
- febrile agglutinin t.
- fecal fat t.
- fecal occult blood t.
- FeNa t
- fermentation t
- ferric chloride t.
- fibrinogen titer t.
- FIGLU excretion t.
- fluorescent antibody t.
- formaldehyde t
- Foshay t.
- Fouchet's t
- Francis' t
- Frei t.
- fructosamine t
- fructose t.
- FTA-ABS t.
- galactose breath t.
- Gastroccult t.
- gel diffusion precipitin t.
- Gerhardt's t.
- Gibson-Cook sweat t.
- Gies' biuret t
- glucose t.
- glucose insulin tolerance t.
- glycogen storage t.

test (*continued*)
    glycosylated hemoglobin t.
    glycosylated hemoglobin t.
    Gmelin's t
    gonadotropin t.
    Gravindex pregnancy t.
    Grigg's t
    guaiac t
    Guthrie t
    Gutzeit's t.
    haptoglobin t.
    Harrison spot t.
    heavy metal screening t.
    hemagglutin t.
    hemoccult t.
    HemoQuant fecal blood t.
    hemosiderin t
    histidine loading t.
    HIVAGEN t.
    HIV antibody t.
    Hoffmann's t
    Hofmeister's t
    Hoppe-Seyler t.
    human chorionic
      gonadotropin injection t.
    HVA t.
    hydroxybutyric t.
    hydrochloric acid t
    hydrogen breath t
    hydrogen peroxide t
    hydrostatic t
    hypochlorite-orcinol t
    hypoxanthine t.
    icterus index t.
    immune adhesion t.
    immunofluorescence t.
    immunoglobulin A, D, G, M
      t.
    immunologic pregnancy t.
    indican t.
    indigo-carmine t.
    indirect bilirubin t.
    indirect Coombs t.
    indole t.
    intradermal t.
    intraesophageal pH t.
    intravenous glucose
      tolerance t. (IVGTT)

test (*continued*)
    iodine t.
    iron binding capacity t.
    islet cell antibody screening
      t.
    Jacquemin's t.
    Jaffe's t.
    Jolles t.
    Jones Cantarow t.
    Jorissen's t.
    Kahn t.
    Katayama t.
    Kentmann's t.
    Kerner's t.
    ketogenic corticoids t.
    kidney function t.
    Kjeldahl's t.
    Knapp's t
    KOH t.
    Kossel's t.
    Külz's t.
    Kunkel t.
    lactic acid t.
    lactic dehydrogenase t.
    Ladendorff t.
    Lang's t
    Lange's t
    LAP t.
    latex agglutination t.
    latex fixation t.
    latex flocculation t.
    LE cell t.
    Lee's t
    leishmaniasis serological t.
    Leo's t.
    lepromin skin t.
    leucine
      aminoaminopeptidase t.
    leukocyte esterase t.
    leukocyte histamine release
      t.
    levulose tolerance t.
    Liebermann-Burchard t
    Liebig's t
    limulus t
    Lindemann's t
    Linder's t
    lipase t.

test (*continued*)

lipoprotein electrophoresis t.
litmus milk t.
liver function t.
long-acting thyroid stimulating hormone t.
Lücke's t.
lupus band t.
lupus erythematosus cell t.
lysozyme t.
Machado-Guerreiro t.
MacLean t
macrophage migration inhibition t.
MacWilliam's t.
magnesium t.
Magpie's t
Malot's t.
Mantoux skin t.
Master 2-step t.
mastic t.
Mayer's t
Mayerhofer's t
melanin t.
mercury t.
metanephrine t.
Mett's (Mette's) t.
Microflow t.
microimmunofluorescent t.
microsomal thyroid antibody t.
migration inhibition t.
Millon's t.
mixed agglutination t.
mobilization t.
Mohr's t
Molisch's t.
Mono-Diff t.
Morelli's t
Mörner's t.
mucin clot t.
multiple puncture tuberculin t.
murexide t.
Napier formed-gel t.
NBT t.
Nencki's t

test (*continued*)

Nessler's t.
niacin t.
Ninhydrin t
nitrate reduction t
nitrites t
nitroprusside t
nitroso-indole-nitrate t.
Obermayer t.
occult blood t.
oleic acid uptake t.
ONPG t.
O&P t.
orcinol t
organic acid t.
osmotic fragility t.
Osterberg's t.
oxidase t.
oxytocin challenge t.
Paget t.
pancreati islet cell antibody t.
Pandy t.
Pap t.
Papaniculaou smear t.
parainfluenza antibody t.
partial thromboplastin time t.
PAS t.
passive cutaneous anaphylaxis t.
passive hemagglutinin t.
patch t.
Paul t.
pentagastrin t.
peptide t
peptone t
Peria t.
periodic acid-Schiff t.
Perls' t
permanganate t
phenacetin t
phenol t
phenolphthalein t.
phenylketonuria t.
phospholipid t.
Piazza t.
picrate t.

test (*continued*)
    pineapple t
    pine wood t
    Piria t.
    pituitary function t.
    P-K t.
    PKU t.
    plant protease t.
    plasmacrit t.
    platelet aggregation t.
    platelet retention t.
    platelet survival t.
    porphyrin t.
    Porter-Silber chromogens t.
    positive whiff t.
    PPD skin t.
    presumptive heterophil t.
    Preyer t.
    prolactin t.
    prostaglandin t.
    protein t.
    proteose t
    prothrombin time t.
    Protocult t.
    provocative chelation t.
    Queckenstedt t.
    Quick Vue chlamydia t.
    rabbit t.
    Rabuteau t.
    RA latex fixation t.
    random plasma glucose t.
    Rapid ANA II t.
    rapid plasma reagin t.
    RapiTex Hp t.
    Raygat t.
    Rees t.
    Reichl t.
    Reinsch t.
    Reiter protein complement-fixation t.
    renal function t.
    resorcinol hydrochloric acid t.
    respiratory synctial virus antigen t.
    Reuss t.
    Rh blocking t.
    rheumatoid factor t.

test (*continued*)
    rhubarb t.
    RISA t.
    Rivalta t.
    Ronchese t.
    Ropes t.
    rose bengal radioactive t.
    Rosenbach-Gmelin t.
    Rosenthal t.
    Rotazyme t.
    Rothera t
    Rous t
    Roussin's t.
    RPR t.
    rubella antibody t.
    Rubner's t
    Ruttan and Hardisty's t.
    Sabin-Feldman dye t.
    saccharimeter t
    Sakaguchi t.
    salicylic acid t.
    Salkowski's t.
    scarification t.
    Schaffer's t.
    schistosomiasis serological t.
    Schönbein's t
    Schroeder's t
    Schulte's t
    Schultze's t
    Schumm's t.
    scatch t.
    sedimentation rate t.
    Selivanoff's (Seliwanow's) t.
    serum alkaline phosphatase t.
    serum amylase t.
    serum globulin t.
    serum protein electrophoresis t.
    sex chromatin t.
    Sia t
    SMAC t.
    SMA-12 profile t.
    Solera's t
    solubility t.
    soybean t

test (*continued*)
 specific gravity t.
 spironolactone t.
 STA t.
 Stamey t.
 standard tube agglutination t.
 starch t
 Staub-Traugott t.
 streptococcal antigen t.
 streptozyme t.
 strychnine t.
 sucrose hemolysis t.
 sugar t
 sulfur t
 Sullivan t.
 sweat t.
 taurine t.
 TCPI Rapid HIV t.
 Teichmann t.
 Tes-Tape urine glucose t.
 thalleioquin t
 thiocyanate t
 Thormählen t
 Thudichum t.
 thyroid suppression t.
 thyroid uptake t.
 TIBC t.
 Tollens, Neuberg, and Schwket's t
 triiodothyronine resin uptake t
 triketohydrindene hydrate t
 Trousseau t
 tryptophan load t
 tyrosine t
 Tyson t
 Tzanck t
 Udránszky t
 Uffelmann t
 Ulrich t
 Ultzmann t
 uracil t
 urea t
 urease t
 uric acid t
 urine concentration t
 urochromogen t

test (*continued*)
 van den Bergh t
 Van Slyke t
 Vitali t
 Vogel and Lee t
 von Maschke t
 von Zeynek and Mencki t
 Wagner t
 Weber t
 Weidel t
 Weisz t
 Weisz permanganate t
 Wenzell t
 Wetzel t
 Weyl t
 Wheeler and Johnson t
 Winckler t
 Wishart t
 Witz t
 Woodbury t
 Wormley t
 Wurster t
 xanthine t
 d-xylose absorption t
 d-xylose tolerance t
 Zaleski t
 Zeisel t

testalgia

testitis

testopathy

testotoxicosis

tetanus
 cephalic t.
 cerebral t.
 neonatal t.
 t. neonatorum

tetany
 gastric t.
 hyperventilation t.
 t. of newborn
 parathyroid t.
 parathyroprival t.

tetartanopia

tetartanopic

tetartanopsia

tetrabromofluorescein

tetrabromophenolphthalein

tetrachromic

tetralogy
    t. of Eisenmenger
    t. of Fallot

tetramethylbenzidine

tetranopsia

tetraparesis

tetraplegia

tetrasomic

tetrasomy

tetraster

tetrastichiasis

thalassanemia

thalassemia

thalleioquin

thamuria

thanatognomonic

thanatoid

thanatology

thanatometer

thanatosis

thaumatropy

thecitis

thecomatosis

thecostegnosis

thelalgia

thelitis

thelorrhagia

thelyblast

thelyblastic

theory
    acidogenic theory
    aging theory of
      atherosclerosis
    Altmann's theory
    cell theory
    contractile ring theory
    encrustation theory
    expanding surface theory
    Kern plasma relation theory
    membrane ionic theory
    metabolic theory of
      atherosclerosis
    overflow theory
    polarization-membrane
      theory
    proteolysis-chelation theory
    proteolytic theory
    sliding filament theory
    spindle elongation theory
    underfilling theory

theque

thermalgesia

thermalgia

thermanalgesia

thermanesthesia

thermhyperesthesia

thermhypesthesia

thermoalgesia

thermoanalgesia

thermoanesthesia

thermohyperalgesia

thermohyperesthesia

thermohypesthesia

thermohypoesthesia

thermoplegia

thesaurocyte

thiasine

thiemia

thioflavine

thioneine

thionine

thiozine

thoracalgia

thoracocyllosis

thoracocyrtosis

thoracodynia

thoracomyodynia

thoracopathy

thoracostenosis

throe

thrombasthenia
  Glanzmann's t.

thromboangiitis

thromboarteritis
  t. purulenta

thromboasthenia

thrombocyst

thrombocystis

thrombocythemia
  essential t.
  hemorrhagic t.
  idiopathic t.
  primary t.

thrombocytolysis

thrombocytopathia

thrombocytopathic

thrombocytopathy
  constitutional t.

thrombocytopenia
  essential t.
  immune t.
  neonatal t.
  neonatal alloimmune t.

thrombocytosis

thrombocytosis (*continued*)
  primary t.
  reactive t.
  secondary t.

thromboembolia

thromboembolism

thromboendarteritis

thromboendocarditis

thrombogenesis

thrombogenic

thromboid

thrombolymphangitis

thrombopathy

thrombopenia

thrombophilia

thrombophlebitis
  iliofemoral t., postpartum
  intracranial t.
  t. migrans
  migratory t.

thrombopoiesis

thrombopoietic

thrombosis (pl. thromboses)
  agonal t.
  atrophic t
  cardiac t
  cerebral t
  coronary t
  creeping t
  deep venous t
  dilatation t
  marantic t
  marasmic t
  mesenteric arterial t
  mesenteric venous t
  placental t.
  plate t
  platelet t.
  portal vein t.
  propagating t.

thrombosis (*continued*)
 puerperal t.
 renal vein t.
 traumatic t.
 venous t.

thrombostasis

thrombotic

thrombus (pl. thrombi)

thrush

thrypsis

Thuja

thymelcosis

thymine-uraciluria

thymion

thymitis

thymohydroquinone

thymokesis

thymol
 t. phthalein

thymolphthalein

thymopathic

thymopathy

thymoprivic

thymoprivous

thymotoxic

thymotoxin

thymus
 t. independent antigen
 t. persistens hyperplastica

thyroadenitis

thyroaplasia

thyrocele

thyroid
 t. antimicrosomal antibody
 t. antithyroid antibody

thyroid (*continued*)
 t. crisis
 t. function test
 t. stimulating hormone-
  relaxing factor TSH RF)
 t. suppression t.
 t. uptake test

thyroiditis
 acute t.
 autoimmune t.
 chronic t.
 chronic lymphadenoid t.
 chronic lymphocytic t.
 chronic sclerosing t.
 de Quervain's t.
 focal lymphocytic t.
 giant cell t.
 giant follicular t.
 granulomatous t.
 Hashimoto's t.
 induced t.
 invasive t.
 ligneous t.
 lymphoid t.
 radiation t.
 Riedel's t.
 sclerosing t.
 subacute granulomatous t.
 subacute lymphocytic t.

thyrointoxication

thyrolytic

thyromegaly

thyroparathyroprivic

thyropathy

thyroprivous

thyroptosis

thyrotoxic
 t. complement-fixation
  factor

thyrotoxicosis
 t. factitia

thyrotrope

thyrotroph

TIBC
    total iron-binding capacity

tibialgia

tic
    convulsive tic
    diaphragmatic tic
    tic douloureux
    facial tic
    tic de Guinon
    tic de sommeil

tick
    t. fever
    t. paralysis

tick-borne
    t-b. encephalitis
    t-b. virus

Tietze syndrome

tigroid striation

Tilden stain

tilmus

time
    activated coagulation t.
    bleeding t.
    cell cycle t.
    clot lysis t.
    clot retraction t.
    gastric emptying t.
    Kaolin clotting t.
    mean circulation t.
    partial thromboplastin t.
    plasma clotting t.
    prothrombin t.
    Russell viper venom
        clotting t.
    serum prothrombin t.
    thermal death t.
    thromboplastin generation
        t.
    whole-blood clotting t.

tinctable

tinction

tinctorial

tintometer

tintometric

tintometry

tiqueur

TIS
    tissue in situ

tissue
    aberrant t.
    adipose t.
    cancellous t.
    chondroid t.
    chromaffin t.
    t. culture
    dartoid t.
    episcleral t.
    epivaginal connective t.
    t. factor
    t. glycogen
    granulation t.
    heterologous t.
    heterotopic t.
    hyperplastic t.
    Kuhnt's intermediary t.
    lardaceous t.
    lymphatic t.
    metanephrogenic t.
    myeloid t.
    tuberculosis granulation t.

titer
    agglutinin t.
    AH t.
    antibody t.
    anti-Rh t.
    antstreptolysin-O t.
    ASO t.
    California encephalitis virus
        t.
    CF antibody t.
    Chlamydia group t.
    cold agglutinin t.
    Coxsackievirus A, B virus t.
    cryptococcal antigen t.
    cysticercosis t.

titer (*continued*)
    eastern equine encephalitis
      virus t.
    fibrin t.
    hemagglutination t.
    influenza A and B t.
    mumps antibody t.
    poliomyelitis I, II, III, t.
    psittacosis t.
    Q fever t
    Salmonella t.

titrant

titrate

titration
    coulometric t.
    potentiometric t.

titremetric

titubant

titubation

Tokelau ringworm

tolerance
    alkali t.
    drug t.
    glucose t.
    immunological t.

o-tolidine

tomaculous

tonaphasia

tongue
    amyloid t.
    bifid t.
    black hairy t.
    cerebriform t.
    cleft t.
    coated t.
    cobble-stone t.
    fern leaf t.
    fissured t.
    furrowed t.
    lobulated t.
    magenta t.
    plicated t.

tongue (*continued*)
    raspberry t.
    Sandwith's bald t.
    strawberry t.

tonicity

tonofibril

tonofilament

tonsillitis
    acute t.
    follicular t.
    herpetic t.
    lacunar t.
    streptococcal t.
    Vincent's t.

tonsillolith

tonsillomycosis

tonsillopathy

tonsillopharyngitis

tonsolith

topagnosia

topagnosis

tophaceous

tophus (pl. tophi)
    auricular t.
    gouty t.
    tophus t.

topoanesthesia

torpid

torpidity

torpor

torsades de pointes

torticollis
    dermatogenic t.
    fixed t.
    labyrinthine t.
    myogenic t.
    reflex t.

tortipelvis

toxanemia

toxemia

toxicemia

toxicity
    aspirin t.
    O2 t.

Toxicodendron

toxicohemia

toxicosis

toxoplasmosis

toxuria

trachealgia

tracheitis

trachelism

trachelismus

trachelitis

trachelocystitis

trachelodynia

tracheloschisis

tracheoaerocele

tracheobronchitis

tracheobronchomegaly

tracheocele

tracheomalacia

tracheopathia

tracheopathy

tracheorrhagia

tracheoschisis

tracheostenosis

trachitis

trachoma
    Arlt's trachoma
    t. virus

trachychromatic

trachyonychia

tragomaschalia

tragophonia

tragophony

tragopodia

trait
    hemoglobin C t.
    sickle cell t.
    thalassemia t.

transduction

transferase

transformation
    asbestos t.
    bacterial t.
    cell t.
    lymphocytic t.
    malignant t.
    nodular t. of the liver

transfusion
    autologous t.
    coagulation factor t.
    exchange t.
    platelet t.
    t. reaction
    reciprocal t.

transgenic mouse

translocation
    autosome t.
    chromosome t.
    insertional t.
    reciprocal t.
    robertsonian t.
    t. trisomy

transmigration

transmogrification

transpeptidase

transplantation
    allogenic t.
    autologous t.
    bone marrow t.

transplantation (*continued*)
    heterotopic t.
    orthotopic t.

transposable element

transposition
    corrected t.
    t. of great arteries
    t. of great vessels

transsynaptic
    t. chromatolysis
    t. degeneration

transthyretin

transudate

transudative inflammation

transvector

transversion mutation

trauma (pl. traumata)

traumatic
    t. anemia
    t. aneurysm
    t. hemolysis

trephocyte

trepopnea

triad
    acute compression t.
    adrenomedullary t.
    Andersen t.
    Beck t.
    Bezold t.
    Carney t.
    Charcot t.
    Currarino t.
    Dieulafoy t.
    Grancher t.
    Hutchinson t.
    Jacod t.
    Kartagener t.
    t.of Luciani
    Osler t.
    t.of retinal cone
    Saint t.

triad (*continued*)
    t.of Schultz
    t.of skeletal muscle
    Virchow t.

tricellular

trichiasis

trichloroacetic acid

trichobezoar

trichocardia

trichoclasia

trichoclasis

trichoglossia

trichohyalin

tricholith

trichoma

trichomatous

trichomegaly

trichomycosis
    t.axillaris
    t. chromatica
    t. favosa
    t. rubra

trichonodosis

trichopathic

trichopathy

trichophytic

trichophytid

trichophytobezoar

trichophytosis

trichopoliodystrophy

trichoptilosis

trichorrhexis nodosa

trichoschisis

trichosis carunculae

trichostasis spinulosa

trichothiodystrophy

trichromacy

trichromatism

trichterbrust

trigonitis

trigonocephalia

trigonocephalic

trigonocephalus

trigonocephaly

triiodothyronine

triketohydrindene hydrate

trinucleate

triorchid

triorchidism

triorchism

triphenylmethane

triploid

triploidy

triplokoria

triplopia

tripoding

triptokoria

trisomia

trisomic

trisomy

tristichia

tritan

tritanomal

tritanomalous

tritanomaly

tritanope

tritanopia

tritanopic

tritanopsia

triticeous

trochocephalia

trochocephaly

trombiculiasis

trombiculidiasis

trombidiiasis

trombidiosis

tropate

trophedema

trophodermatoneurosis

trophoedema

trophoneurosis
    facial t.
    lingual t.
    t. of Romberg

trophoneurotic

trophonosis

trophopathia

trophopathy

trophoplast

trophospongium

tropia

tropic acid

tropochrome

trough
    peak and t.

trypanid

trypanosomid

tryptophanuria

tubatorsion

tuber

tubercle
    anatomical t.
    Babè t.
    caseous t.
    dissection t.
    fibrous t.
    Ghon tubercle
    hard tubercle
    hyaline t.
    sebaceous t.

tubercular

tuberculate

tuberculated

tuberculation

tuberculid
    nodular t.
    papular t.
    rosacea-like t.

tuberculin
    albumose-free t.
    alkaline t.
    t. filtrate
    Koch old t.
    t. precipitation
    purified protein derivative
        of t.
    t. reaction

tuberculitis

tuberculization

tuberculocele

tuberculoderma

tuberculoid

tuberculoma

tuberculosis
    acute miliary t.
    adult t.
    aerogenic t.
    anthracotic t.
    attenuated t.
    basal t.

tuberculosis (*continued*)
    central nervous system t.
    cerebral t.
    childhood-type t.
    cutaneous t.
    t. cutis
    t. cutis luposa
    t. orificialis
    t. cutis verrucosa
    dermal t.
    disseminated t.
    endobrachial t.
    extrapulmonary t.
    gastrointestinal t.
    hilus t.
    inhalation t.
    laryngeal t.
    miliary t.
    open t.
    papulonecrotic t.
    pericardial t.
    postprimary t.
    primary t.
    pulmonary t.
    reinfection t.
    secondary t.
    t. of serous membranes
    t. skin test
    tracheobronchial t.

tuberculum

tuberosis

tuberous

tubiferous

tuborrhea

tubotorsion

tubule
    attenuated t.
    collecting t.

tubulocyst

tubulopathy

tubulorrhexis

tubulovesicle

tubulovesicular

tularemia

tumefacient

tumefaction

tumentia

tumescence

tumeur
- t. perlée
- t. pileuse

tumor
- acinar cell t.
- acinic t.
- acoustic nerve t.
- acute splenic t.
- adrenocorticoid rest t.
- adenomatoid odontogenic t.
- adrenal t.
- t. angiogenesis
- benign epithelial breast t.
- Brenner t.
- Brooke t.
- t. burden
- Burkitt t.
- t. of Capella
- carcinoid t.
- cavernous t.
- chemoreceptor t.
- chondromatous giant cell t.
- chromaffin t.
- dendritic cell t.
- dermoid t.
- ductus deferens t.
- eccrine t.
- eighth nerve t.
- endobronchial t.
- endodermal sinus t.
- erectile t.
- Ewing t.
- extrarenal rhabdoid t.
- false t.
- fecal t.
- fibroid t.
- germ cell t.
- giant cell t.

tumor (*continued*)
- glomus jugulare t.
- gonadal stromal t.
- granulation t.
- heterologous t.
- hilar cell t.
- homologous t.
- islet cell t.
- Koenen's t.
- t. lienis
- Leydig cell t.
- Lindau's t.
- malignant mixed mesodermal t.
- margaroid t.
- t. marker
- mast cell t.
- melanotic neuroctodermal t.
- metastatic t.
- t. necrosis
- pancreatic t.
- pearly t.
- phyllodes t.
- Pindborg t.
- plasma cell t.
- Pott's puffy t.
- prostatic t.
- Recklinghausen t.
- renal t.
- renomedullary interstitial cell t.
- rete cell t.
- retinal anlage t.
- Sertoli cell t.
- t. staging
- stercoral t.
- t. suppressor gene
- teratoid t.
- theca cell t.
- thymic t.
- transitional t.
- Triton t.
- ulcerogenic t.
- Warthin t.
- Wilms t.
- Yaba t.
- yolk sac t.
- Zollinger-Ellison t.

tumoral calcinosis

tumor-associated rejection
  antigen (TARA)

tumor-specific
    t-s. antigen
    t-s. transplantation antigen

tumultus

tungiasis

tungsten

tunica albuginea

turbidimeter

turbidimetric

turbidimetry

turgescence

turgescent

turgid

turista

turmschädel

turricephaly

tussiculation

twinning

tyloma

tylosis
    t. ciliaris
    t. palmaris et plantaris

tylotic

tympania

tympanism

tympanites

tympanitic

tympanous

tympany
    Skoda's t.

type and crossmatch

typhlectasis

typhlitis

typhlodicliditis

typhlosis

typing

tyroid

tyromatosis

tyrosinemia
    hepatorenal t.
    hereditary t.
    neonatal t.

tyrosinosis

tyrosinuria

tyrosis

tyrosyluria

tysonitis

U

U6 riboprobe

UA
    urinalysis

uarthritis

ubiquinol

U-cell lymphoma

Uganda S virus

ulcer
    acute hemorrhagic u.
    amebic u.
    amputating u.
    aphthous u.
    atheromatous u.
    atonic u.
    Barrett's u.
    burrowing phagedenic u.
    Buruli u.
    catarrhal corneal u.
    chancroidal u.
    chronic u.
    concealed u.
    corneal u.
    Cruveilhier's u.
    Curling u.
    Cushing's u.
    Cushing-Rokitansky u.
    decubitus u.
    dendritic u.
    diabetic u.
    Dieulafoy u.
    diphtheritic u.
    duodenal u.
    Fenwick-Hunner u.
    fistulous u.
    focal u.
    follicular u.
    gastric u.
    groin u.
    gouty u.
    gummatous u.
    hemorrhagic u.
    herpetic u.
    Hunner's u.

ulcer (*continued*)
    hypertensive ischemic u.
    hypopyon u.
    jejunal u.
    Kocher's dilatation u.
    Lipschütz u.
    lupoid u.
    marginal u.
    Marjolin u.
    Meleney's u.
    Meleney's chronic
      undermining u.
    Mooren's u.
    neurogenic u.
    neurotrophic u.
    penetrating u.
    penetrating u. of foot
    peptic u.
    perambulating u.
    perforating u.
    phagedenic u.
    plantar u.
    pneumococcus u.
    pressure u.
    round u.
    Saemisch's u.
    sea anemone u.
    serpiginous corneal u.
    simple u.
    sloughing u.
    stasis u.
    stercoraceous u.
    stercoral u.
    stomal u.
    stress u.
    submucous u.
    tanner's u.
    trophic u.
    trophoneurotic u.
    undermining burrowing u.
    varicose u.

ulcera

ulcerate

ulceration

ulcerative

ulcerocavernous

ulcerogangrenous

ulcerogenic

ulceromembranous

ulcerous

ulegyria

ulerythema
   u. ophryogenes

uloglossitis

ulorrhagia

ultracentrifugation

ultracentrifuge

ultrafilter

ultrafiltrate

ultrafiltration

ultramicropipet

ultramicroscope

ultramicroscopic

ultramicroscopy

ultramicrotome

ultraphagocytosis

ultrastructure

ultravisible

umber

UMP synthase deficiency

uncarthrosis

unconscious

undernutrition

understain

undertoe

unguis

unicollis

uninephric

uninuclear

uninucleated

unipolar

unit
   alexin u.
   Allen Doisy u.
   androgen u.
   Angstrom u.
   antitoxin u.
   antivenene u.
   atomic mass u.
   Bethesda u.
   biological standard u.
   Bodansky u.
   Bowers-McComb u.
   British thermal u.
   chorionic gonadotropin u.
   Clauberg u.
   complement u.
   diphtheria anitoxin u.
   Ehrlich u.
   electromagnetic u.
   enzyme u.
   estradiol benzoin u.
   estrone u.
   hemolysis u.
   Holzknecht u.
   Hounsfield u.
   Jenner-Kay u.
   Karmen unit
   King unit
   King-Armstrong u
   u. of mass
   MKS u.
   Oxford u.
   u. of penicillin
   pantothenic acid u.
   pepsin u.
   progesterin u.
   prolactin u.
   protein nitrogen u.
   riboflavin u.
   skin test u.

unit (*continued*)
 Somogyi u.
 Svedberg flotation u.
 tetanus antitoxin u.
 u. of thyrotropic activity
 turbidity reducing u.
 u. of wavelength
 v. of weight

univalent antibody

univariate analysis

unmedullated

unmyelinated

Unna-Pappenheim stain

uptake
 absolute iodine u.
 triiodothyronine resin u.
 radioactive iodine u.

uracrasia

uracratia

uranin

uraniscochasma

uraniscolalia

uranoplegia

uranoschisis

uranoschism

uranostaphyloschisis

urapostema

urarthritis

urate

uratemia

uratic

uratohistechia

uratoma

uratosis

uraturia

urea
 u. nitrogen

ureametry

urecchysis

uredema

urelcosis

uremia

uremic

uremigenic

ureometry

ureteralgia

ureterectasia

ureterectasis

ureteritis
 u. cysticus
 u. glandularis

ureterocele

ureteroduodenal

ureteroenteric

ureterointestinal

ureterolith

ureterolithiasis

ureteropathy

ureterophlegma

ureteropyelitis

ureteropyosis

ureterorectal

ureterorrhagia

ureterostenosis

ureterostoma

ureterouterine

ureterovaginal

urethralgia

urethratresia

urethremphraxis

urethrism

urethritis
u. cystica
u. glandularis
follicular u.
gouty u
granular u.
nongonococcal u. (NGU)
nonspecific u.
u. petrificans
posterior u.
prophylactic u.
simple u.

urethroblennorrhea

urethrocele

urethrocystitis

urethrodynia

urethroperineal

urethrophraxis

urethrophyma

urethrorectal

urethrorrhagia

urethrorrhea

urethroscrotal

urethrospasm

urethrostaxis

urethrostenosis

urethrotrigonitis

urethrovaginal

urhidrosis

uricacidemia

uricaciduria

uricemia

uricocholia

uricometer
Ruhemann's u.

uricosuria

Uricult

urinacidometer

urinaemia

urine
black u
chylous u.
cloudy u
crude u.
u. cytology
diabetic u.
dyspeptic u.
febrile u.
u. fungus culture
gouty u.
honey u.
milky u.
nebulous u.
u. osmolality
residual u.
u. sediment crystal

urinemia

urinidrosis

urinocryoscopy

urinoglucosometer

urinoma

urinometer

urinometry

urinoscopy

urinothorax

uriposia

uroacidimeter

uroammoniac

uroazotometer

urobenzoic acid

urobilinemia

urobilinogenemia

urobilinogenuria

urobilinoid

urobilinoiden

urobilinuria

urocanase deficiency

urocele

urocheras

urochezia

urocinetic

uroclepsia

urocrisia

urocriterion

urocystitis

urodialysis

urodynia

uroedema

uroerythrin

uroflavin

urofuscin

urofuscohematin

urogravimeter

urohematonephrosis

urohematoporphyrin

urokinetic

urolith

urolithiasis

urolithic

urolithology

uromelanin

urometer

urometric

urometry

uroncus

uronephrosis

uropathogen

uropathy
    obstructive u.

uropenia

uropepsinogen

urophanic

urophein

urophosphometer

uroplania

uroporphyria

uropsammus

uropyonephrosis

uropyoureter

urosaccharometry

uroscheocele

uroschesis

uroscopic

uroscopy

urosemiology

urosepsis

uroseptic

urosis

urospectrin

urostalagmometry

urostealith

urothelial

urothelium

urotoxia

urotoxic

urotoxicity

urotoxin

urotoxy

uroureter

uroxin

urticant

urticaria
    acute u.
    aquagenic u.
    u. bullosa
    bullous u.
    cholinergic u.
    chronic u.
    cold u.
    colonic u.
    contact u.
    giant u.
    heat u.
    light u.
    u. medicamentosa
    u. multiformis endemica
    papular u.
    u. pigmentosa
    pressure u.
    solar u.
    u. solaris

urticarial

urticarious

urticate

Usher syndrome

uteralgia

uterodynia

uterolith

uterosclerosis

UTI
    urinary tract infection

utriculitis

uveitic

uveitis
    Förster's u.
    granulomatous u.
    heterochromic u.
    lens-induced u.
    nongranulomatous u.
    phacoantigenic u.
    phacotoxic u.
    sympathetic u.
    toxoplasmic u.
    tuberculous u.

uveomeningitis

uveoparotid

uveoscleritis

uvula

uvulitis

uvuloptosis

V

V
   V antigen
   factor V

vacemic cell

vaccinia
   v. gangrenosa
   progressive v.
   v. virus

vaccinia-immune globulin

vacciniform

vacuolar

vacuolate

vacuolated

vacuolation

vacuole
   autophagic v.
   condensing v.
   digestive v.
   heterophagic v.
   plasmocrine v.
   rhagiocrine v.
   water v.

vacuolization

vacuome

vagina
   congenital absence of v.

vaginismus

vaginitis (pl. vaginitides)
   adhesive v.
   atrophic v.
   candidal v.
   desquamative inflammatory
      v.
   diphtheritic v.
   emphysematous v.
   senile v.
   v. testis
   trichomonas v.

vaginocele

vaginodynia

vaginomycosis

vaginopathy

vaginosis
   bacterial v.

vagotonia

vagotonic

vagotony

valinemia

value
   absolute v.
   acetyl v.
   acid v.
   buffer v.
   globular v.
   iodine v.
   normal v.
   predictive v.
   reference v.
   threshold limit v.
   valence v.

vanillism

vanillylmandelic acid

vanilmandelic acid

variant
   L-phase v.
   migraine v.
   petit mal v.

varication

variceal

varicella
   v. gangrenosa

varices

variciform

varicoblepharon

varicocele
    ovarian v.
    pelvic v.
    tubo-ovarian v.
    utero-ovarian v.

varicoid

varicomphalus

varicophlebitis

varicose
    v. aneurysm

varicosis (pl. varicoses)

varicosity

varicula

variegate porphyria

variola
    v. benigna
    v. hemorrhagica
    v. maligna
    v. pemphigosa
    v. verrucosa

varix (pl. varices)
    anastomotic v.
    aneurysmal v.
    arterial v.
    cirsoid v.
    esophageal v.
    lymph v.
    v. lymphaticus

vasculitis
    Churg-Strauss v.
    granulomatous cerebral v.
    hypersensitivity v.
    hypocomplementemic v.
    leukocytoclastic v.
    livedo v.
    necrotizing v.
    nodular v.
    pulmonary v.
    rheumatoid v.
    segmented hyalinizing v.
    systemic v.
    urticarial v.

vasculotoxic

vasoneuropathy

vasoneurosis

vasoparesis

vasospasm

vasospastic

vasovagal

vasovesiculitis

Vecta stain

veil
    aqueduct v.
    Jackson's v.

vein
    aqueous v.
    varicose v.

venectasia

venereal
    v. disease
    v. disease – gonorrhea
    V. Disease Research
      Laboratory (VDRL)
    v. lymphogranuloma
    v. ulcer
    v. wart

venin

Venn diagram

venofibrosis

venom
    antisnake v.
    kokoi v.
    Protac v.

veno-occlusive

venosclerosis

venostasis

venous
    v. claudication
    v. congestion
    v. hematocrit

venous (*continued*)
  v. thrombosis

ventriculitis

ventriculoencephalitis
  cytomegalovirus v.

ventriculomegaly

ventroptosia

ventroptosis

venulitis
  cutaneous necrotizing v.

verotoxin

verruca (pl. verruccae)
  v. acuminata
  v. digitata
  v. filiformis
  v. glabra
  v. mollusciformis
  v. necrogenica
  v. peruana
  v. plana
  v. plana juvenilis
  v. plana senilis
  v. plantaris
  seborrheic v.
  v. simplex
  v. vulgaris

verrucae

verruciform

verrucose

verrucosis

verrucous
  v. carcinoma
  v. endocarditis
  v. papilloma
  v. vegetation

verruga

verumontanitis

vesicant

vesication

vesicatory

vesicle
  acrosomal v.
  archoplasmic v.
  concentrating v.
  germinal v.
  intermediate v.
  matrix v.
  olfactory v.
  pinocytotic v.
  plasmalemmal v.
  Purkinje v.
  secretory v.
  synaptic v.
  transfer v.
  transitional v.
  transport v.

vesicoabdominal

vesicocele

vesicocervical

vesicocolic

vesicocolonic

vesicoenteric

vesicointestinal

vesicoperineal

vesicopustule

vesicouterovaginal

vesicovaginal

vesicovaginorectal

vesicular

vesiculated

vesiculation

vesiculiform

vesiculitis

vesiculocavernous

vesiculopapular

vesiculopustular

vesiculotympanic

vesiculotympanitic

vestibular anus

vestibulitis

vestigial

vesuvine

viable cell count

vibex

vibices

vicine

videomicroscopy

villin

villitis

villonodular

villositis

villus (pl. villi)
    v. of choroid plexus

vinculin

violaceous

violet
    cresyl v. acetate
    cresyl v.
    cresylecht v.
    crystal v.
    Hofmann's v.
    iodine v.
    Lauth's v.
    methyl v.
    methylene v.
    gentian v.
    hexamethyl v.

viremia

virilescence

virilism
    adrenal v.

virilization

virolactia

viruria

visceralgia

visceromegaly

viscerotome

viscerotomy

viscometer

viscometry

viscosimeter
    Ostwald v.
    Stormer v.

viscosimetry

vitanition

vitiatin

vitiation

vitiligines

vitiliginous

vitiligo
    v. iridis

vitium

vitreous
    detached v.
    primary persistent
      hyperplastic v.

vitritis

voix
    v. de Polichinelle

volumetric

volumette

volutin

volutrauma

volvulate

volvulus
    v. neonatorum

vomit

vomit (*continued*)
    Barcoo v.
    bilious v.
    black v.
    coffee-ground v.

vomitus
    v. cruentus
    v. matutinus

vortex
    Fleischer's vortex
    vortex lentis

vulvismus

vulvitis
    atrophic v.
    diabetic v.

vulvitis (*continued*)
    eczematiform v.
    erosive v.
    leukoplakic v.
    phlegmonous v.
    plasma cell v.
    v. plasmocellularis
    pseudoleukoplakic v.
    ulcerative v.

vulvopathy

vulvorectal

vulvovaginitis
    Candida v.
    senile v.
    candidal v.

Wako NEFA test kit

Wallenberg syndrome

wallerian degeneration

walleye

Walsh average

WAMPOLE ISOLATER blood
   culture system

Wang test

Warburg theory

warfarin assay

wart
   acuminate w.
   anatomical w.
   common w.
   digitate w.
   filiform w.
   genital w.
   Hassall-Henle w.
   mosaic w.
   necrogenic w.
   plane w.
   plantar w.
   postmortem w.
   prosector's w.
   seborrheic w.
   telangiectatic w.
   tuberculous w.
   venereal w.

wasserhelle

wasting
   salt w.

water brash

wen

wheal

Webb antigen

Wegener
   W. granulomatosis

Wegener (*continued*)
   W. syndrome

Weigert-Gram stain

weight
   atomic w.
   gram-molecular w.
   molar w.
   molecular w.

Welcozyme HIV 1&2 ELISA
   antibody test

whitlockite

whitlow
   herpetic w.
   thecal w.

Whitmore-Jewett tumor staging
   system

whooping cough

whorl
   bone w.

Wilder stain for reticulum

Wilkins-Chigren agar

Wilms tumor

withering crypt appearance

Witkop disease

WMR
   work metabolic rate

Wohlegemuth unit

wound
   avulsed w.
   blowing w.
   sucking w.

Wratten filter

wrist
   SLAC w.
   tennis w.

wryneck

X

xanchromatic

xanthelasma

xanthelasmatosis

xanthene

xanthin

xanthinuria

xanthinuric

xanthism

xanthiuria

xanthochromatic

xanthochromia
   x. striata palmaris

xanthochromic

xanthocyanopsia

xanthoderma

xanthoerythrodermia
   x. perstans

xanthokyanopy

xanthoma
   craniohypophyseal x.
   diabetic x.
   disseminated x.
   eruptive x.
   x. multiplex
   x. palpebrarum
   planar x.
   plane x.
   x. planum
   x. striatum palmare
   x. tendinosum
   tendinous x.
   tuberoeruptive x.
   x. tuberosum
   x. tuberosum multiplex
   tuberous x.
   craniohypophysial x.

xanthomatosis

xanthomatosis (*continued*)
   biliary
      hypercholesterolemic x.
   x. bulbi
   cerebrotendinous x.
   chronic idiopathic x.
   x. corneae
   x. generalisata ossium
   x. iridis
   primary familial x.
   Wolman x.

xanthomatous

xanthopia

xanthoproteic acid

xanthoprotein

xanthopsia

xanthosis

xanthurenic acid

xanthuria

xanthyl

xenomenia

xenophthalmia

xerocyte

xerocytosis

xeroderma

xerodermatic

xerodermia

xerodermoid

xeroma

xeromenia

xeromycteria

xerophthalmia

xerophthalmus

xerosis

xerosis (*continued*)
 x. conjunctivae
 conjunctival x.
 x. corneae
 corneal x.
 x. cutis
 x. generalisata
 x. parenchymatosa
 x. superficialis

xerostomia

xerotic

xiphodynia

xiphoiditis

xylene

xylidine

xylol

Y

Y
    Y. body
    Y. chromatin
    Y. chromosome

yaws

y-axis

yeast
    baker's y.
    y. extract agar
    y. fungus

yellow
    acridine y.
    alizarin y.
    y. atrophy of liver
    y. corallin

yellow (*continued*)
    y. fever
    y. hepatization
    hydrazine y.
    Leipzig y.
    martius y.
    metaline y
    methyl y.
    titan y.

yield
    quantum y.

yolk

y. sac carcinoma

Young syndrome

ytterbium

z-axis

zeiosis

zeism

zeismus

Zenker
Z. degeneration
Z. diverticulum
Z. fixative

zenkerism

zenkerize

zeoscope

Ziehl stain

zinc
z. assay
z. flocculation test
z. formalin
z. phosphide
z. sulfate centrifugal
flotation technique
z. turbidity test

zincalism

zoacanthosis

zonal necrosis

zonate

zone
active z.
antibody excess z.
biokinetic z.
ependymal z.
epileptogenic z.
z. of exclusion
Golgi z.
grenz z.

zone (*continued*)
hyperesthetic z.
juxtanuclear z.
keratogenous z.
mantle z.
marginal z.
Nitabuch z.
nuclear z.
z. of oval nuclei
z. of partial preservation
pellucid z.
z. of round nuclei
transformation z.
Turck's z.
Weil's basal z.

zonesthesia

zonulitis

zooblast

zoosperm

zoster
herpes z.
ophthalmic z.

zuckergussdarm

zuckergussleber

zygodactyly

zygomycosis
rhinocerebral z.

zygotene

zygotoblast

zymogen granule

zymogram

zymoplastic substance

zymosan

Appendix A: Bacteria

Abiotrophia
    A. adiacens
    A. defectiva

Acanthanamoeba
    A. castellanii
    A. culbertsoni
    A. hartmannella
    A. hatchetti
    A. keratitis
    A. polyphaga
    A. rhysodes

Acanthia lectularia

Acanthobdella

Acanthocephala

Acanthocheilonema
    A. perstans
    A. streptocera

Acarus
    A. folliculorum
    A. gallinae
    A. hordei
    A. rhizoglypticus hyacinthi
    A. scabiei
    A. siro

Acaulium

Achillea

Acholeplasma
    A. laidlawii

Achorion
    A. violaceum

Achromobacter group B
    Achromobacter group E

Acidaminococcus
    A. fermentans

Acidovorax
    A. delafieldii
    A. temperans

Acinetobacter

Acinetobacter (*continued*)
    A. anitratus
    A. baumannii
    A. calcoaceticus
    A. calcoaceticus anitratus
    A. calcoaceticus lwoffi
    A. genomospecies 3
    A. haemolyticus
    A. johnsonii
    A. junii
    A. lwoffii
    A. parapertussis

Acladium

Aconitum

Acremonium

Acrotheca
    A. pedrosoi

Acrothesium
    A. floccosum

Actinobacillus
    A. actinomycetemcomitans
    A. equuli
    A. hominis
    A. lignieresii
    A. mallei
    A. pseudomallei
    A. suis
    A. ureae

Actinobaculum schaalii

Actinomadura
    A. africana
    A. madurae
    A. pelletieri

actinoides
    Thysanosoma a.

Actinomyces
    A. bernardiae
    A. bovis
    A. congolensis
    A. eriksonii

Actinomyces (*continued*)
- A. europaeus
- A. georgiae
- A. gerencseriae
- A. graevenitzii
- A. israelii
- A. meyeri
- A. muris
- A. muris-ratti
- A. naeslundii
- A. necrophorus
- A. neuii
- A. odontolyticus
- A. pyogenes
- A. radingae
- A. rhusiopathiae
- A. turicensis
- A. vinaceus
- A. viscosus

Actinoplanes

Actinopoda

Acuaria spiralis

Adansonia

Adiantum

Aerobacter
- A. aerogenes
- A. cloacae
- A. liquefaciens
- A. subgroup A, B, C

Aerococcus
- A. caviae
- A. hydrophila
- A. jandaei
- A. media
- A. schubertii
- A. salmonicida
- A. trota
- A. urinae
- A. veronii biovar sobria
- A. veronii biovar veronii
- A. viridans 1
- A. viridans 2
- A. viridans 3

Aeromonas

Aeromonas (*continued*)
- A. hydrophila
- A. liquefaciens
- A. punctata
- A. salmonicida

Afipia
- A. broomeae
- A. clevelandensis
- A. felis
- A. genomospecies 1
- A. genomospecies 2

Agamodistomum
- A. ophthalmobium

Agamomermis culicis

Agamonema

Agamonematodum
- A. migrans

Agarbacterium

Agaricus

agouti

Agrobacterium

Ajellomyces
- A. capsulatum
- A. dermatitidis
- A. dermatitis

Alcaligenes
- A. bookeri
- A. bronchisepticus
- A. denitrificans
- A. faecalis
- A. faecalis type II
- A. marshalli
- A. odorans
- A. piechaudii
- A. recti

Alectorobius talaje

Aletris

Alginomonas

Allescheria boydii

Allodermanyssus
   A. sanguineus

Alloiococcus otitis

Alocinma

Alphavirus

Alstonia

Alternaria
   I. tenuis

Amanita
   A. muscaria
   A. phalloides
   A. virosa

ambiguus
   Passalurus a.

Amblyomma

Ambrosia

Amidostomum anseris

Amoeba
   A. buccalis
   A. coli
   A. coli mitis
   A. dentalis
   A. dysenteriae
   A. histolytica
   A. meleagridis
   A. urogenitalis
   A. verrucosa

Amoebotaenia

Amycolata
   A. autotrophica

Anaerobiospirillum
   A. succiniciproducens
   A. thomasii

Anaerorhabdus
   A. furcosus

Anaplasma

Anatrichosoma

Ancylostoma
   A. braziliense

Ancylostoma (*continued*)
   A. caninum
   A. duodenale

Angiostrongylus
   A. cantonensis

Anguillula

Anisakis
   A. marina

Ankylostoma

anomalus
   Hoplopsyllus a.

Anopheles
   A. maculipennis

Anoplocephala

anseris
   Amidostomum a.

Anthomyia
   A. canicularis
   A. incisura

apiospermum
   Monosporium a.
   Scedosporium a.

Apium

Apocynum

Arachis hypogaea (AH)

Arachnia
   A. propionica

Arcanobacterium
   A. haemolyticum

Arcobacter
   A. butzleri
   A. cryaerophilus

Argas
   A. persicus
   A. reflexus   .

Arizona
   A. hinshawii
   A. organism

Armigeres
   A. obturbans

Armillifer
   A. armillatus
   A. moniliformis

Arthrobacter
   A. cumminsii
   A. woluwensis

Arthroderma

Arthographis
   A. langeroni

Artyfechinostomum

Ascaridia

Ascaris
   A. alata
   A. canis
   A. lumbricoides
   A. mystax
   A. pneumonitis
   A. suum

Ascarops
   A. strongylina

Aspergillus
   A. auricularis
   A. barbae
   A. bouffardi
   A. candidus
   A. concerntricus
   A. fisherii
   A. flavus
   A. fumigatus
   A. giganteus
   A. glaucus
   A. gliocladium
   A. mucoroides
   A. nidulans
   A. niger
   A. ochraceus
   A. parasiticus
   A. pictor
   A. repens
   A. terreus
   A. versicolor

Aspiculuris tetraptera

Asterococcus

Atelosaccharomyces

Atopobium
   A. minutum
   A. parvulum
   A. rimae

Atrax
   A. robustus

Auchmeromyia

Aurococcus

Aviadenovirus

Avipoxvirus

avium-intracellulare
   Mycobacterium a.-i. (MAC, MAI)

Azotobacter

Babesia
   B. microti

Babesiella

Bacillus
   B. aerogenes capsulatus
   B. aertrycke
   B. alvei
   B. ambiguus
   B. anthracis
   B. botulinus
   B. brevis
   B. bronchisepticus
   B. cereus
   B. cereus var. mycoides
   B. circulans
   B. coagulans
   B. coli
   B. diphtheriae
   B. dysenteriae
   B. enteritidis
   B. faecalis alcaligenes
   B. firmus
   B. influenzae
   B. larvae

Bacillus (*continued*)
    B. laterosporus
    B. leprae
    B. licheniformis
    B. macerans
    B. mallei
    B. megaterium
    B. necrophorus
    B. oedematiens
    B. oedematis maligni
    B. oedematis maligni No. II
    B. pertussis
    B. pestis
    B. pneumoniae
    B. polymyxa
    B. proteus
    B. pseudomallei
    B. pumilus
    B. pyocyaneus
    B. sphaericus
    B. stearothermophilus
    B. subtilis
    B. suipestifer
    B. tetani
    B. thuringiensis
    B. tuberculosis
    B. tularense
    B. typhi
    B. typhosus
    B. welchii
    B. whitmori

Bacterium

Bacteroides
    B. caccae
    B. capillosus
    B. coagulans
    B. corrodens
    B. distasonis
    B. eggerthii
    B. forsythus
    B. fragilis
    B. macacae
    B. melaninogenicus
    B. ochraceus
    B. ovatus
    B. pneumosintes
    B. putredinis

Bacteroides (*continued*)
    B. ruminicola
    B. serpens
    B. splanchnicus
    B. stercoralis
    B. tectum
    B. thetaiotaomicron
    B. uniformis
    B. ureolyticus
    B. vulgatus

Balantidium
    B. coli

Bartonella
    B. bacilliformis
    B. clarridgeiae
    B. elizabethae
    B. henselae
    B. quintana

Basidiobolus
    B. haptosporus

Baylisascaris

Bdellonyssus
    B. bacoti

Beauvaria

Belascaris

Belneatrix
    B. alpica

Bergeyella
    B. zoohelcum

Bertiella
    B. studeri

Besnoitia

bieneusi
    Enterocytozoon b.

Bifidobacterium
    B. adolescentis
    B. angulatum
    B. bifidum
    B. breve
    B. catenulatum
    B. denticolens

Bifidobacterium (*continued*)
- B. dentium
- B. eriksonii
- B. gallicum
- B. infantis
- B. inopinatum
- B. longum
- B. pseudocatenulatum
- B. pseudolongum

Bilharzia

Bilophila
- B. wadsworthia

Biomphalaria
- B. glabrata

Bithynia

Blastocystis
- B. hominis

Blastoschizomyces
- B. brasiliensis
- B. capitatus
- B. coccidioides
- B. dermatitidis

Blatta

Blattella

Bodo
- B. caudatus
- B. saltanas
- B. urinaria

Boletus

Boophilus
- B. annulatus

Bordetella
- B. bronchiseptica
- B. hinzii
- B. holmesii
- B. parapertussis
- B. pertussis
- B. trematum

Borrelia
- B. burgdorferi
- B. duttonii

Borrelia (*continued*)
- B. hermsii
- B. hispanica
- B. parkeri
- B. persica
- B. recurrentis
- B. turicatae
- B. venezuelensis

Bothriocephalus

Bothrops
- B. atrox *serine proteinase*

Botryomyces

Bovicola

boydii
- Allescheria b.
- Pseudallescheria b.

Brachyspira aalborgi

Branhamella
- B. catarrhalis

brasiliensis
- Paracoccidioides b.

Brevibacterium
- B. casei
- B. epidermidis

Brevundimonas
- B. diminuta
- B. vesicularis

Brucella
- B. abortus
- B. bronchiseptica
- B. canis
- B. melitensis
- B. suis

Brugia
- B. malayi
- B. microfilariae

Budvicia
- B. aquatica

Bulimus
- B. fuchsianus

Bulinus

Bunostomum

Burkholderia
    B. cepacia
    B. gladioli
    B. mallei
    B. pseudomallei

Buttiauxella
    B. noackiae

Butyrivibrio
    B. crossotus
    B. fibrisolvens

CDC Alcaligenes-like group 1
    CDC group DF-3
    CDC group DF-3-like
    CDC group EF-4a
    CDC group EF-4b
    CDC group EO-2
    CDC group EO-3
    CDC group F-1
    CDC group G-1
    CDC group G-2
    CDC group I
    CDC group IIc
    CDC group IIg
    CDC group IV c-2
    CDC group Ic
    CDC group NO-1
    CDC group O-1
    CDC group O-2
    CDC group WO-1

calcitrans
    Stomoxyus c.

Callatomonas
    C. turbata

Calliphora
    C. vomitoria

Callitroga

Calvatia
    C. gigantea

Calymmatobacterium
    C. donovania
    C. granulomatis

Campylobacter
    C. concisus
    C. fetus intestinalis
    C. fetus jejuni
    C. gracilis
    C. hyointestinalis
    C. lari
    C. mucosalis
    C. pylori
    C. rectus
    C. sputorum
    C. upsaliensis

Candida
    C. aaseri
    C. albicans
    C. catenulata
    C. ciferrii
    C. colliculosa
    C. dubliniensis
    C. etchellsii
    C. famata
    C. glabrata
    C. guilliermondii
    C. haemulonii
    C. humicola
    C. inconspicua
    C. intermedia
    C. kefyr
    C. krusei
    C. lambica
    C. lipolytica
    C. lusitaniae
    C. magnoliae
    C. maris
    C. melibiosica
    C. membranaefaciens
    C. norvegensis
    C. parapsilosis
    C. pelliculosa
    C. pulcherrima
    C. rugosa
    C. silvae
    C. stellatoidea
    C. tropicalis
    C. viswanathii
    C. zeylanoides

Canavalia

caninum
    Diphylidium c.

Canis

Capillaria
    C. hepactica
    C. philippinenisis

capillatus
    Solenopotes c.

Capnocytophaga
    C. canimorsus
    C. cynodegmi
    C. gingivalis
    C. granulosa
    C. haemolytica
    C. ochracea
    C. sputigena

Capripoxvirus

capsulata
    Emmonsiella c.

capsulatum
    Ajellomyces c.
    Histoplasma c.

Cardiobacterium
    C. hominis

Carica
    C. papaya

carinii
    Pneumocystis c.

Carpoglyphus
    C. passularum

casei
    Philopia c.
    Piophila c.

Castellanella
    C. castellani

Castellania

Catalpa

catanella
    Gonyaulax c.

Catenabacterium

cati
    Notoedres c.

Caulobacter

Cedecea
    C. davisae
    C. lapagei
    C. neteri

Cellfalcicula

Cellulomonas
    C. hominis

Cellvibrio
    C. mixtus

Centrocestus

Centruroides

Cephaelis

Cephalomyia

Cephalosporium
    C. falciforme
    C. granulomatis

Ceratophyllus

Cercomonas

Cercopithecus

Cerithidea

Cetraria

ceylonica
    Haemadipsa c.

Chabertia

Chaetomium

Chenopodium

Cheyletiella
    C. parasitovorax

Chilomastix
    C. mesnili

Chlamydia
    C. oculogenitalis

Chlamydia (*continued*)
- C. pneumoniae
- C. psittaci
- C. trachomatis

Chlamydophrys

Chlamydozoon

Chlorobacterium

Chlorobium

Chlorochromatium

Choanotaenia infundibulum

Choleraesuis

Chorioptes

Chromobacterium
- C. violaceum

Chromohalobacter marismortui

Chryseobacterium
- C. indologenes
- C. meningosepticum

Chryseomonas luteola

Chrysomyia

Chrysops

Chrysosporium parvum

Cicuta

Cillobacterium

Cimex lectularius

Citellis

Citrobacter
- C. amalonaticus
- C. braakii
- C. diversus
- C. farmeri
- C. freundii
- C. koseri
- C. sedlakii
- C. werkmanii
- C. youngae

Cladorchis watsoni

Cladothrix

Clathrochloris

Clathrocystis

Claviceps purpurea

Clitocybe

Clonorchis sinensis

Clostridium
- C. aminovalericum
- C. aurantibutyricum
- C. baratii
- C. barkeri
- C. beijerinckii
- C. bifermentans
- C. botulinum
- C. butyricum
- C. cadaveris
- C. carnis
- C. celatum
- C. cellobioparum
- C. chauvoei
- C. clostridiiforme
- C. cochlearium
- C. cocleatum
- C. difficile
- C. fallax
- C. felsineum
- C. ghonii
- C. glycolicum
- C. haemolyticum
- C. hastiforme
- C. histolyticum
- C. indolis
- C. innocuum
- C. irregulare
- C. leptum
- C. limosum
- C. malenominatum
- C. mangenotii
- C. nexile
- C. novyi A
- C. novyi B
- C. oceanicum
- C. orbiscindens
- C. oroticum
- C. paraputrificum

Clostridium (*continued*)
C. perfringens
C. putrifaciens
C. putrificum
C. ramosum
C. sardiniense
C. sartagoforme
C. scatologenes
C. septicum
C. sordellii
C. sphenoides
C. spiroforme
C. sporogenes
C. sporosphaeroides
C. subterminale
C. symbiosum
C. tertium
C. tetani
C. tyrobutyricum
C. welchii

Cnephia

Coccidioides
C. immitis

Cochliomyia
C. hominivorax

Coenurus

Collyriclum

Comamomas
C. acidivorans
C. testosteroni

Conidiobolus
C. incongruus

Coniosporium

Conium

Cooperia

Coprinus

Copromastix
C. prowazeki

Copromonas
C. subtilis

Cordylobia
C. anthropophaga

Coronavirus

corticale
Cryptostroma c.

Corynebacterium
C. accolens
C. acnes
C. afermentans
C. amycolatum
C. aquaticum
C. argentoratense
C. auris
C. bovis
C. coyleae
C. diphtheriae
C. genitalium
C. glucuronolyticum
C. imitans
C. jeikeium
C. kutscheri
C. macginleyi
C. matruchotii
C. minutissimum
C. mycetoides
C. propinquum
C. pseudodiphthericum
C. pseudogenitalium
C. pseudotuberculosis
C. renale group
C. striatum
C. ulcerans
C. urealyticum
C. xerosis

Coryzavirus

costaricensis
Morerastrongylus c.

Councilmania

Cowdria ruminantium

Coxiella
C. brunetii

Craigia

Crenosoma vulpis

Crithidia

Crotalus

cruzi
　Schizotrypanum c.

Cryptococcus
　C. albidus 1
　C. albidus 2
　C. curvatus
　C. gastricus
　C. kuetzingii
　C. laurentii
　C. luteolus
　C. neoformans
　C. terreus
　C. uniguttulatus

Cryptocystis trichodectis

Cryptosporidium

Cryptostroma corticale

Ctenocephalides
　C. canis

culbertsoni
　Acanthamoeba c.

Culex

culicis
　Agamomermis c.

Culicoides

Culiseta melanura

Cunninghamella elegans

Curvularia

Cuterebra

Cyathostoma

Cyathostomum

Cyclops

Cyclospora

Cysticercus
　C. bovis
　C. cellulosae
　C. fasciolaris
　C. ovis
　C. tenuicollis

Cytauxzoon

Dactylaria

Damalinia

Dasyprocta

Davainea

davtiani
　Teladorsagia d.

Debaryomyces
　D. hansenii
　D. hominis
　D. neoformans

Dematium

Demodex
　D. folliculorum

dentatus
　Stephanurus d.

Dependovirus

Dermacentor
　D. andersoni
　D. occidentalis
　D. reticulatus
　D. variabilis

Dermacentroxenus
　D. akari
　D. australis
　D. conori
　D. orientalis
　D. rickettsi
　D. sibericus

Dermanyssus gallinae

dermatitidis
　Ajellomyces d.
　Blastomyces d.

Dermatobia
　D. hominis

Dermatophagoides
　pteronyssinus

Dermatophilus
　D. congolensis
　D. penetrans

Desmodus

destruens
    Hyphomyces d.

Dialister

Diaptomus

Dibrothriocephalus

Dichelobacter
    D. nodosus

Dicrocoelium
    D. dendriticum

Dictycaulus
    D. viviparus

Didelphis

Dientamoeba fragilis

Digitalis

Digramma
    D. brauni

Dimastigamoeba

Dinobella
    D. ferax

Dioctophyma
    D. renale

Dipetalonema
    D. perstans
    D. streptocerca

Diphyllobothrium
    D. latum

Diplococcus
    D. constellatus
    D. magnus
    D. morbillorum
    D. mucosus
    D. palepneumoniae
    D. plagarumbello
    D. pneumoniae

Diplogaster

Diplogonoporus
    D. brauni
    D. grandis

Dipus sagitta

Dipylidium caninum

Dirofilaria
    D. conjunctivae
    D. immitis
    D. repens
    D. tenuis

Distoma

Distomum

Dolosigranulum pigrum

Donovania
    D. granulomatis

Dracunculus
    D. medinensis

Drechslera hawaiiensis

Drepanospira

Drosophilia

Duboisia

Duttonella

Eberthella
    E. typhi

echidninus
    Laelaps e.

Echidnophaga gallinacea

Echinochasmus

Echinococcus
    E. granulosus
    E. multilocularis

Echinostoma
    E. ilocanum
    E. linoensis
    E. malayanum
    E. perfoliatum
    E. revolutum

E. coli
    Escherichia coli

Edwardsiella
    E. tarda
    E. tarda biogroup 1

Ehrlichia

Eikenella
    E. corrodens

Eimeria

Elaeophora
    E. schneideri

elizabethae
    Bartonella e.

Embadomonas

Emmonsiella capsulata

Empedobacter brevis

Encephalitozoon

Endamoeba

Endodermophyton

Endolimax
    E. nana

Endomyces
    E. albicans
    E. capsulatus
    E. epidermatidis
    E. epidermidis
    E. geotrichum

Entamoeba
    E. buccalis
    E. coli
    E. gingivalis
    E. hartmanni
    E. histolytica
    E. nana
    E. polecki
    E. tetragena
    E. tropicalis

Entemopoxvirus

Enteric
    E. group 58
    E. group 60
    E. group 68

Enteritidis
    E. salmonella

Enterobacter
    E. aerogenes
    E. agglomerans
    E. alvei
    E. amnigenus biogroup 1
    E. amnigenus biogroup 2
    E. asburiae
    E. cancerogenus
    E. cloacae
    E. gergoviae
    E. hafniae
    E. hormaechei
    E. kobei
    E. liquefaciens
    E. sakazakii

Enterobius
    E. vermicularis

Enterococcus
    E. avium
    E. casseliflavus
    E. durans
    E. faecalis
    E. faecium
    E. flavescens
    E. gallinarum
    E. malodoratus
    E. mundtii
    E. raffinosus

Enterocytzoon
    E. bieneusi

Enteromonas
    E. hominis

Enterovirus

Entoloma sinuatum

Entomomophthora
    E. coronata

Eperythrozoon

Epidermophyton
    E. floccosum
    E. inguinale
    E. rubrum

Escherichia
    E. coli

Escherichia (*continued*)
 E. coli, inactive
 E. fergusonii
 E. hermanii
 E. vulneris

equi
 Rhodococues e.

equorum
 Parascaris e.

Erysipelothrix
 E. insidiosa
 E. rhusiopathiae

Erythrobacillus

Erythrobacter longus

Escherichia (Esch.)
 E. aurescens
 E. coli (EC, *E. coli*)
 E. coli *enterotoxin*
 E. dispar *var.* ceylonensis
 E. dispar *var.* madampensis

esulenta
 Gyromitra e.
 Helvella e.

Eubacterium
 E. aerofaciens
 E. alactolyticum
 E. biforme
 E. brachy
 E. combesii
 E. contortum
 E. cylindroides
 E. dolichum
 E. endocarditis
 E. eligens
 E. exiguum
 E. formicigenerans
 E. hadrum
 E. hallii
 E. lentum
 E. limosum
 E. minutum
 E. moniliforme
 E. nitritogenes
 E. nodatum

Eubacterium (*continued*)
 E. parvum
 E. ramulus
 E. rectale
 E. saburreum
 E. saphenum
 E. siraeum
 E. tenue
 E. timidum
 E. tortuosum
 E. ventriosum

Euglena
 E. gracilis

Euparyphium

europaeus
 Ulex e.

Eurotium
 E. malignum

Eusimulium

Eustrongylus

Eutrombicula
 E. alfreddugesi

Ewingella americana

Exophiala
 E. jeanselmei
 E. mycetoma
 E. werneckii

expansa
 Moniezia e.

Exserohilum longirostratum

Facklamia hominis

faecalis
 Vibrio f.

Fannia
 F. canicularis
 F. scalaris

Fasciola
 F. gigantica
 F. hepatica

Fascioloides magna

Fasciolopsis
F. buski

felis
Afipia f.

Ferribacterium

Fibrobacter succinogenes

Filaria
F. bancrofti
F. conjunctivae
F. demarquayi
F. hominis oris
F. juncea
F. labialis
F. lentis
F. loa
F. lymphatica
F. medinensis
F. ozzardi
F. palpebralis
F. philippinensis
F. sanguinis
F. tucumana
F. volvulus

Filaroides

Filobasidiella
F. bacillisporus
F. neoformans

Filovirus

Flavimonas oryzihabitans

Flavivirus

Flavobacterium
F. meningosepticum
F. IIe
F. IIh
F. IIi

follicilorum
Simonea f.

Fonsecaea
F. compactum
F. dermatitidis
F. jeanselmei
F. pedrosoi

fragilis
Dientamoeba f.

Francisella
F. philomiragia
F. (Pasteurella) tularensis
F. tularensis

Fusarium
F. moniliforme

Fusiformis
F. necrophorus

Fusobacterium
F. aquatile
F. fusiforme
F. glutinosum
F. gonidiaformans
F. mortiferum
F. naviforme
F. necrogenes
F. necrophorum
F. nucleatum
F. perfoetens
F. plauti-vincentii
F. prausnitzii
F. russii
F. symbiosum
F. varium

Gadus

Gaffkya

gallinacea
Echidnophaga g.

gallinae
Dermanyssus g.

Gardnerella
G. vaginalis

Gastrodiscoides hominis

Gastrodiscus hominis

Gastrophilus

Gastrospirillum hominis

Gedoelstia

genavense
Mycobacterium g.

Gemella
    G. haemolysans
    G. morbillorum

Geodermatophilus

Geophilus

Geotrichum
    G. candidum
    Endomyces g.
    G. penicillatum

Giardia
    G. intestinalis
    G. lamblia

Gigantorhynchus

Gilardi Rod Group 1

Globidium

Globicatella sanguis

Globocephalus

Glossina

Glyciphagus
    G. buski
    G. domesticus

Glycophagus

Glycyphagus
    G. domesticus

Gnathostoma
    G. spinigerum

Gongylonema
    G. pulchrum

Gonyaulax catanella

Gordius
    G. aquaticus
    G. robustus

Gordona
    G. aichiensis
    G. bronchialis
    G. rubropertincta
    G. sputi
    G. terrae

gougerotii
    Sporotrichum g.

Graphium

Gregarina

Grisonella ratellina

Gymnoascus

Gymnodinium

Gyromitra esculenta

Habronema

Hadrurus

Haemadipsa ceylonica

Haemagogus

Haemaphysalis
    H. concinna
    H. leporis-palustris
    H. spinigera

Haematopinus

Haemobartonella

Haecoccidium

Haemodipsus vetricosus

Haemogregarina

Haemonchus
    H. contortus
    H. placei

Haemophilus
    H. aegyptius
    H. aphrophilus
    H. ducreyi
    H. haemolyticus
    H. influenzae
    H. parahaemolyticus
    H. parainfluenzae
    H. paraphrophilus
    H. segnis

Haemoproteus

Hafnia
    H. alvei

Halteridium

Hansenula
   H. jadinii
   H. polymorpha

Haplorchis

Hartmannella

hatchetti
   Acanthamoeba h.

Haverhillia
   H. moniliformis
   H. multiformis

Hebeloma

Helcococcus kunzii

Helicobacter
   H. cinaedi
   H. fenneliae
   H. pullorum
   H. pylori
   H. westmeadii

helmintheca
   Neorickettsia h.

Helminthosporium

Heloderma

Helophilus

Helvella
   H. esculenta

Hemispora stellata

Hemobartonella

Hendersonula toruloidea

henselae
   Bartonella h.
   Rochalimaea h.

Hepatocystis

Hepatozoon

Hermetia
   H. illucens

Herpetomonas

Herpetomonas (*continued*)
   H. donovani
   H. furunculosa
   H. tropica

Heterakis

Heterobilharzia

Heterodera
   H. radicicola

Heterodoxus spiniger

Heterophyes
   H. heterophyes
   H. katsuradai

Hexamita

Hippelates

Hippeutis

Hippobosca

Hirudo
   H. aegyptiaca
   H. medicinalis

Histomonas meleagridis

Histoplasma
   H. capsulatum
   H. farciminosus

Holophyra coli

Homalomyia

hominis
   Gastrodiscoides h.
   Gastrodiscus h.
   Octomitus h.

Hoplopsyllus anomalus

Hyalomma
   H. variegatum

Hydatigeria
   H. infantis
   H. taeniaeformis

Hydrotaea

Hylemyia

Hymenolepis
   H. diminuta
   H. nana

Hyostrongylus rubidus

Hyphomyces destruens

Hyphopichia burtonii

Hypoderma
   H. bovis

hypogaea
   Arachis h. (AH)

Indiella

Inermicapsifer
   I. madagascariensis

Inocybe

insidiosum
   Pythium i.

intestinalis
   Lamblia i.
   Septata i.

Iodamoeba
   I. bütschlii

Ipomoea

Iridovirus

irritans
   Siphoma i.

Isoparorchis
   I. trisimilitubis

Isospora
   I. belli
   I. hominis

Ixodes
   I. bicornis
   I. cavipalpus
   I. cookei
   I. dammini
   I. frequens
   I. holocyclus
   I. pacificus
   I. persulcatus

Ixodes (*continued*)
   I. rasus
   I. ricinus
   I. scapularis
   I. spinipalpis

Jatropha

Johnsonella ignava

Kingella
   K. dinitrificans
   K. kingae
   K. orale

Klebsiella
   K. friedländeri
   K. group 47
   K. oxytoca
   K. planticola
   K. pneumoniae
   K. rhinoscleromatis

Kloeckera
   K. apis
   K. japonica

Kluyvera
   K. ascorbata
   K. cryocrescens

Knemidokoptes

Kurthia
   K. gibsonii
   K. zopfii

Lachesis

Lactarius

Lactobacillus
   L. acidophilus
   L. brevis
   L. buchneri
   L. bulgaris
   L. casei
   L. catenaformis
   L. crispatus
   L. fermentum
   L. gasseri
   L. jensenii
   L. johnsonii

Lactobacillus (*continued*)
    L. leichmannii
    L. paraplantarum
    L. plantarum
    L. reuteri
    L. salivarius
    L. uli

Lactococcus
    L. cremoris
    L. garvieae
    L. lactis
    L. plantarum

Laelaps echidninus

Lagochilascaris
    L. minor

Lamblia intestinalis

Lasiohelea

Latrodectus
    L. bishopi
    L. geometricus
    L. mactans

Lautropia mirabilis

Laverania

Leclercia adecarboxylata

lectularia
    Acanthia l.

lectularius
    Cimex l.

Legionella
    L. bozemanii
    L. jordanis
    L. longbeachae
    L. pneumophila

Leischmania
    L. braziliensis
    L. caninum
    L. donovani
    L. infantum
    L. nilotica
    L. peruviana
    L. tropica

Leminorella
    L. grimontii
    L. richardii

Lentzea albidocapillata

leonina
    Toxascaris l.

leporipoxvirus

Leptoconops

Leptomonas

Leptopsylla
    L. segnis

Leptospira
    L. australis
    L. autumnalis
    L. biflexa
    L. canicola
    L. grippotyphosa
    L. hebdomidis
    L. hyos
    L. icterohaemorrhagiae
    L. interrogans
    L. pomona

Leptothrix

Leptotrichia
    L. buccalis

Leptotrombidium
    L. akamushi
    L. deliense

Leucocytozoon

Leuconostoc
    L. citreum
    L. lactis
    L. mesenteroides
    L. pseudomesenteroides

Leukocytozoon

Leukosporidium

Leukovirus

Limnatis nilotica

Linguatula
    L. serrata

Lingonathus

Liponyssus

Listerella

Listeria
> L. grayi
> L. innocua
> L. ivanovii
> L. monocytogenes
> L. seeligeri
> L. welshimeri

Lithobius

Loa
> L. loa

Loboa loboi

loboi
> Loboa l.

longior
> Tyroglyphus l.

longirostratum
> Exserohilum l.

longispiculata
> Nematodirella l.

Lophophora

Loxosceles
> L. laeta
> L. reclusa

Loxoterma ovatum

Lucilia

lupi
> Spirocerca l.

Lutzomyia

Lycoperdon

Lymantria

Lymnaea

Lyponyssus

Lyssavirus

Lytta

Macaca

Macracanthorhynchus
> M. hirudinaceus

Macrobdella

Macromonas
> M. bipunctata
> M. mobilis

macrorchis
> Prosthogonimus m.

Madurella
> M. grisea
> M. mycetomi

magna
> Fascioloides m.

MAI
> Mycobacterium avium-
>   intracellulare

Malassezia
> M. furfur
> M. macfadyani
> M. ovalis
> M. pachydermatis
> M. tropica

Malleomyces
> M. mallei
> M. malleomyces
> M. pseudomallei
> M. whitmori

Mallophaga

Mansonella
> M. ozzardi

mansoni
> Oxyspirura m.
> Schistosoma m.

Mansonia

Mansonoides

Margaropus

Marshallagia marshalli

marshalli
> Marshallagia m.

Mastadenovirus

Mastophora

Mecistocirrus

Megalopyge

Megamonas hypermegas

Megaselia

Megasphera

Melanoides

Melanolestes
    M. picipes

melanura
    Culiseta m.

meleagridis
    Histomonas m.

Melophagus

Menopon

Mentha

Mesocestoides
    M. variabilis

Metagonimus
    M. ovatus
    M. yokogawai

Metastrongylus
    M. elongatus

Methanobacterium

Methanococcus

Metopium

Metorchis

Microbacterium
    M. arborescens
    M. imperiale

Micrococcus
    M. kristinae
    M. luteus
    M. sedentarius

Microfilaria

Microfilaria (*continued*)
    M. bancrofti
    M. streptocerca

Microsporon

Microsporum
    M. audouinii
    M. canis
    M. felineum
    M. ferrugineum
    M. fulvum
    M. furfur
    M. gallinae
    M. gypseum
    M. lanosum
    M. nanum
    M. persicolor
    M. vanbreuseghemi

Microtrombidium

Microtus

Micrurus

Miescheria

Mima
    M. polymorpha

Mitsuokella multiacidus

Miyagawanella

Mobiluncus
    M. curtisii
    M. mulieris

Moellerella wisconsensis

Moniezia expansa

Monilia

Moniliformis
    M. moniliformis

Mononchus

Monosporium apiospermum

Monostoma

Monotricha

Moraxella

Moraxella (*continued*)
- M. atlantae
- M. bovis
- M. catarrhalis
- M. lacunata
- M. lincolnii
- M. nonliquefaciens
- M. osloensis
- M. phenylpyruvica

Morbillivirus

Morerastrongylus costaricensis

Morganella
- M. morganii

Mortierella

Mucor

Mucuna

Muellerius capillaris

Multiceps
- M. multiceps

multipapillosa
- Parafilaria m.

Musca
- M. domestica

Mycobacterium
- M. abscessus
- M. africanum
- M. aichiense
- M. asiaticum
- M. aurum
- M. avium
- M. bovis
- M. branderi
- M. celatum
- M. chelonae
- M. confluentis
- M. conspicuum
- M. duvalii
- M. flavescens
- M. fortuitum
- M. gadium
- M. gastri
- M. genavense

Mycobacterium (*continued*)
- M. gilvum
- M. gordonae
- M. haemophilum
- M. hassiacum
- M. interjectum
- M. intermedium
- M. intracellulare
- M. kansasii
- M. lentiflavum
- M. leprae
- M. malmoense
- M. marinum
- M. mucogenicum
- M. neoaurum
- M. nonchromogenicum
- M. obuense
- M. perigrinum
- M. rhodesiae
- M. scrofulaceum
- M. shimoidei
- M. simiae
- M. smegmatis
- M. species
- M. szulgai
- M. terrae
- M. thermoresistibile
- M. triplex
- M. triviale
- M. tuberculosis
- M. ulcerans
- M. vaccae
- M. xenopi

Mycocandida

Mycoplana
- M. bullata
- M. dimorpha

Mycoplasma
- M. buccale
- M. faucium
- M. felis
- M. fermentans
- M. genitalium
- M. hominis
- M. lipophilum
- M. orale

Mycoplasma (*continued*)
    M. penetrans
    M. pneumoniae
    M. primatum
    M. salivarium
    M. spermatophilum

Myrmecia

Myroides odoratimimus

Myxococcidium stegomyiae

Myzomyia

Myzorhynchus

Naegleria

Nannizzia

Nanophyetus salmincola

Necator
    N. americanus

Neisseria
    N. canis
    N. cinera
    N. elongata
    N. flavescens
    N. gonorrhoeae
    N. lactamica
    N. meningitidis
    N. mucosa
    N. polysaccharea
    N. sicca
    N. subflava
    N. weaveri

Nematodirella longispocilata

Nematodirus

Neoascaris vitulorum

Neorickettsia helmintheca

Neotestudina rosati

Neurospora

Nicotiana

Nigrospora

Nippostrongylus

Nitrobacter

Nitrocystis

Nocardia
    N. asteroides
    N. brasiliensis
    N. caviae
    N. farcinica
    N. leishmanii
    N. lutea
    N. madurae
    N. nova
    N. otitidiscaviarum
    N. pseudobrasiliensis
    N. transvalensis

Nocardiopsis dassonvillei

Noguchia
    N. granulosus

Nosema

Nosopsyllus
    N. fasciatus

Notoedres cati

Nucleophaga

Nuttallia

Nyctotherus

Nyssorhynchus

Ochrobacterum anthropi

Ochromyia
    O. anthropophaga

Octomitus hominis

Octomyces
    O. etiennei

Odontobutis

Oerskovia xanthineolytica

Oesophagotomum
    O. apiostomum
    O. bifurcum
    O. stephanostomum

Oestrus

Oestrus (*continued*)
    O. hominis
    O. ovis

Oligella
    O. ureolytica
    O. urethralis

Onchocerca
    O. caecutiens
    O. cervicalis
    O. lienalis
    O. volvulus

Oncocerca

Oncomelania

Oncorhynchus

Onthophagus

Oospora

Opisthorchis
    O. felineus
    O. noverca
    O. viverrini

Orbivirus

Ornithobilharzia

Ornithodoros
    O. coriaceus

Orinthonyssus

Orthopodomyia

Orthopoxvirus

Ostertagia

Otobius

Otodectes

Otomyces
    O. hageni
    O. purpureus

ovarii
    Pseudomyxoma o.

ovatum
    Loxotrema o.

Oxyspirura mansoni

Oxytrema

Oxyuris
    O. incognita
    O. vermicularis

Paecilomyces

Paederus

Palaemonetes

Paludina

Pangonia

Panstrongylus

Pantoea agglomerans

Papaver

Papillomavirus

Parabuthus

Parachordodes

Paracoccidioides brasiliensis

Paracolobactrum
    P. aerogenoides
    P. arizonae
    P. coliforme
    P. intermedium

Parafilaria multipapillosa

Parafossarulus

Paragonimus
    P. africans
    P. caliensis
    P. heterotremus
    P. kellicotti
    P. mexicanus
    P. westermani

Paragordius
    P. cintus
    P. tricuspidatus
    P. varius

Paramecium
    P. coli

Paramoeba

Paramphistomum

Paramyxovirus

Paraponera

Parapoxvirus

Parasa

Parasaccharomyces
P. ashfordi

Parascaris equorum

Parastrongylus

Parvovirus
P. B 19

parvum
Chrysosporium p.

Paryphostomum
P. sufrartyfex

Pasteurella
P. aerogenes
P. bettyae
P. canis
P. dagmatis
P. enterocolitica
P. gallinarum
P. haemolytica
P. multocida
P. pestis
P. pneumotropica
P. pseudotuberculosis
P. septica
P. stomatis
P. tularensis
P. volantium

Pectobacterium
P. carotovorum

Pediculoides verticosus

Pediculus
P. humanus
P. humanus capitus
P. humanus corporis
P. inguinalis
P. pubis

Pediococcus
P. acidilactici
P. equinus
P. pentosaceus

penetrans
Sarcopsylla p.
Tunga p.

Penicillium
P. barbae
P. bouffardi
P. minimum
P. montoyai
P. notatum
P. patulum
P. spinulosum

Pentastoma
P. constrictum
P. denticulatum
P. taenioides

Pentatrichomonas
P. ardin delteili

Peptococcus
P. anaerobius
P. asaccharolyticus
P. constellatus
P. magnus
P. niger
P. prevotii

Peptostreptococcus
P. anaerobius
P. asaccharolyticus
P. harei
P. hydrogenalis
P. indolicus
P. livorii
P. lacrimalis
P. lactolyticus
P. magnus
P. micros
P. octavius
P. prevotii
P. productus
P. tetradius
P. vaginalis

Periplaneta

Pestivirus

Petriellidium
P. boydii

Phaenicia sericata

Phialophora
P. compactum
P. dermatitidis
P. gougerotii
P. jeanselmei
P. mutabilis
P. parasitica
P. repens
P. richardsia
P. spinifera
P. verrucosa

Philopia casei

Phlebotomus
P. argentipes
P. chinensis
P. intermedius
P. macedonicum
P. noguchi
P. papatasii
P. sergenti
P. verrucarum
P. vexator

Phlebovirus

Phobetron

Phoma
P. hibernica

Phormia regina

Photorhabdus luminescens

Phthirus
P. pubis

Physa

Physaloptera
P. caucasica
P. mordens

Physocephalus sexalatus

Physopsis

Phytobdella

Pichia
P. carsonii
P. etchellsii
P. farinosa
P. membranaefaciens

Piedraia
P. hortae

Pila

Piophila casei

Pirenella

Piroplasma

Pityrosporon
P. orbiculare
P. ovale
P. versicolor

Pityrosporum
P. furfur
P. orbiculare
P. ovale

Plagiorchis

Plantago

Pleisiomonas shigelloides

Pleospora

Plesiomonas

Pneumocystis
P. carnii
P. pneumoniae

pneumoniae
Chlamydia p.
Pneumocystis p.

Pneumovirus

Pogonomyrmex

Polistes

Pollenia

Polydesmus

Polyomavirus

polyphaga
Acanthamoeba p.

Polyplax

Polyplis

Pomatiopsis

Porocephalus
P. armillatus
P. clavatus
P. constrictus
P. denticulatus

Porphyromonas
P. asaccharolytica
P. catoniae
P. endontalis
P. gingivalis
P. levii

Porthetria

Potamon

Prevotella
P. bivia
P. buccae
P. buccalis
P. corporis
P. dentalis
P. denticola
P. disiens
P. enoeca
P. heparinolytica
P. intermedia
P. loescheii
P. melaninogenica
P. nigrescens
P. oralis
P. oris
P. oulorum
P. ruminocola
P. tannerae
P. veroralis
P. zoogleoformans

Prionurus

Probstymayria vivipara

Propionibacterium
P. acnes
P. avidum
P. granulosum
P. lymphophilum
P. propionicum

Proprioniferax innocua

Prosthogonimus macrorchis

Proteus
P. inconstans
P. mirabilis
P. morganii
P. OC-19
P. penneri
P. rettgeri
P. stuartii
P. vulgaris

Protostrongylus rufescens

Prototheca
P. ciferrii
P. filamenta
P. wickerhamii
P. zopfii

Providencia
P. alcalifaciens
P. providenciae
P. rettgeri
P. rustigianii
P. stuartii

Prowazekia

Psammolestes

Pselaphephilia

Pseudallescheria boydii

Pseudamphistomum
P. truncatum

Pseudogordius

Pseudohazis

Pseudomonas
P. acidovorans
P. aeruginosa
P. alcaligenes

Pseudomonas (*continued*)
P. cepacia
P. diminuta
P. eisenbergii
P. fluorescens
P. fragi
P. kingii
P. mallei
P. maltophilia
P. mendocina
P. monteilii
P. multivorans
P. nonliquefaciens
P. paucimobilis
P. pertucinogena
P. pseudoalcaligenes
P. pseudomallei
P. putida
P. putrefaciens
P. pyocyanea
P. stutzeri
P. syncyanea
P. testosteroni
P. thomasii
P. viscosa

Pseudmonilia

Pseudomyxoma
P. ovarii

Pseudoramibacter alactolyticus

Pseudostertagia bullosa

Pseudothelphusa

Psilocybe

Psorergates

Psorophora

Psoroptes

Psychrobacter immobilis

Pthirus

Pulex
P. irritans

Pullularia
P. pullulans

Puntius

purpurea
Claviceps p.

purpureus
Rhinoestrus p.

putrescentiae
Tyrophagus p.

Pyemotes tritici

Pyrazus

Pyrenochaeta romeroi

pyriformis
Tetrahymena p.

Pythium insidiosum

quintana
Bartonella q.

Rahnella aquatilis

Raillietina
R. celebensis
R. demerariensis

Ralstonia pickettii

ratellina
Grisonella r.

Rattus

Reduvius

regina
Phormia r.

Reovirus

Retortamonas
R. intestinalis

Rettgerella rettgeri

Rhabditis
R. hominis

Rhabdomonas

Rhinocladiella

Rhinocladium

Rhinoestrus purpereus

Rhinosporidium seeberi

Rhinovirus

Rhipocentor

Rhipicephalus
R. sanguineus

Rhizobium

Rhizoglyphus
R. parasiticus

Rhizopus
R. arrhizus
R. equinus
R. niger
R. nigricans
R. prolixus
R. rhizopodoformis

Rhodnius

Rhodococcus
R. equi
R. obuensis

Rhodophyllus sinuatus

Rhodotorula
R. minuta
R. rubra 1
R. rubra 2
R. glutinis

Rhombomys

rhysodes
Acanthamoeba r.

Rickettsia
R. akamushi
R. akari
R. australis
R. burnetti
R. canada
R. conorii
R. diaporica
R. mooseri
R. muricola
R. nipponica
R. orientalis
R. pavlovskii

R. prowazekii
R. quintana
R. rickettsii
R. sibirica
R. tsutsugamushi
R. tyhpi
R. wolhynica

Rikenella microfusus

Rochalimaea
R. henselae
R. quintana

romeroi
Pyrenochaeta r.

rosati
Neotestudina r.

Roseomonas
R. cervicalis
R. fauriae
R. genomospecies 4
R. genomospecies 5
R. genomospecies 6
R. gilardii

Rothia dentocariosa

rubidus
Hyostrongylus r.

Rubivirus

rufescens
Protostrongylus r.

ruminantium
Cowdria r.

Ruminobacter
R. amylophilus

Russula emetica

Sabethes

Saccharomonospora viridis

Saccharomyces
S. albicans
S. anginae
S. apiculatus
S. cantliei

Schizosaccharomyces

Schizotrypanum cruzi

schneideri
Elaeophora s.

Sclerostoma

Scolopendra

Scopulariopsis
S. americana
S. aureus
S. blochi
S. brevicaulis
S. cinereus
S. koningi
S. minimus

Scutigera

Sebaldella termitidis

seeberi
Rhinosporidium s.

Segmentina

Selenomonas
S. aretemidis
S. dianae
S. flueggei
S. infelix
S. noxia
S. sputigena

Semisulcospina

Septata
S. intestinalis

sericata
Phaenicia s.

Sericopelma
S. communis

Serpulina pilosicoli

Serratia
S. ficaria
S. fonticola
S. indica
S. kiliensis
S. liquefaciens

Serratia (*continued*)
S. marcescens
S. odorifera
S. plymuthica
S. rubidaea

Setaria

sexalatus
Phsyocephalus s.

Shewanella
S. alga
S. putrifaciens

Shigella
S. alkalescens
S. ambigua
S. arabinotarda
S. boydii
S. ceylonensis
S. dipar
S. dysenteriae
S. etousae
S. flexneri
S. madampensis
S. newcastle
S. paradysenteriae
S. parashigae
S. schmitzii
S. sonnei
S. wakefield

Sibine

Siderobacter

Siderocapsa

Siderococcus

simicola
Pneumonyssus s.

Simonea folliculorum

Simonsiella muelleri

Simulium

sinensis
Clonorchis s.

sinuatum
Entoloma s.

Saccharomyces (*continued*)
  S. capillitii
  S. carlsbergensis
  S. cerevisiae 1
  S. cerevisiae 2
  S. coprogenus
  S. epidermica
  S. galacticolus
  S. glutinis
  S. hominis
  S. lemonneri
  S. mellis
  S. mycoderma
  S. neoformans
  S. pastorianus
  S. telluris

Saccharopolyspora
  rectivirgula

sagitta
  Dipus s.

Saksenaea

salmincola
  Nanophyetus s.
  Troglotrma s.

Salmonella
  S. arizonae
  S. bongori
  S. cholerae-suis
  S. derby
  S. enteritidis
  S. gallinarum
  S. hirschfeldii
  S. indiana
  S. infantis
  S. minnesota
  S. montevideo
  S. muenchen
  S. newington
  S. oranienburg
  S. paratyphi
  S. pullorum
  S. schottülleri
  S. sendai
  S. thompson
  S. typhi

Salmonella (*continued*)
  S. typhimurium
  S. typhisuis
  S. typhosa
  S. virginia

Salmonella-Shigella (SS)

Salvia
  S. horminium
  S. sclarea

Sanguisuga

Sappinea
  S. diploidea

Saprospira

Sarcina
  S. ventriculi

Sarcinosporon inkin

Sarcocystis

Sarcophaga
  S. carnaria
  S. dux
  S. fuscicauda
  S. haemorrhoidalis
  S. nificornis
  S. rubicornis

Sarcopsylla penetrans

Sarcoptes scabiei

scabiei
  Sarcoptes s.

Scaurus

Scedosporium apiospermum

Scheloribates

Schistosoma
  S. haematobium
  S. intercalatum
  S. japonicum
  S. mansoni

Schizoblastosporion

Schizophyllum commune

Schizosaccharomyces

Schizotrypanum cruzi

schneideri
Elaeophora s.

Sclerostoma

Scolopendra

Scopulariopsis
S. americana
S. aureus
S. blochi
S. brevicaulis
S. cinereus
S. koningi
S. minimus

Scutigera

Sebaldella termitidis

seeberi
Rhinosporidium s.

Segmentina

Selenomonas
S. aretemidis
S. dianae
S. flueggei
S. infelix
S. noxia
S. sputigena

Semisulcospina

Septata
S. intestinalis

sericata
Phaenicia s.

Sericopelma
S. communis

Serpulina pilosicoli

Serratia
S. ficaria
S. fonticola
S. indica
S. kiliensis
S. liquefaciens

Serratia (*continued*)
S. marcescens
S. odorifera
S. plymuthica
S. rubidaea

Setaria

sexalatus
Phsyocephalus s.

Shewanella
S. alga
S. putrifaciens

Shigella
S. alkalescens
S. ambigua
S. arabinotarda
S. boydii
S. ceylonensis
S. dipar
S. dysenteriae
S. etousae
S. flexneri
S. madampensis
S. newcastle
S. paradysenteriae
S. parashigae
S. schmitzii
S. sonnei
S. wakefield

Sibine

Siderobacter

Siderocapsa

Siderococcus

simicola
Pneumonyssus s.

Simonea folliculorum

Simonsiella muelleri

Simulium

sinensis
Clonorchis s.

sinuatum
Entoloma s.

Siphona irritans

Siphunculina

Sisyrosea

Solenopotes capillatus

Solenopsis

Sparganum
  S. proliferum

Spelotrema

Sphaerophorus
  S. necrophorus

Sphingobacterium
  S. mizutae
  S. multivorum
  S. spiritivorum
  S. thalpophilum
  S. yabuuchiae

Sphingomonas paucimobilis

spiniger
  Heterodoxus s.

spiralis
  Acuaria s.

Spirillum
  S. minor
  S. minus

Spirocerca lupi

Spirochaeta
  S. daxensis
  S. eurystrepta
  S. marina
  S. plicatilis
  S. stenostrepta

Spirometra

Sporobolomyces
  S. roseus
  S. salmonicolor

Sporothrix
  S. schenckii

Sporotrichum
  S. beurmanni

Sporotrichum (*continued*)
  S. gougerotii
  S. schenckii

stagnora

Stamnosoma

Staphylococcus
  S. aureus
  S. auricularis
  S. capitis
  S. caprae
  S. carnosus
  S. cohnii
  S. epidermidis
  S. haemolyticus
  S. hominis
  S. hyicus
  S. intermedius
  S. lugdunensis
  S. pasteuri
  S. pulvereri
  S. saccharolyticus
  S. saprophyticus
  S. schleiferi
  S. simulans
  S. warneri
  S. xylosus

Stasisia

Stegobium

Stegomyia

stegomyiae
  Myxococcidium s.

Stelangium

Stellantchasmus

Stenotrophomonas
  S. africana
  S. maltophilia

Stephanofilaria stilesi

Stephanurus dentatus

Sterculia

Sterigmatomyces
  S. elviae
  S. halophilus

stilesi
Stephanofilaria s.

Stomatococcus mucilaginosus

Stomoxys calcitrans

Strengeria

Streptobacillus
S. moniliformis
S. pseudotuberculosis
Streptococcus
S. acidominimus
S. agalactiae
S. anginosus
S. bovis
S. canis
S. constellatus
S. cricetus
S. crista
S. dysgalactiae
S. equi
S. gordonii
S. hansenii
S. iniae
S. intermedius
S. microaerophilic
S. mitis
S. mutans
S. oralis
S. pleomorphus
S. pneumoniae
S. porcinus
S. pyogenes
S. rattus
S. salivarius
S. sanguis
S. sobrinus
S. uberis
S. vestibularis
S. viridans
S. zooepidemicus
S. zymogenes

Streptomyces
S. madurae
S. paraguayensis
S. somaliensis

Streptothrix

strongylina
Ascarops s.

Strongyloides
S. fulleborni
S. stercoralis

Strongylus

Succinivibrio
S. dextrinosolvens

Superstitionia

Sutterella wadsworthensis

Suttonella indologenes

Syncephalastrum

Syngamus
S. laryngeus
S. trachea

Synosternus
S. pallidus

Syphacia
S. obvelata

Tabanus

Taenia
T. africana
T. bremneri
T. canina
T. confusa
T. diminuta
T. echinococcus
T. lata
T. murina
T. nana
T. philippina
T. saginata
T. solium
T. taeniaeformis

taeniaeformis
Hydatigera t.

Taeniarhynchus

Taeniorhynchus

talaje
Alectorobius t.

Tamulus

Tatlockia micdadei

Tatumella ptyseos

Teladorsagia davtiani

Tenebrio

Ternidens
　T. diminutus

Tetrahymena pyriformis

tetraptera
　Aspiculuris t.

Tetratrichomonas
　T. buccalis
　T. hominis

Thaumetopoea

Theileria

Thelazia
　T. callipaeda

Thermoactinomyces
　T. candidus
　T. sacchari
　T. vulgaris

Thermolospora viridis

Thiara

Thysanosoma actinoides

Tissierella praeacuta

Tityus serrulatus

Torula
　T. capsulatus
　T. histolytica

toruloidea
　Hendersonula t.

Torulopsis
　T. glabrata

Toxascaris leonina

Toxocara
　T. canis
　T. cati
　T. mystax

Toxoplasma
　T. gondii
　T. pyrogenes

Trachybdella bistriata

Treponema
　T. amylovorum
　T. buccale
　T. calligyrum
　T. carateum
　T. denticola
　T. genitalis
　T. macrodentium
　T. maltophilum
　T. medium
　T. microdentium
　T. minutum
　T. mucosum
　T. pallidum
　T. pectinovorum
　T. pertenue
　T. phagedenis
　T. pintae
　T. refringens
　T. scoliodontum
　T. socranskii
　T. vincentii

Triatoma

Tricercomonas

Trichinella
　T. spiralis

Trichobilharzia

Trichocephalus
　T. trichiura

Trichodectes

trichodectis
　Cryptocystis t.

Tricholoma
　T. pardinum

Tricholomapardinum

Trichomonas
　T. buccalis
　T. hominis

Trichomonas (*continued*)
    T. intestinalis
    T. pulmonalis
    T. tenax
    T. vaginalis

Trichophyton
    T. concentricum
    T. crateriforme
    T. epilans
    T. equinum
    T. ferrugineum
    T. gallinae
    T. glabrum
    T. gourvilii
    T. gypseum
    T. megninii
    T. mentagrophytes
    T. purpureum
    T. rosaceum
    T. sabouraudi
    T. schoenleinii
    T. simii
    T. sulfureum
    T. tonsurans
    T. verrucosum
    T. violaceum

Trichopleuris

Trichoprosopon

Trichosporon
    T. beigelii
    T. cutaneum
    T. giganteum
    T. pedrosianum
    T. pullulans

Trichostrongylus
    T. axei
    T. brevis
    T. colubriformis
    T. instabilis
    T. orientalis
    T. probolurus
    T. vitrinus

Trichothecium
    T. roseum

Trichuris
    T. trichiura

Tricula

Triodontophorus
    T. diminutus

Triphleps insidiosus

tritici
    Pyemotes t.

Troglotrema salmincola

Trombicula
    T. akamushi
    T. alfreddugesi
    T. autumnalis
    T. deliensis
    T. irritans
    T. pallida
    T. scutellaris
    T. tsalsahuatl
    T. vandersandi

Tropheryma whippelii

Tropicorbis

Trypanoplasma

Trypanosoma
    T. ariarii
    T. brucei
    T. castellani
    T. cruzi
    T. gambiense
    T. hominis
    T. nigeriense
    T. rangeli
    T. rhodesiense
    T. ugandense

Tsukamurella
    T. inchonensis
    T. paurometabola
    T. pulmonis
    T. tyrinosolvens

Tunga penetrans

Turbatrix
    T. aceti

Turicella otitidis

Tyroglyphus
    T. longior
    T. siro

Tyrophagus putrescentiae

Tyzzeria

Ulex
    U. europaeus

Uncinaria
    U. americana
    U. duodenalis

Ureaplasma
    U. urealyticum

Uronema caudatum

Ustilago
    U. maydis
    U. zeae

Vaginulus plebeius

vasorum
    Haemostrongylus v.

Veillonella
    V. alcalescens
    V. discoides
    V. orbiculus
    V. parvula
    V. reniformis
    V. vulvovaginitidis

Vejovis

Vena

ventricosus
    Haemodipsus v.
    Pediculoides v.

Verticillium
    V. graphii

Vesiculovirus

Vibrio
    V. alginolyticus
    V. carchariae
    V. cholerae

Vibrio (*continued*)
    V. cincinnatiensis
    V. damsela
    V. fluvialis
    V. furnissii
    V. hollisae
    V. metschnikovii
    V. mimicus
    V. natiensis
    V. niger
    V. parahaemolyticus
    V. proteus
    V. septicus
    V. sputorum
    V. tyrogenus
    V. vulnificus

Vicia
    V. graminea

vitulorum
    Neoascaris v.

Viviparus

Volutella
    V. cinerescens

Volvox

Vorticella

vulpis
    Crenosoma v.

Wangiella

watsoni
    Cladorchis w.
    Watsonius w.

Watsonius watsoni

Weeksella virosa

Weissella paramesenteroides

Wohlfartia
    W. magnifica
    W. opaca
    W. vigil

Wolinella succinogenes

Wuchereria

Appendix B: Normal Values

Reference Values for the Interpretation of Laboratory Tests*

Reference Intervals for Hematology

Test	Conventional Units	SI Units
Acid hemolysis (Ham test)	No hemolysis	No hemolysis
Alkaline phosphatase, leukocyte	Total score 14–100	Total score 14–100
Cell counts		
Erythrocytes		0/L
Males	4.6–6.2 million/mm^3	4.6–6.2 × 10^{12}/L
Females	4.2–5.4 million/mm^3	4.2–5.4 × 10^{12}/L
Children (varies with age)	4.5–5.1 million/mm^3	4.5–5.1 × 10^{12}/L
Leukocytes, total	4500–11,000/mm^3	4.5–11.0 × 10^9/L
Leukocytes, differential counts†		
Myelocytes	0%	0/L
Band neutrophils	3–5%	150–400 × 10^6/L
Segmented neutrophils	54–62%	3000–5800 × 10^6/L
Lymphocytes	25–33%	1500–3000 × 10^6/L
Monocytes	3–7%	300–500 × 10^6/L
Eosinophils	1–3%	50–250 × 10^6/L
Basophils	0–1%	15–50 × 10^6/L
Platelets	150,000–400,000/mm^3	150–400 × 10^9/L
Reticulocytes	25,000–75,000/mm^3 (0.5–1.5% of erythrocytes)	25–75 × 10^9/L
Coagulation tests		
Bleeding time (template)	2.75–8.0 min	2.75–8.0 min
Coagulation time (glass tube)	5–15 min	5–15 min
D-Dimer	<0.5 μg/mL	<0.5 mg/L
Factor VIII and other coagulation factors	50–150% of normal	0.5–1.5 of normal
Fibrin split products (Thrombo-Wellco test)	<10 μg/mL	<10 mg/L

Appendix B: Normal Values

Reference Values for the Interpretation of Laboratory Tests*

Reference Intervals for Hematology

Test	Conventional Units	SI Units
Acid hemolysis (Ham test)	No hemolysis	No hemolysis
Alkaline phosphatase, leukocyte	Total score 14–100	Total score 14–100
Cell counts		
Erythrocytes		
Males	4.6–6.2 million/mm³	4.6–6.2 × 10¹²/L
Females	4.2–5.4 million/mm³	4.2–5.4 × 10¹²/L
Children (varies with age)	4.5–5.1 million/mm³	4.5–5.1 × 10¹²/L
Leukocytes, total	4500–11,000/mm³	4.5–11.0 × 10⁹/L
Leukocytes, differential counts†		0/L
Myelocytes	0%	0/L
Band neutrophils	3–5%	150–400 × 10⁶/L
Segmented neutrophils	54–62%	3000–5800 × 10⁶/L
Lymphocytes	25–33%	1500–3000 × 10⁶/L
Monocytes	3–7%	300–500 × 10⁶/L
Eosinophils	1–3%	50–250 × 10⁶/L
Basophils	0–1%	15–50 × 10⁶/L
Platelets	150,000–400,000/mm³	150–400 × 10⁹/L
Reticulocytes	25,000–75,000/mm³ (0.5–1.5% of erythrocytes)	25–75 × 10⁹/L
Coagulation tests		
Bleeding time (template)	2.75–8.0 min	2.75–8.0 min
Coagulation time (glass tube)	5–15 min	5–15 min
D-Dimer	<0.5 µg/mL	<0.5 mg/L
Factor VIII and other coagulation factors	50–150% of normal	0.5–1.5 of normal
Fibrin split products (Thrombo-Wellco test)	<10 µg/mL	<10 mg/L

Reference Intervals for Hematology (continued)

Test	Conventional Units	SI Units
Fibrinogen	200–400 mg/dL	2.0–4.0 g/L
Partial thromboplastin time, activated (aPTT)	20–35 s	20–35 s
Prothrombin time (PT)	12.0–14.0 s	12.0–14.0 s
Coombs' test		
Direct	Negative	Negative
Indirect	Negative	Negative
Corpuscular values of erythrocytes		
Mean corpuscular hemoglobin (MCH)	26–34 pg/cell	26–34 pg/cell
Mean corpuscular volume (MCV)	80–96 μm^3	80–96 fL
Mean corpuscular hemoglobin concentration (MCHC)	32–36 g/dL	320–360 g/L
Haptoglobin	20–165 mg/dL	0.20–1.65 g/L
Hematocrit		
Males	40–54 mL/dL	0.40–0.54
Females	37–47 mL/dL	0.37–0.47
Newborns	49–54 mL/dL	0.49–0.54
Children (varies with age)	35–49 mL/dL	0.35–0.49
Hemoglobin		
Males	13.0–18.0 g/dL	8.1–11.2 mmol/L
Females	12.0–16.0 g/dL	7.4–9.9 mmol/L
Newborns	16.5–19.5 g/dL	10.2–12.1 mmol/L
Children (varies with age)	11.2–16.5 g/dL	7.0–10.2 mmol/L
Hemoglobin, fetal	<1.0% of total	<0.01% of total
Hemoglobin A_{1c}	3–5% of total	0.03–0.05 of total

Reference Intervals for Hematology (*continued*)

Test	Conventional Units	SI Units
Hemoglobin A_2	1.5–3.0% of total	0.015–0.03 of total
Hemoglobin, plasma	0.0–5.0 mg/dL	0.0–3.2 μmol/L
Methemoglobin	30–130 mg/dL	19–80 μmol/L
Sedimentation rate (ESR)		
Wintrobe: Males	0–5 mm/h	0–5 mm/h
Females	0–15 mm/h	0–15 mm/h
Westergren: Males	0–15 mm/h	0–15 mm/h
Females	0–20 mm/h	0–20 mm/h

*From William Z. Borer, Reference Values for the Interpretation of Laboratory Tests. *In* Robert E. Rakel (ed.): Conn's Current Therapy 2000. Philadelphia, W.B. Saunders Company, 2000.
†Conventional units are percentages; SI units are absolute counts.

Reference Intervals* for Clinical Chemistry (Blood, Serum, and Plasma)

Analyte	Conventional Units	SI Units
Acetoacetate plus acetone		
Qualitative	Negative	Negative
Quantitative	0.3–2.0 mg/dL	30–200 μmol/L
Acid phosphatase, serum (thymolphthalein monophosphate substrate)	0.1–0.6 U/L	0.1–0.6 U/L
ACTH (see Corticotropin)		
Alanine aminotransferase (ALT) serum (SGPT)	1–45 U/L	1–45 U/L
Albumin, serum	3.3–5.2 g/dL	33–52 g/L
Aldolase, serum	0.0–7.0 U/L	0.0–7.0 U/L
Aldosterone, plasma		
Standing	5–30 ng/dL	140–830 pmol/L
Recumbent	3–10 ng/dL	80–275 pmol/L
Alkaline phosphatase (ALP), serum		
Adult	35–150 U/L	35–150 U/L
Adolescent	100–500 U/L	100–500 U/L
Child	100–350 U/L	100–350 U/L
Ammonia nitrogen, plasma	10–50 μmol/L	10–50 μmol/L
Amylase, serum	25–125 U/L	25–125 U/L
Anion gap, serum, calculated	8–16 mEq/L	8–16 mmol/L
Ascorbic acid, blood	0.4–1.5 mg/dL	23–85 μmol/L
Aspartate aminotransferase (AST) serum (SGOT)	1–36 U/L	1–36 U/L
Base excess, arterial blood, calculated	0 ± 2 mEq/L	0 ± 2 mmol/L
Bicarbonate		
Venous plasma	23–29 mEq/L	23–29 mmol/L
Arterial blood	21–27 mEq/L	21–27 mmol/L

Reference Intervals* for Clinical Chemistry (Blood, Serum, and Plasma) (Continued)

Analyte	Conventional Units	SI Units
Bile acids, serum	0.3–3.0 mg/dL	0.8–7.6 μmol/L
Bilirubin, serum		
Conjugated	0.1–0.4 mg/dL	1.7–6.8 μmol/L
Total	0.3–1.1 mg/dL	5.1–19.0 μmol/L
Calcium, serum	8.4–10.6 mg/dL	2.10–2.65 mmol/L
Calcium, ionized, serum	4.25–5.25 mg/dL	1.05–1.30 mmol/L
Carbon dioxide, total, serum or plasma	24–31 mEq/L	24–31 mmol/L
Carbon dioxide tension (P_{CO_2}), blood	35–45 mm Hg	35–45 mm Hg
β-carotene, serum	60–260 μg/dL	1.1–8.6 μmol/L
Ceruloplasmin, serum	23–44 mg/dL	230–440 mg/L
Chloride, serum or plasma	96–106 mEq/L	96–106 mmol/L
Cholesterol, serum or ethylenediaminetetraacetic acid (EDTA) plasma		
Desirable range	<200 mg/dL	<5.20 mmol/L
Low-density lipoprotein (LDL) cholesterol	60–180 mg/dL	1.55–4.65 mmol/L
High-density lipoprotein (HDL) cholesterol	30–80 mg/dL	0.80–2.05 mmol/L
Copper	70–140 μg/dL	11–22 μmol/L
Corticotropin (ACTH), plasma, 8 AM	10–80 pg/mL	2–18 pmol/L
Cortisol, plasma		
8 AM	6–23 μg/dL	170–630 nmol/L
4 PM	3–15 μg/dL	80–410 nmol/L
10 PM	<50% of 8 AM value	<50% of 8 AM value
Creatine, serum		
Males	0.2–0.5 mg/dL	15–40 μmol/L
Females	0.3–0.9 mg/dL	25–70 μmol/

Reference Intervals* for Clinical Chemistry (Blood, Serum, and Plasma) (*continued*)

Analyte	Conventional Units	SI Units
Creatine kinase (CK), serum		
Males	55–170 U/L	55–170 U/L
Females	30–135 U/L	30–135 U/L
Creatine kinase MB isoenzyme, serum	<5% of total CK activity	<5% of total CK activity
<5.0 ng/mL by immunoassay	<5.0 ng/mL by immunoassay	
Creatine, serum	0.6–1.2 mg/dL	50–110 μmol/L
Estradiol-17β, adult		
Males	10–65 pg/mL	35–240 pmol/L
Females		
Follicular	30–100 pg/mL	110–370 pmol/L
Ovulatory	200–400 pg/mL	730–1470 pmol/L
Luteal	50–140 pg/mL	180–510 pmol/L
Ferritin, serum	20–200 ng/mL	20–200 μg/L
Fibrinogen, plasma	200–400 mg/dL	2.0–4.0 g/L
Folate, serum	3–18 ng/mL	6.8–41 nmol/L
Erythrocytes	145–540 ng/mL	330–1220 nmol/L
Follicle-stimulating hormone (FSH), plasma		
Males	4–25 mU/mL	4–25 U/L
Females, premenopausal	4–30 mU/mL	4–30 U/L
Females, postmenopausal	40–250 mU/mL	40–250 U/L
Gamma-glutamyltransferase (GGT), serum	5–40 U/L	5–40 U/L
Gastrin, fasting, serum	0–100 pg/mL	0–100 mg/L
Glucose, fasting, plasma or serum	70–115 mg/dL	3.9–6.4 nmol/L
Growth hormone (hGH), plasma, adult, fasting	0–6 ng/mL	0–6 μg/L
Haptoglobin, serum	20–165 mg/dL	0.20–1.65 gm/L

Reference Intervals* for Clinical Chemistry (Blood, Serum, and Plasma) (continued)

Analyte	Conventional Units	SI Units
Immunoglobulins, serum (see table of Reference Intervals for Tests of Immunologic Function)		
Iron serum	75–175 µg/dL	13–31 µmol/L
Iron binding capacity, serum		
Total	250–410 µg/dL	45–73 µmol/L
Saturation	20–55%	0.20–0.55
Lactate		
Venous whole blood	5.0–20.0 mg/dL	0.6–2.2 mmol/L
Arterial whole blood	5.0–15.0 mg/dL	0.6–1.7 mmol/L
Lactate dehydrogenase (LD), serum	110–220 U/L	110–220 U/L
Lipase, serum	10–140 U/L	10–140 U/L
Lutropin (LH), serum		
Males	1–9 U/L	1–9 U/L
Females		
Follicular phase	2–10 U/L	2–10 U/L
Midcycle peak	15–65 U/L	15–65 U/L
Luteal phase	1–12 U/L	1–12 U/L
Postmenopausal	12–65 U/L	12–65 U/L
Magnesium, serum	1.3–2.1 mg/dL	0.65–1.05 mmol/L
Osmolality	275–295 mOsm/kg water	275–295 mOsm/kg water
Oxygen, blood, arterial, room air		
Partial pressure (Pao_2)	80–100 mm Hg	80–100 mm Hg
Saturation (Sao_2)	95–98%	95–98%
pH, arterial blood	7.35–7.45	7.35–7.45
Phosphate, inorganic, serum		
Adult	3.0–4.5 mg/dL	1.0–1.5 mmol/L

Reference Intervals* for Clinical Chemistry (Blood, Serum, and Plasma) (Continued)

Analyte	Conventional Units	SI Units
Child	4.0–7.0 mg/dL	1.3–2.3 mmol/L
Potassium		
Serum	3.5–5.0 mEq/L	3.5–5.0 mmol/L
Plasma	3.5–4.5 mEq/L	3.5–4.5 mmol/L
Progesterone, serum, adult		
Males	0.0–0.4 ng/mL	0.0–1.3 mmol/L
Females		
Follicular phase	0.1–1.5 ng/mL	0.3–4.8 mmol/L
Luteal phase	2.5–28.0 ng/mL	8.0–89.0 mmol/L
Prolactin, serum		
Males	1.0–15.0 ng/mL	1.0–15.0 µg/L
Females	1.0–20.0 ng/mL	1.0–20.0 µg/L
Protein, serum, electrophoresis		
Total	6.0–8.0 g/dL	60–80 g/L
Albumin	3.5–5.5 g/dL	35–55 g/L
Globulins		
Alpha$_1$	0.2–0.4 g/dL	2.0–4.0 g/L
Alpha$_2$	0.5–0.9 g/dL	5.0–9.0 g/L
Beta	0.6–1.1 g/dL	6.0–11.0 g/L
Gamma	0.7–1.7 g/dL	7.0–17.0 g/L
Pyruvate, blood	0.3–0.9 mg/dL	0.03–0.10 mmol/L
Rheumatoid factor	0.0–30.0 IU/mL	0.0–30.0 kIU/L
Sodium, serum or plasma	135–145 mEq/L	135–145 mmol/L
Testosterone, plasma		
Males, adult	300–1200 ng/dL	10.4–41.6 nmol/L

Reference Intervals* for Clinical Chemistry (Blood, Serum, and Plasma) (*Continued*)

Analyte	Conventional Units	SI Units
Thyroglobulin		
Females, adult	20–75 ng/dL	0.7–2.6 nmol/L
Pregnant females	40–200 ng/dL	1.4–6.9 nmol/L
Thyroglobulin	3–42 ng/mL	3–42 μg/L
Thyrotropin (hTSH), serum	0.4–4.8 μIU/mL	0.4–4.8 mIU/L
Thyrotropin-releasing hormone (TRH)	5–60 pg/mL	5–60 ng/L
Thyroxine (FT_4), free, serum	0.9–2.1 ng/dL	12–27 pmol/L
Thyroxine (T_4), serum	4.5–12.0 μg/dL	58–154 nmol/L
Thyroxine-binding globulin (TBG)	15.0–34.0 μg/mL	15.0–34.0 mg/L
Transferrin	250–430 mg/dL	2.5–4.3 g/L
Triglycerides, serum, 12-h fast	40–150 mg/dL	0.4–1.5 g/L
Triiodothyronine (T_3), serum	70–190 ng/dL	1.1–2.9 nmol/L
Triiodothyronine uptake, resin (T_3RU)	25–38%	0.25–0.38
Urate		
Males	2.5–8.0 mg/dL	150–480 μmol/L
Females	2.2–7.0 mg/dL	130–420 μmol/L
Urea, serum or plasma	24–49 mg/dL	4.0–8.2 nmol/L
Urea nitrogen, serum or plasma	11–23 mg/dL	8.0–16.4 nmol/L
Viscosity, serum	1.4–1.8 × water	1.4–1.8 × water
Vitamin A, serum	20–80 μg/dL	0.70–2.80 μmol/L
Vitamin B_{12}, serum	180–900 pg/mL	133–664 pmol/L

*Reference values may vary, depending on the method and sample source used.

Reference Intervals for Therapeutic Drug Monitoring (Serum)

Analyte	Therapeutic Range	Toxic Concentrations	Proprietary Name(s)
Analgesics			
Acetaminophen	10–20 µg/mL	>250 µg/mL	Tylenol Datril
Salicylate	100–250 µg/mL	>300 µg/mL	Aspirin Bufferin
Antibiotics			
Amikacin	25–30 µg/mL	Peak >35 µg/mL Trough >10 µg/mL	Amikin
Gentamicin	5–10 µg/mL	Peak >10 µg/mL Trough >2 µg/mL	Garamycin
Tobramycin	5–10 µg/mL	Peak >10 µg/mL Trough >2 µg/mL	Nebcin
Vancomycin	5–35 µg/mL	Peak >40 µg/mL Trough >10 µg/mL	Vancocin
Anticonvulsants			
Carbamazepine	5–12 µg/mL	>15 µg/mL	Tegretol
Ethosuximide	40–100 µg/mL	>150 µg/mL	Zarontin
Phenobarbital	15–40 µg/mL	40–100 ng/mL	Luminal (varies widely)
Phenytoin	10–20 µg/mL	>20 µg/mL	Dilantin
Primidone	5–12 µg/mL	>15 µg/mL	Mysoline
Valproic acid	50–100 µg/mL	>100 µg/mL	Depakene
Antineoplastics and Immunosuppressives			
Cyclosporine	50–400 ng/mL	>400 ng/mL	Sandimmune

Reference Intervals for Therapeutic Drug Monitoring (Serum) *(Continued)*

Analyte	Therapeutic Range	Toxic Concentrations	Proprietary Name(s)
Methotrexate, high dose, 48-h	Variable	>1 μmol/L 48 h after dose	
Tacrolimus (FK-506), whole blood	3–10 μg/mL	>15 μg/L	Prograf
Bronchodilators and Respiratory Stimulants			
Caffeine	3–15 ng/mL	>30 ng/mL	Elixophyllin
Theophylline (aminophylline)	10–20 μg/mL	>20 μg/mL	Quibron
Cardiovascular Drugs			
Amiodarone (obtain specimen more than 8 h after last dose)	1.0–2.0 μg/mL	>2.0 μg/mL	Cordarone
Digitoxin (obtain specimen 12–24 h after last dose)	15–25 ng/mL	>35 ng/mL	Crystodigin
Digoxin (obtain specimen more than 6 h after last dose)	0.8–2.0 ng/mL	>2.4 ng/mL	Lanoxin
Disopyramide	2–5 μg/mL	>7 μg/mL	Norpace
Flecainide	0.2–1.0 ng/mL	>1 ng/mL	Tambocor
Lidocaine	1.5–5.0 μg/mL	>6 μg/mL	Xylocaine
Mexiletine	0.7–2.0 ng/mL	>2 ng/mL	Mexitil
Procainamide	4–10 μg/mL	>12 μg/mL	Pronestyl
Procainamide plus *N*-acetyl-*p*-aminophenol (NAPA)	8–30 μg/mL	>30 μg/mL	
Propranolol	50–100 ng/mL	Variable	Inderal
Quinidine	2–5 μg/mL	>6 μg/mL	Cardioquin
			Quinaglute
Tocainide	4–10 ng/mL	>10 ng/mL	Tonocard

Reference Intervals for Therapeutic Drug Monitoring (Serum) (*Continued*)

Analyte	Therapeutic Range	Toxic Concentrations	Proprietary Name(s)
Psychopharmacologic Drugs			
Amitriptyline	120–150 ng/mL	>500 ng/mL	Elavil
			Triavil
Bupropion	25–100 ng/mL	Not applicable	Wellbutrin
Desipramine	150–300 ng/mL	>500 ng/mL	Norpramin
Imipramine	125–250 ng/mL	>400 ng/mL	Tofranil
Lithium			Lithobid
(obtain specimen 12 h after last dose)	0.6–1.5 mEq/L	>1.5 mEq/L	Aventyl
Nortriptyline	50–150 ng/mL	>500 ng/mL	Pamelor

Reference Intervals* for Clinical Chemistry (Urine)

Analyte	Conventional Units	SI Units
Acetone and acetoacetate, qualitative	Negative	Negative
Albumin		
Qualitative	Negative	Negative
Quantitative	10–100 mg/24 h	0.15–1.5 μmol/d
Aldosterone	3–20 μg/24 h	8.3–55 nmol/d
δ-Aminolevulinic acid (δ-ALA)	1.3–7.0 mg/24 h	10–53 μmol/d
Amylase	<17 U/h	<17 U/h
Amylase/creatinine clearance ratio	0.01–0.04	0.01–0.04
Bilirubin, qualitative	Negative	Negative
Calcium (regular diet)	<250 mg/24 h	<6.3 nmol/d

Reference Intervals for Therapeutic Drug Monitoring (Serum) (*Continued*)

Analyte	Therapeutic Range	Toxic Concentrations	Proprietary Name(s)
Catecholamines			
Epinephrine	<10 μg/24 h		<55 nmol/d
Norepinephrine	<100 μg/24 h		<590 nmol/d
Total free catecholamines	4–126 μg/24 h		24–745 nmol/d
Total metanephrines	0.1–1.6 mg/24 h		0.5–8.1 μmol/d
Chloride (varies with intake)	110–250 mEq/24 h		110–250 mmol/d
Copper	0–50 μg/24 h		0.0–0.80 μmol/d
Cortisol, free	10–100 μg/24 h		27.6–276 nmol/d
Creatine			
Males	0–40 mg/24 h		0.0–0.30 mmol/d
Females	0–80 mg/24 h		0.0–0.60 mmol/d
Creatinine	15–25 mg/kg/24 h		0.13–0.22 mmol/kg/d
Creatine clearance (endogenous)			
Males	110–150 mL/min/1.73 m^2		110–150 mL/min/1.73 m^2
Females	105–132 mL/min/1.73 m^2		105–132 mL/min/1.73 m^2
Cystine or cysteine	Negative		Negative
Dehydroepiandrosterone			
Males	0.2–2.0 mg/24 h		0.7–6.9 μmol/d
Females	0.2–1.8 mg/24 h		0.7–6.2 μmol/d
Estrogens, total			
Males	4–25 μg/24 h		14–90 nmol/d
Females	5–100 μg/24 h		18–360 nmol/d
Glucose (as reducing substance)	<250 mg/24 h		<250 mg/d

Reference Intervals* for Clinical Chemistry (Urine) (Continued)

Analyte	Conventional Units	SI Units
Hemoglobin and myoglobin, qualitative	Negative	Negative
Homogentisic acid, qualitative	Negative	Negative
17-Ketogenic steroids		
Males	5–23 mg/24 h	17–80 μmol/d
Females	3–15 mg/24 h	10–52 μmol/d
17-Hydroxycorticosteroids		
Males	3–9 mg/24 h	8.3–25 μmol/d
Females	2–8 mg/24 h	5.5–22 μmol/d
5-Hydroxyindoleacetic acid		
Qualitative	Negative	Negative
Quantitative	2–6 mg/24 h	10–31 μmol/d
17-Ketosteroids		
Males	8–22 mg/24 h	28–76 μmol/d
Females	6–15 mg/24 h	21–52 μmol/d
Magnesium	6–10 mEq/24 h	3–5 mmol/d
Metanephrines	0.05–1.2 ng/mg creatinine	0.03–0.70 mmol/mmol creatinine
Osmolality	38–1400 mOsm/kg water	38–1400 mOsm/kg water
pH	4.6–8.0	4.6–8.0
Phenylpyruvic acid, qualitative	Negative	Negative
Phosphate	0.4–1.3 g/24 h	13–42 mmol/d
Porphobilinogen		
Qualitative	Negative	Negative
Quantitative	<2 mg/24 h	<9 μmol/d

Reference Intervals* for Clinical Chemistry (Urine) *(Continued)*

Analyte	Conventional Units	SI Units
Porphyrins		
Coproporphyrin	50–250 µg/24 h	77–380 nmol/d
Uroporphyrin	10–30 µg/24 h	12–36 nmol/d
Potassium	25–125 mEq/24 h	25–125 mmol/d
Pregnanediol		
Males	0.0–1.9 mg/24 h	0.0–6.0 µmol/d
Females		
Proliferative phase	0.0–2.6 mg/24 h	0.0–8.0 µmol/d
Luteal phase	2.6–10.6 mg/24 h	8–33 µmol/d
Postmenopausal	0.2–1.0 mg/24 h	0.6–3.1 µmol/d
Pregnanetriol	0.0–2.5 mg/24 h	0.0–7.4 µmol/d
Protein, total		
Qualitative	Negative	Negative
Quantitative	10–150 mg/24 h	10–150 mg/d
Protein/creatinine ratio	<0.2	<0.2
Sodium (regular diet)	60–260 mEq/24 h	60–260 mmol/d
Specific gravity		
Random specimen	1.003–1.030	1.003–1.030
24-hour collection	1.015–1.025	1.015–1.025
Urate (regular diet)	250–750 mg/24 h	1.5–4.4 mmol/d
Urobilinogen	0.5–4.0 mg/24 h	0.6–6.8 µmol/d
Vanillylmandelic acid (VMA)	1.0–8.0 mg/24 h	5–40 µmol/d

*Values may vary depending on the method used.

Reference Intervals for Toxic Substances

Analyte	Conventional Units	SI Units
Arsenic, urine	<130 μg/24 h	<1.7 μmol/d
Bromides, serum, inorganic	<100 mg/dL	<10 mmol/L
Toxic symptoms	140–1000 mg/dL	14–100 mmol/L
Carboxyhemoglobin, blood:	Saturation	
Urban environment	<5%	<0.05
Smokers	<12%	<0.12
Symptoms		
Headache	>15%	>0.15
Nausea and vomiting	>25%	>0.25
Potentially lethal	>50%	>0.50
Ethanol, blood	<0.05 mg/dL	<1.0 mmol/L
	<0.005%	
Intoxication	>100 mg/dL	>22 mmol/L
	>0.1%	
Marked intoxication	300–400 mg/dL	65–87 mmol/L
	0.3–0.4%	
Alcoholic stupor	400–500 mg/dL	87–109 mmol/L
	0.4–0.5%	
Coma	>500 mg/dL	>109 mmol/L
	>0.5%	
Lead, blood		
Adults	<25 μg/dL	<1.2 μmol/L
Children	<15 μg/dL	<0.7 μmol/L
Lead, urine	<80 μg/24 h	<0.4 μmol/d
Mercury, urine	<30 μg/24 h	<150 nmol/d

Reference Intervals for Tests Performed on Cerebrospinal Fluid

Test	Conventional Units	SI Units
Cells	<5/mm^3, all mononuclear	<5 × 10^6/L, all mononuclear
Protein electrophoresis	Albumin predominant	Albumin predominant
Glucose	50–75 mg/dL	2.8–4.2 mmol/L
	(20 mg/dL less than in serum)	(1.1 mmol less than in serum)
IgG		
Children under 14	<8% of total protein	<0.08 of total protein
Adults	<14% of total protein	<0.14 of total protein
IgG index*	0.3–0.6	0.3–0.6
CSF/Serum IgG ratio		
CSF/Serum albumin ratio		
Oligoclonal banding on electrophoresis	Absent	Absent
Pressure, opening	70–180 mm H$_2$O	70–180 mm H$_2$O
Protein, total	15–45 mg/dL	150–450 mg/L

Abbreviation: CSF = cerebrospinal fluid.

Reference Intervals for Tests of Gastrointestinal Function

Test	Conventional Units
Bentiromide test	6-h urinary arylamine excretion greater than 57% excludes pancreatic insufficiency
β-Carotene, serum	60–260 ng/dL
Fecal fat estimation	
Qualitative	No fat globules seen by high-power microscope
Quantitative	<6 g/24 h (>95% coefficient of fat absorption)
Gastric acid output	
Basal	
Males	0.0–10.5 mmol/h
Females	0.0–5.6 mmol/h
Maximum (after histamine or pentagastrin)	
Males	9.0–48.0 mmol/h
Females	6.0–31.0 mmol/h
Ratio: basal maximum	
Males	0.0–0.31
Females	0.0–0.29
Secretin test, pancreatic fluid	
Volume	>1.8 mL/kg/h
Bicarbonate	>80 mEq/L
D-Xylose absorption test, urine	>20% of ingested dose excreted in 5 h

Reference Intervals for Tests of Immunologic Function

Test	Conventional Units	SI Units
Complement, Serum		
C3	85–175 mg/dL	0.85–1.75 gm/L
C4	15–45 mg/dL	150–450 mg/L
Total hemolytic (CH_{50})	150–250 U/mL	150–250 U/mL
Immunoglobulins, Serum, Adult		
IgG	640–1350 mg/dL	6.4–13.5 g/L
IgA	70–310 mg/dL	0.70–3.1 g/L
IgM	90–350 mg/dL	0.90–3.5 g/L
IgD	0.0–6.0 mg/dL	0.0–60 mg/L
IgE	0.0–430 ng/dL	0.0–430 µg/L

Lymphocyte Subsets, Whole Blood, Heparinized

Antigen(s) Expressed	Cell Type	Percentage	Absolute Cell Count
CD3	Total T cells	56–77%	860–1880
CD19	Total B cells	7–17%	140–370
CD3 and CD4	Helper-induced cells	32–54%	550–1190
CD3 and CD8	Suppressor-cytotoxic cells	24–37%	430–1060
CD3 and DR	Activated T cells	5–14%	70–310
CD2	E rosette T cells	73–87%	1040–2160
CD16 and CD56	Natural killer (NK) cells	8–22%	130–500
Helper/suppressor ratio: 0.8–1.8			

Reference Values for Semen Analysis

Test	Conventional Units	SI Units
Volume	2–5 mL	2–5 mL
Liquefaction	Complete in 15 min	Complete in 15 min
pH	7.2–8.0	7.2–8.0
Leukocytes	Occasional or absent	Occasional or absent
Spermatozoa		
Count	$60–150 \times 10^6$/mL	$60–150 \times 10^6$/mL
Motility	>80% motile	>0.80 motile
Morphology forms	80–90% normal forms	>0.80–0.90 normal
Fructose	>150 mg/dL	>8.33 mmol/L